1/2008   not weeded

Health:
What Is It Worth?
(PPS-23)

Pergamon Titles of Related Interest

Catalano   *Health, Behavior and the Community: An Ecological Perspective*

Fritz   *Combatting Nutritional Blindness in Children: A Case Study of Technical Assistance in Indonesia*

Gartner/Greer   *Consumer Education in the Human Services*

Geismar/Geismar   *Families in an Urban Mold: Policy Implications of an Australian-U.S. Comparison*

Morris   *Measuring the Condition of the World's Poor: The Physical Quality of Life Index*

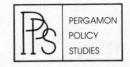

PERGAMON
POLICY
STUDIES

Health:
What Is It Worth?
Measures of Health Benefits

Edited by
Selma J. Mushkin
David W. Dunlop

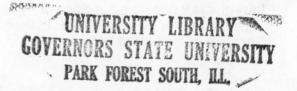
Pergamon Press

NEW YORK • OXFORD • TORONTO • SYDNEY • FRANKFURT • PARIS

Pergamon Press Offices:

U.S.A.   Pergamon Press Inc., Maxwell House, Fairview Park,
                     Elmsford, New York 10523, U.S.A.

U.K.   Pergamon Press Ltd., Headington Hill Hall,
                     Oxford OX3 OBW, England

CANADA   Pergamon of Canada, Ltd., 150 Consumers Road,
                     Willowdale, Ontario M2J, 1P9, Canada

AUSTRALIA   Pergamon Press (Aust) Pty. Ltd., P O Box 544,
                     Potts Point, NSW 2011, Australia

FRANCE   Pergamon Press SARL, 24 rue des Ecoles,
                     75240 Paris, Cedex 05, France

FEDERAL REPUBLIC Pergamon Press GmbH, 6242 Kronberg/Taunus,
OF GERMANY   Pferdstrasse 1, Federal Republic of Germany

Library of Congress Cataloging in Publication Date

Main entry under title:
Health, what is it worth?

   (Pergamon policy studies)
   'Derived from a series of papers presented at a
two-day conference at Georgetown University in
September 1977.'
   Bibliography: p.
   Includes index.
   1. Medical research—Economic aspects—Congresses.
2. Health status indicators—Congresses. 3. Medical
research—Cost effectiveness—Congresses. 4. Medical
care—Evaluation—Congresses. 5. Social values—
Congresses. I. Mushkin, Selma J., 1913-
II. Dunlop, David W. [DNLM: 1. Cost benefit
analysis—Congresses. 2. Economics, Medical—
Congresses. 3. Health—Congresses. 4. Health
resources—Economics—Congresses. W74 H4365 1977]
R850.A2H4   1979   362.1   79-4532
ISBN 0-08-023898-X

This volume is produced under a grant (HS02939-01) from the
National Center for Health Services Research, USDHEW, and
a grant from the Milbank Memorial Fund.

Printed in the United States of America

Contributors

Shaul Ben-David
Professor of Economics
University of New Mexico

James W. Bush
Division of Health Policy
University of California
    at San Diego

Milton M. Chen
San Diego State University
        and
Division of Health Policy
University of California
    at San Diego

Edward H. Clarke
Woodrow Wilson International
    Center for Scholars
Smithsonian Institution

Thomas D. Crocker
Professor of Economics
University of Wyoming

Paul M. Densen
Center for Community Health
    and Medical Care
Harvard University

Nancy S. Dorfman
Charles River Associates
Cambridge

David W. Dunlop
Department of Family and
    Community Health and
    Division of Health Care
    Administration and
    Planning
Meharry Medical College
        and
Department of Economics
Vanderbilt University

Linda N. Edwards
National Bureau of
    Economic Research

Gregory W. Fischer
Public Policy Studies
Duke University

Michael Grossman
National Bureau of
    Economic Research

Ellen W. Jones
Center for Community Health
    and Medical Care
Harvard University

Allen Kneese
Professor of Economics
University of New Mexico

Joseph Lipscomb
Institute of Policy
    Sciences and Public
    Affairs
Duke University

Barbara J. McNitt
Center for Community Health
    and Medical Care
Harvard University

Selma J. Mushkin
Public Services Laboratory
Georgetown University

Solomon Schneyer
Division of Program
    Analysis
National Institutes of
    Health

v

William Schulze
Department of Economics
University of Southern California

John E. Ware, Jr.
The Rand Corporation

Shih-Yen Wu
Department of Economics
University of Iowa

JoAnne Young
Southern Illinois University

Contents

Preface

This present volume is derived from a series of papers presented at a two-day conference at Georgetown University in September 1977. The conference, then titled "Functional Health Status and Biomedical Research and Technology," was made possible by grants from the National Center for Health Services Research and the Milbank Memorial Fund. These two organizations have also funded the publication of this book. We are grateful to NCHSR and the Milbank Memorial Fund not only for their financial aid, but also for their helpful suggestions in the development of the conference and the preparation of the manuscript for this volume. In particular, we are indebted to Linda Siegenthaler of the Economic Analysis Branch of the Division of Health Services Research and Analysis at NCHSR, and to Richard V. Kasius of Milbank.

We thank the authors of the papers presented here for their patience at the delay in bringing their efforts into print. We have endeavored to do no disservice to their presentation by the exigencies of editing for publication and apologize for any inadvertent error.

The proceedings of the conference and the preparation of the volume of papers were much enhanced by the thoughtful comments of the panels of discussants who participated in the conference. They are:

Martin Bailey (University of Maryland)
Glenn Blomquist (Illinois State University)
Ralph C. d'Arge (University of Wyoming)
Harvey Garn (The Urban Institute)
Paul M. Gertman (Boston University Medical Center)
Peter Goldschmidt (Policy Research, Inc., Baltimore)
Teh-wei Hu (State College, Pa.)
Herbert E. Klarman (New York University)
Alma L. Koch (University of California)
Steven Lipson (Georgetown University)
Carl Richard Neu (Congressional Budget Office)

Mancur Olson (University of Maryland)
Anne Scitovsky (Palo Alto Medical Research
    Foundation)
Marcelo Selowsky (The World Bank)
David Siskie (Office of Management and Budget)
David Syss (Federal Reserve Board)
Milton Weinstein (Harvard School of Public Health)
Donald E. Yett (University of Southern California)

Frank H. Sandifer of the Public Services Laboratory,
Georgetown University, was of great assistance in the research
and writing of the Introduction to the book. Laurel Rabin
was a conscientious and meticulous editor. Cynthia Resnick
of the Public Services Laboratory staff not only contributed
to the editing of several papers, but was invaluable in the
onerous task of proofreading. Violet Gunther was responsible
for the overall editing and production of the manuscript.
And lastly, we must give very special thanks to Alva Wood for
the monumental task of typing--which she performed not only
with excellence, but with unfailing patience and good humor.

NOTE.—In this volume, the pronoun "he" (unless referring to
    a specific person) is used in the generic sense, mean-
    ing a person rather than a male.

                                  Selma J. Mushkin
                                  David W. Dunlop
                                  Editors

Foreword

Several years ago, the Public Services Laboratory of
Georgetown University, with support from the Milbank Memorial
Fund, convened a conference to consider consumer incentives
for health care. Four years later, the Milbank Memorial Fund
was pleased to join with the National Center for Health
Services Research to enable the Public Services Laboratory
to present a conference on Functional Health Status and
Biomedical Research and Technology, whose proceedings are
contained in this volume. Although the two conferences were
disparate in their topics and their sponsors intended no sub-
stantive linkage, they do serve to mark a change in the cli-
mate in which health policy questions are considered. At the
first conference, the assumption that medical care was a
valued and necessary service was not challenged. The later
conference dealt with medical care and biomedical research
as they were becoming subject to a growing public skepticism
concerning their benefits and to increasing legislative
scrutiny and question in the allocation of the public dollars.

This conference could be viewed as a response to these
changes in the political environment in which health policy
is being developed. Its central purpose was to create a
forum for the discussion of some of the newer concepts and
methods for addressing the related issues of setting
priorities for and allocating resources to biomedical research
and of measuring the health status of populations to whom the
findings of research are applied. Scholars from economics,
psychology, sociology, public health, and biostatistics concerned with these questions were able to submit some methodological and conceptual developments from their disciplines
to a critical multi-disciplinary examination and assessment.

It is not unfair to the contributors to this volume
to suggest that they have not presented many definitive
answers to the complex set of questions being considered.
What they have done is to bring us progress reports on some

promising research initiatives, but it is progress of which
other scholars, government, and even foundations, should be
aware.

It is my privilege to commend the unique contribution
of Selma J. Mushkin to the success of this conference of
which she was the chief architect. Her identification of
the conference themes and her wide knowledge of the significant work in progress pertinent to these themes enabled
her to convene the assembly of scholars whose papers are the
substance of this volume. She was assisted in this by
David W. Dunlop who participated in the earlier conference
on health incentives and has a very thoughtful paper in this
volume. He was co-sponsor of the recent conference and is
co-editor of the book.

Richard V. Kasius
Milbank Memorial Fund

Introduction

Today, a great scepticism surrounds the use of resources for health care and research to advance medical knowledge. Originating as it does in the vital statistics of the
past few decades, the scepticism is fostered by what appears
to be a failure of medical care (and biomedical advances embodied in that care) to improve life expectancy. For over a
decade, death rates remained unchanged despite the billions
spent for medical care and research. Indeed, McKeown (1976)
and McKinlay and McKinlay (1977) have assessed historic improvements in mortality and found little relation between biomedical science and death-rate reduction. Up until the down-
turn of age-adjusted death rates in 1975 and some further reductions in 1976, the data gave some credence to the notion
that limits had been reached on the health impact of medical
care and research (figure 1).

Despite the recent reductions in death rates, there
continue to be nagging doubts about medicine and science as
contributing to the improvements. Instead, better living
habits and reduced speed limits are cited as primary determinants. Moreover, iatrogenic disease has taken on great
importance in the public mind as a cause of death and disability. Almost every day, the press reports some charge of
erroneous diagnoses or harmful medication. Illich (1976) has
perhaps led the way in his emphasis, which may be stated
thus: The doctoring you receive may be bad for your health.

Besides mortality, or life expectancy-rates, the other
usual measure of the population's health is disability. Since
death rates have not changed markedly in recent years, despite
massive health expenditures, are disability rates on the decline, reflecting improved health? On the surface at least,
the answer is no. With the exception of work-loss days, all
the customary indexes of disability have increased over the
last couple of decades, as shown in figure 2. (Note, however,
that 1957 should not be used as a benchmark for comparison

1

Figure 1.   Age-Adjusted Death Rates, 1900-76.

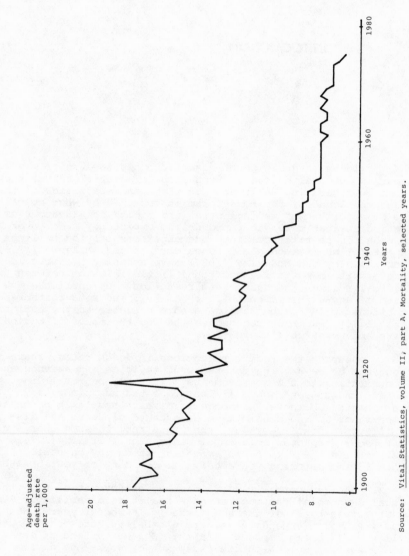

Age-adjusted
death rate
per 1,000

Source: Vital Statistics, volume II, part A, Mortality, selected years.

Figure 2. <u>Changes in Measures of Disability, 1957-76</u>.

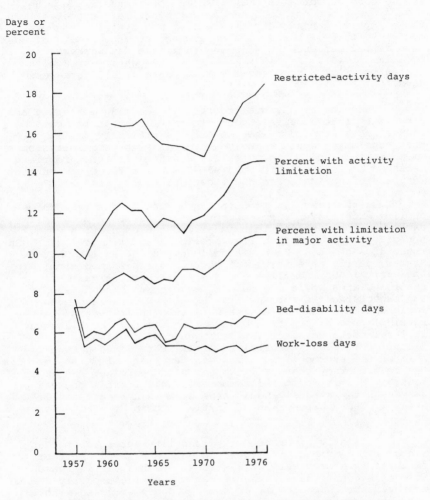

Days or
percent

Restricted-activity days

Percent with activity
limitation

Percent with limitation
in major activity

Bed-disability days

Work-loss days

Years

Source: Derived from various issues of <u>Vital and Health Statistics</u>,
         series 10, which reports data from the National Health Sur-
         vey and is published by the National Center for Health
         Statistics, Public Health Service, U.S.DHEW. The reader
         is cautioned that there have been some changes in methods
         over the years, which may affect the comparability of the
         numbers, and the unusually large size of work-loss days
         and bed-disability days for 1957 is probably primarily due
         to the very severe flu epidemic that year. Data reported
         for 1957-65 are actually fiscal year data for fiscal
         1958-66, while 1966-76 data are on a calendar basis.
         Also, 1960 values for work loss, bed-days, and restricted-
         activity days have been estimated based on annual varia-
         tions in these categories due to acute illnesses only.

since it was a year of extremely high influenza rates.) And
the measure of work-loss days, while not increasing as the
others have, has not declined as one might have expected. In
fact, it has changed very little over many years. For example, in 1928-31 there were on average about 5.2 days of work
loss a year per worker, adjusted to a five-day work week
(Collins, 1940). For 1976, the National Center for Health
Statistics (1977) reported a similar rate of 5.2 work-loss
days.

The lack of obvious progress in reducing mortality and
disability rates could lead one to conclude that the outcome
of resources devoted to health care is pitifully small. Yet
that conclusion would be only as valid as the statistics on
which it is based. Are mortality and disability appropriate
measures of health improvements? Do they reflect the current
purposes of medical care and recent biomedical research?

Death rates (or some variant, such as survival rates
or life expectancy) were appropriate criteria of program impact when the diseases that imperiled the population were
typhoid, cholera, diphtheria, smallpox, and tuberculosis. But
these diseases have been virtually wiped out in the United
States, partly as a result of past progress in medicine. In
the early 1900s, families could expect that one-quarter of
their children would die before reaching adulthood. Today
the expectation is for survival of all children and even
young adults. Indeed, adults well into their forties have a
survival probability from one year to the next so high that
it is almost a certainty. The absence of continuing,
dramatic declines in mortality rates is in large part a result of the enormous gains made in the past. It also reflects
the contemporary changes in emphasis of medicine. An important aim now is to make life more livable for all those who
survive but previously would have died as a result of illnesses. That purpose was of little concern 75 or 100 years
ago.

Similarly, increases in disability rates (or the absence of significant declines) do not necessarily reflect
failures in health care or research. Rather, it is reasonable to suggest that the increases are at least partly due to
improvements in medicine, as those who are stricken with a
serious disease now are more likely to survive and live on
with a temporary or permanent impairment. This phenomenon
has been labeled a "failure of success" by Gruenberg (1977)
and others. It is particularly relevant in connection with
such a measure as the percentage of the population with major
activity limitation. Furthermore, other important factors
may be largely responsible for the lack of apparent progress
in some of the disability statistics (especially work-loss
days and restricted-activity days). Among them are higher
education and income levels, greater sick-pay coverage, and
changing attitudes toward work.

All of this is intended to suggest that alternative measures of health progress are needed to replace the earlier exclusive reliance on mortality and morbidity. These early statistics were developed mainly as general indicators of the health of the nation or community, but they do not capture the essential impacts of current and recent biomedical advances. Nor are they adequate criteria for evaluation or needs-assessment.

Given the considerable progress in the past, most health policies (including research activities) are aimed at alleviating disease conditions or providing half-way technologies that do not necessarily cure a disease but, rather, allow a person with the disease to function. Thus, major research institutes deal mainly with chronic diseases, such as heart disease, cancer, and chronic obstructive lung disease. The aim of applied biomedical research appears to be to treat and control those chronic diseases.

Valuing Health Benefits

In addition to the question of how health progress should be measured, there also is considerable debate over how the benefits of health programs are valued. The growing pressures for accountability in government are resulting in widespread application of measurements of the value of human life and limb. The application of analysis in policy decisions is compelling the formulation of objectives of health programs and criteria for assessing progress toward achieving them, as well as costing out alternative policies and measuring effectiveness. The increasing use of evaluations to examine the record of achievement toward defined objectives is accelerating the acquisition of measurement information.

The application of investment concepts to health program calculations has long been the subject of much concern. Valuation of human life in crass dollar terms raises ethical and emotional questions, as well as conceptual ones. Nevertheless, despite opposition to such measurements, political pressures for some kind of valuation have prevailed, so that by the mid-1960s, cost-benefit calculations were frequently applied to health programs. In the process, the "pricing" of health benefits has relied on measuring the gains in production--present and future--from reductions in disability or death.

More recently, however, this "human capital" approach has been challenged on conceptual grounds. It has been charged that the notion of human capital does not fit the basic concept of consumer satisfaction. For example, it does not fully reflect the desire of individuals to improve their own chances of surviving an illness when it strikes.

Furthermore, the human capital approach understates the value
of the old, the young, women, and persons in minority groups.
The understatement results from several facets of conventional
valuations.

First, value is determined by attachment to the
workforce--wages reflect the marginal product of labor. Thus,
those who have retired and will no longer earn wages are assigned no value by this type of capital accounting. Similarly, women who are housewives have no attachment to the
workforce as defined. (Mostly in recognition of the problem
of a "no value" count, more or less arbitrary decisions have
been made to assess the value of housewife services.) For
women workers and minority workers, it is not workforce attachment that creates the value issue but rather the relative
level of earnings. Those who have low earnings come to be
assigned a low value. The value question is exacerbated in
the case of children and youth by the discounting of future
earnings.

Secondly, the appropriate rate of discount for the
stream of future earnings is unclear. Some recommended the
rate at which commercial capital is borrowed; others use a
pure time-preference rate. The discount rate has an ap-
preciable effect on the computed values: The higher the rate,
the lower the amount assigned to earnings postponed for long
terms. Thus, the value of children drops sharply when relatively high rates are applied. Yet, in social and ethical
terms, high values are placed on children and young persons.

There are many other technical questions involved in
human capital computation, such as (1) trends in workforce
participation rates at different ages and for males and
females, (2) the productivity growth outlook, and (3) earning patterns over a working lifetime.

Because of such problems as these--both conceptual and
practical--alternative methods of valuing health benefits
have been advanced. The calculation method for traditional
valuations considers the cost or gain for society as a whole.
Alternative approaches start from the perspective of individual preferences or choices in the use of scarce resources.
Instead of quantification in terms of the present values of
future earnings of those potentially in the workforce, the
newer methods aim for quantification in terms of consumer
preferences, that is, the relative willingness to pay for
probable health benefits from the resources available.

Previous work by economists yields a review of the
criticisms of human capital investment measurements and a
formalization of concepts that underlie the emphasis on the
alternative measure, based on consumer preferences or willingness to pay. Unobtrusive measurements of consumer
preference also have been outlined, including (a) property

values in hazardous areas, (b) pain-killer expenditures,
(c) smoking expenditures, which suggest little risk aversion
on the part of consumers, (d) risk of death or disability on
the job and wage-rate differentials in relation to risk, and
(e) court awards in negligence cases.

Other health service researchers have been developing
measures of "health status," "functional status," and
"quality of life" to be used as effectiveness criteria for
health program evaluation or as social indicators in needs
assessment. A synthesis of these related research endeavors
is necessary. Exchange between those developing health or
functional status measures and those pursuing methods of
quantifying consumer preferences or willingness to pay is an
important step for advancing present research work and defining an agenda for new research. Papers were requested from
Conference participants with the intent of contributing to
earlier discussions of alternative approaches to measurement
and using the research already completed as a springboard for
new advances in quantifying the benefits of human resource
programs in general and health programs in particular.

Measures of Health Status

In the opening paper, Chen and Bush review the rapidly
expanding literature on alternative measures of health status
with respect to their public policy usefulness. They develop
a taxonomy to determine how each health status index may be
used for specific resource allocation decisions in the health
sector. Primary attention is given to measures of functional
health change as opposed to measures that focus on the occurrence of death. Chen and Bush's view, as developed in this
paper, is that there are a number of potential measures of
health status, and that determining which measure is appropriate for use depends on the specific resource allocation
decision being addressed. The Chen, Bush paper essentially
sets the stage for the presentations that follow by outlining
what is happening in the area of functional health status
measurement.

The paper on assessing long-term care by Jones, McNitt,
and Densen provides an appropriate extension of the Chen,
Bush discussion by describing the operational use of a particular set of functional status indicators. The research
reported in the paper developed a patient assessment procedure for use in long-term care facilities. Status indicators derived from assessment and reassessment of patient
conditions are usable in decisions about placement and
planning of care, in quantifying changes in patient status,
and in studying patient outcomes.

Valuing Health and Health Benefits

Following the opening papers on health status measurement is a collection of papers dealing with various conceptual
and operational aspects of valuing health benefits. In the
first of these, Nancy Dorfman reviews each of the frequently
discussed methods of valuing a health benefit (lifesaving)
and outlines significant problems with all of them. Dorfman
concludes that none of the currently available methods of
valuation is satisfactory. She prefers to "refrain from
placing a dollar sign on lives saved," until a sounder basis
for such valuations is developed.

In the second paper, Edward Clarke reviews the theoretical approach that he has pioneered to determine the social
value of public goods via the demand-revealing process. He
points out that the demand-revealing process would permit
each individual to state his willingness to pay for biomedical research--"presumably the amount that would compensate him for increased risk of death or decline in functional
health status" if the research were not undertaken.

The next two papers reflect attempts to overcome some
of the basic conceptual and practical difficulties in assessing consumers' willingness to pay for health benefits.
Joseph Lipscomb describes a health planning model to determine
an "efficient allocation of inputs among competing medical
care programs which would on average lead to maximum improvement in population health status." In Lipscomb's theoretical
formulation, changes in health status would be valued according to a procedure which would reveal consumer preferences
by using a willingness-to-pay voting scheme. The theoretical model is specified with a mathematical programming
structure and assumes that many variables of interest have a
semi-Markovian format that reflects the movements between
various health states. Lipscomb is using his theoretical
framework in an empirical test of alternative programmatic
resource allocations available to the Indian Health Service.

Following the discussions of theoretical approaches to
valuing health benefits, papers by Ware and Young and
Gregory Fischer explore some of the serious practical difficulties in assessing consumer preferences, emphasizing the
psychological aspects. Ware and Young are concerned with
the value that persons place on the concept of health within
the context of their hierarchies of values or ideals. They
describe a survey method for estimating the value of health
in relation to other personal values (e.g., accomplishment,
exciting life) and identify general dimensions of persons'
value orientation.

Fischer concentrates particularly on the problems inherent in the survey method of determining consumers' valuation of health improvements. The complexity of considerations
involved in responding to survey questions result in inconsistent behavior, and data thus obtained are unlikely to be
reliable. The paper investigates the problem confronting an
individual when asked to make probabilistic tradeoffs between
present and future consumption and future health status.
Fischer suggests that a measurement strategy for deriving
consumer willingness to pay should be based on the principles
of decision analysis.

Returns to Biomedical Investments

Two papers are included in this section, one by
Shih-Yen Wu and another by Schulze, Ben-David, Crocker, and
Kneese. Wu examines methods of measuring social returns to
innovations. Using the example of pharmaceutical innovations
for purposes of the presentation, Wu critiques the human
capital and the consumer surplus approaches to measuring the
value of benefits and finds them lacking. He develops an alternative approach drawing on Lancaster's reformulation of
the utility function--"the traditional demand analysis based
upon the utility of goods cannot cope with either a change
in the quality of goods or a change in the number of goods
consumed." Satisfaction is derived from the characteristics
of the goods rather than the goods themselves.

Schulze develops a methodology, following on a
cost of risk concept, for measuring the benefits of
cancer prevention programs which reduce the environmental exposure to carcinogens. He is critical of
decisions made in cancer research to focus on cure,
following contraction of the disease, rather than on
prevention strategies in the areas of air and water
pollution and nutrition. The paper develops estimates
of the benefits from such a cancer prevention program
by assessing the changes in incremental risk of death,
using regression techniques. The authors conclude
that the potential benefits from reduced risk (valued
by the extra wage costs workers demand as compensation
for risk) can be substantial.

Health Resource Allocations

Clearly, one especially important use of health status
measures and valuation of health benefits is in guiding decisions about health policies and resources. In the first
paper of this section, Solomon Schneyer of the National Institutes of Health examines factors that affect resource
allocations in biomedical research. He describes the
relative efficacy of the political process in determining
the value of research on one health problem compared to

others. It is not surprising to find the differences in research funding for cancer and heart disease when political
decision makers obviously consider pain and suffering in conjunction with mortality rates. Schneyer suggests that the
political process, as it now operates, is the only feasible
way of making difficult resource decisions in health until
further methodological advances are made in valuing the returns to biomedical research investments.

David Dunlop analyzes current and prospective biomedical resource allocations for diabetes in relation to their
potential benefits. He focuses on the extent to which the
diabetes research program of NIH addresses the major problems
that could lead to reductions in the incidence of disease,
deaths, and functional health status losses. In this
analysis of present and planned funding, Dunlop finds that
the current research emphasis does not incorporate consumer
preferences explicitly and that funding decisions are largely
"supply side" determined. Dunlop deals with how functional
health status indicators and measures of consumers' willingness to pay can be used in making and analyzing resource allocation decisions. In his conclusion, he notes also that
"well over half the diabetic population do not follow treatment regimes with which they have been provided." He suggests that a portion of the resources for research on chronic
diseases be used to study "consumer behavior and its role as
a determinant of functional health status."

The primary emphasis in the Edwards and Grossman paper
is on functional health status--more specifically on intellectual development as an indicator of health status.
Their conceptual basis is that "enhanced intellectual development is an important source of benefits from investments in
children's health." Edwards and Grossman have been engaged
in a comprehensive theoretical and empirical analysis of
factors affecting children's development and measurement of
the outcomes of child health programs. In this paper, they
discuss their analytic approach and preliminary findings.
Of particular note, they describe how the information they
have developed can be used in making hard choices in "allocating scarce resources among competing programs with respect to children."

In the final paper of this compendium, Selma Mushkin
attempts to draw upon the kinds of work presented in the previous papers to illustrate operational uses of both health
status and willingness-to-pay measures. She outlines the
desired characteristics of health status measures and valuations of health benefits. Using the example of health status
measures she helped to develop in an evaluation plan for lung
disease, Mushkin describes how such measures can be used to
guide health policies and decisions. She extends the discussion to valuation of consumer preferences, or willingness
to pay, and describes an application of some of the recent
theoretical work on demand-revealing processes of valuation.

REFERENCES

Collins, Selwyn D.
    1940   "Cases and days of illness among males and
              females with special reference to confinement
              to bed." Public Health Reports 55(2):47-93.

Gruenberg, Ernest M.
    1977   "The failures of success." Milbank Memorial
              Fund Quarterly 55(4) (Winter):3-24.

Illich, Evan
    1976   Medical Nemesis (The Expropriation of Health).
              New York: Random House, Inc.

McKeown, T.
    1976   The Role of Medicine: Dream, Mirage, or Nemesis.
              London: Nuffield Provincial Hospitals Trust.

McKinlay, J. B. and S. M. McKinlay
    1977   "The questionable contribution of medical mea-
              sures to the decline of mortality in the United
              States in the twentieth century." Milbank
              Memorial Fund Quarterly 55(3):405-428.

National Center for Health Statistics
    1977   "Current estimates from the health interview
              survey, United States - 1976." Vital and
              Health Statistics, series 10, no. 119,
              U.S.DHEW publication no. (PHS) 78-1547,
              Hyattsville, Md.

Measure of
Health Status

1 Health Status Measures, Policy, and Biomedical Research

Milton M. Chen
James W. Bush

why study measures of h/s

The increased public spending on health care (including the proliferation of organizational, diagnostic, and therapeutic innovation) has given added impetus for the development of health status measurement to assess the gains derived from this increase. We shall focus on reviewing recent advances in health status measurement and their possible use in public policy making. (A bibliography on current research on health status measurement is published by the National Center for Health Statistics in its publication Clearinghouse on Health Indexes.)

tasks of measuring h/s

today

Measurement of health status has come to be described in terms of several important related tasks: (a) defining a set of health states that describe the array of conditions prevalent in the population, (b) incorporating prognosis and its duration into the overall construct, (c) developing a set of weights to reflect the relative scale of health states, and (d) integrating mortality and other indicators into a health status indicator, a composite index, or indexes. This paper presents various health status measures, analyzing them for their completeness in addressing these tasks as well as for their public policy uses.

HEALTH OR FUNCTION STATES

The definition of health states, as reflected in health statistics, has expanded over the years. Mortality statistics represent one of the oldest measures still in wide use today. Restricted-activity days, bed-disability days, and work-loss days came into use later as a supplement to mortality data. Today, it is recognized that a health status measure that is sensitive in detecting health changes requires a detailed set of states. However, too large a number of states will tax the ability and the attention span of the analyst, decision makers, and the population at large. A

consolidation of the states, based on internal consistency
and relative desirability, is required.

function/
dysfunction

Many recent works have focused on the function/
dysfunction aspect of health status (Katz, 1963; Patrick,
Bush, and Chen, 1973; Gilson, 1975). The function aspect of
health states can best be defined as conformity to society's
norms of physical and mental states, including performance
of activities usual for an individual's social role. The
dysfunction aspect includes pain and other symptoms considered deviations from norms of well-being, even when there
is no social role performance. Health states may consist of
a series of classifications ranging from optimum function to
various levels of dysfunction, including the total dysfunction state, death. Moreover, these health states may include some loosely defined aspects of "quality of life"
(Berg, 1976) involving mental health and other aspects of
health. Different health status measures encompass different
aspects of health states, some aspects more heavily represented than others. Most recent health status measures include items relating to the physical and mental abilities involved in, for example, communicating and working. The selection of items to be included depends on whether the health
state measurement is for economic, sociological, or medical
evaluation. For instance, to investigate the economic and
social impact of health state change, we need to include
items such as work, blindness, and depression.

If the health status measures do not cover important
aspects of function or quality of life in sufficient detail,
the resulting valuation, economic or non-economic, of health
services and biomedical research will give a misleading result. In a study of the PKU program, for example (Bush,
Chen, and Patrick, 1973), more than half of the benefit in
health units computed came from improved functional capacity.

Using function states has several advantages: (1) It
does not require extensive medical examination and testing in
classifying individuals and can be used to assess the health
status of individuals who do not enter the health care
system. (2) It conforms to the theoretical construct of
health (Parsons, 1958). (3) It can be understood easily,
without special medical training, by the majority of the
population. (4) It can be used to evaluate the impact of,
for example, rehabilitation medicine, prospective medicine,
and home health care. (5) It can be used to assess the impact on the health status of a sick person's family and
friends. (6) It facilitates the evaluation of health services and biomedical advances across diseases and population
groups. The prevalence of chronic disease requires the use
of more sensitive indicators, such as health state measures,
since the disease history involves a long presymptomatic
stage with gradual change in functional ability. The use of
health states, on the other hand, introduces complexity in

data collection, prognostic estimation, ability versus performance assessment, and the weighting of multiple states relative to each other.

PROGNOSIS

Prognosis can best be described in terms of transition probabilities among function states. The usual mortality rate represents the probability of moving to death from the state of life in a two-state model of death and life. Diseases are generally regarded as "serious" or "not serious," depending on both the value of associated health states and the transition probabilities. Prognosis has been couched in vague terms, such as life threatening and likelihood of long or short-term disability. A more precise quantification for monitoring and evaluation purposes is to use health state expectancies parallel to life expectancy.

Prognosis determines the time to be spent in each health state. A table of health state expectancies can be derived that distributes life expectancy among the various health states. In common with the current life table, the health state expectancies table can serve as a convenient summary of current transition patterns (showing how these patterns would persist over life in a synthetic cohort). Differences in health state expectancies with and without a given health program or biomedical advance would constitute the first approximate measure of the return, or outcome, of activities under evaluation.

WEIGHTING HEALTH STATES

As the number of states increases, the need to weight these states becomes progressively greater. Although many policy makers may prefer to assign their own weights in program evaluation, making weighting unnecessary, they may still find weighting useful; it enables policy makers to have a set of weights, representing relative numbers in each state, derived from a sample survey of the population. The weighting is less important when we are dealing with the use of health state measures as social indicators of change; the weighting is more important when health state measures are used as criteria for decision making in program evaluation.

In the fact of uncertainty, ordinal ranking of states will be of little value, hence the measurement calls for an interval (ratio) scale. Various methods have been used in deriving weights: (1) arbitrary scoring, (2) weighting by probability of death, (3) psychometric scaling, (4) von Neumann-Morgenstern utility measurement, and (5) economic valuation.

Arbitrary scoring would assign points to each state. This procedure has been widely used and it is up to the analyst to demonstrate that the resulting scores correlate with some determinants of health. Weighting by probability of death has been proposed by Chiang (1976); each health state is scaled by its respective probability of death. The resulting scale would not necessarily correspond to relative preference for that state.

Psychometric scaling has a long history in attitude and value measurement (Nunnally, 1967). A large number of states will preclude the use of paired comparison developed by Thurston (1959). Category rating obtained from ratings given to a set of stimuli, according to some variable property, is the most frequently obtained interval scale. These methods, variously labeled equal-appearing intervals or category-ratings, require a respondent to assign each stimulus to one of several categories, with the instructions that all categories are to be interpreted as psychologically equal. Another widely used psychometric technique involves the construction of a ratio scale through numerical estimation of the magnitude of the variable property (for example, desirability or willingness to pay) for each stimulus in the set. The crux of this subjective estimation method--magnitude estimation--is the assumption that the respondent can assess and assign numerical values that have ratio meaning.

The von Neumann-Morgenstern (1944) utility measurement is useful in deriving weights for health states (Torrance, 1972). The essence of the method consists of the standard lottery scheme where the subjects are asked to evaluate their preference between the certainty option and lottery option. Based on the expected utility hypothesis, utility for various states can be derived.

Economic weighting of various function states may take the form of human capital valuation or willingness to pay. Economic valuation has the advantage of being measured in dollars that can be compared to the cost directly. Human capital valuation has been developed extensively over the years (Dublin and Lotka, 1946; Weisbrod, 1961; Mushkin, 1962; Rice and Cooper, 1967). Willingness to pay has a more recent focus (Dorfman, 1979; Acton, 1973; Mishan, 1971; Schelling, 1968). Willingness to pay may take different forms. One form involves the analysis of actual public decisions to ascertain the implicit willingness to pay. Data sources include various public programs, court compensation cases, premium wage on risky occupations, real estate valuation in unsafe environment, or hypothetical questionnaires. The interview technique, using the probability of reducing risks, has been applied by Acton (1973) in an interesting experiment. When a fairly large number of health states with

multiple movements of probability is involved, the practicality of using the interview technique is questionable.

Composite Index   *Status Index vs, status Indicators*

     If we apply a set of weights to the set of health
states, we will obtain a scalar number as a composite index.
We shall use health status index in this context and refer to
unweighted individual measures simply as health status indicators. Both the individual indicators and the composite indexes can serve as effectiveness measures or social indicators. For example, the U.S. publication Social Indicators
lists several types of health indicators by such population
characteristics as mortality, disability, and restricted
activity days (U.S. Office of Management and Budget, 1973).
A composite index serves the useful purpose of summarizing,
in a single measure, the health of a population.

SINGLE INDICATORS--MORTALITY AND MORBIDITY

     As mentioned briefly earlier, this paper reviews
health status measures in terms of (1) the array of health
conditions covered, (2) the value-weighting scheme used, if
any, and (3) the incorporation of prognosis (Chen,
Bush, Zaremba, 1975). The taxonomy we shall use consists
of grouping various measures according to these indicators;
we will then evaluate their possible public policy use.
The order in which they are reviewed corresponds closely
to their historical development.

Mortality and Life Expectancy Indicators

     Mortality covers a single health condition, that is,
life (or death). With such a single measure, no weighting
scheme is necessary to contrast it with other functional or
dysfunctional health states. The prognostic element can be
incorporated in the mortality index by a simple computation
of rate.

     The mortality index represents the most prominent
traditional measure of health status. Death indicates the
complete dysfunction of a person at present and in the future
and is presumably unambiguous. Whether expressed as crude or
adjusted rate, mortality statistics have been developed by
biostatistics and related areas primarily as a measure for
population monitoring and for program evaluation. Even
today, a mortality index is widely used by economists and
actuaries as a starting point in benefit evaluation. Mortality by causes or by population characteristics are important yardsticks in health decision making. For example,
the allocation of research funds to disease categories may

be partially based on mortality rates associated with diseases. Other deficiencies in health, such as blindness,
pain, disfigurement, mental retardation, capacity to chew,
which will interfere with a person's functional capacity,
may also be important in the allocation system.

     As acute infectious diseases have been brought under
control, however, the proportion of individuals with chronic
debilitating diseases has increased, and the usual mortality
indexes have become insensitive as measures of program impact. Many biomedical research activities and findings result in the so-called halfway technology that does not improve mortality significantly. These activities and findings
may make significant contributions in terms of improving
other aspects of health, for example, reducing pain, discomfort, mental retardation, and disfigurement. They do not
extend life; they make life more livable. Between the 1950s
and the early 1970s, the mortality rates of the United States
have changed very little; yet various important halfway
technologies and treatments have been developed to improve
the health status of the individuals in the population
(Gordon and Fisher, 1975). It would be grossly incomplete
and inaccurate if only mortality rates were used to evaluate
payoffs from biomedical research and health services. In the
same vein, it would be grossly inadequate to evaluate the
productivity of physicians in terms of mortality alone.
In the study of the cost-effectiveness of a PKU screening and
treatment program (Bush and others, 1973), it was found
that approximately two-thirds of the benefit in terms of
total health improvement were non-mortality-related.

     The use of age or disease-specific mortality rates,
such as infant mortality and cancer death rates, would probably ease the problem of insensitivity somewhat, but no
complete escape is possible. Changes in mortality are still
mostly useful, however, in health planning in developing
countries and for some subgroups in the U.S. population, such
as the migrant workers and the American Indian population.
For example, the Pan American Health Organization (Ahumada,
1965) developed an index for the impact that various disease
categories have on mortality rates. The model, which has
been widely studied and used in Latin America for planning
public health programs, takes the following form:

     $P = MIV/C$

where

P = priority of the disease for public health action, in
    units of weighted preventable deaths/unit cost

M = ratio of the disease-specific mortality rate to the
    mortality rate from all causes

I = number of deaths resulting from the disease, weighted by a set of arbitrary coefficients that are inversely proportional to age

V = vulnerability of the disease, that is, percentage of deaths considered by medical experts to be preventable

C = production cost of the health program (set of activities).

The factor V represents an expert judgment of the general responsiveness of the disease to control. The product MIV is, in essence, an effectiveness measure that takes into account both the relative impact of the disease on the population and its probable responsiveness to a set of treatments (activities). As a ratio of effectiveness over cost, P provides a ranking of diseases in terms of their priority for public health action.

Morbidity Indicators

Traditional morbidity measures consist, basically, of counts of diseases, disability, and utilizations. Disease counts are useful to clinicians so they can make prognostic and treatment decisions; disease counts in a population may be a crude index of health status if the relative seriousness of diseases in terms of dysfunction and prognosis can be established. The relative valuation of diseases depends on the judgment of prognosis, as well as the desirability of standardized health dimensions, such as function/dysfunction, pain, and discomfort. The dilemma of comparing diseases has been aptly pointed out by Moriyama (1968): "How [can] one [equate] a case of coryza with a case of primary lung cancer, or a case of congenital anomaly with a case of senile psychosis?" In a Gallup Poll (1975), the sample of respondents identified cancer as the most feared disease. Without further study to delineate the underlying factors, such as prognosis and pain, no further inference can be made for public policy uses. The validity and reliability of disease counts, to this date, are troublesome even with the available advanced diagnostic technologies. The problem in comparing disease counts is compounded by the differential effectiveness of treatments applied. A serious disease at a particular point in time or space may not be serious at another point.

Various disability measures have been in use for a number of years. In particular, the national health survey conducted by the National Center for Health Statistics (1964 and 1977) has, since the early 1960s, collected yearly data on days of restricted-activity, bed-disability, and work-loss; the data have not shown any significant decrease or increase between the early 1960s and 1970s. In a way, most disability measures are more sensitive than the mortality rate; however, as a group, they suffer several main deficiencies: (1) They

are not mutually exclusive and collectively exhaustive.
(2) They are not sufficiently sensitive.   (3) They lack an
underlying theoretical construct.   Disability measures need
to be integrated with mortality to be complete.   Without a
weighting scheme, various disability measures simply become
loosely connected, with no coherent element to unify them.

Utilization rates (count of health care activities),
such as physician visits and cases treated, are frequently
used as a health status measure.   Utilization has serious
defects, since it does not necessarily correlate positively
with the effectiveness of a service and may even be inversely
related.   Highly effective therapies that cure the patient
(for example, appendectomy) involve no further utilization.
But partially effective therapies, such as those in chronic
disease that prevent mortality but do not cure the patient,
result in greater utilization over time for treatment to keep
the patient comfortable and functioning.   Frequently, the
more ineffective the therapy, the longer the hospital stay.
This is especially true in terminal illnesses where the
imminent outcome is death, but large amounts of resources may
be expended on palliative and symptomatic treatment.   Not
even the inverse relation is consistent, for a patient who
enters a critical care unit with a myocardial infarction and
dies shortly thereafter has a brief hospital stay, but the
therapy was totally ineffective.   Thus, in health services,
it is crucial to distinguish the count of patients who receive a course of treatment from the effectiveness of the
treatment in terms of health status improvement.

COMBINED INDICATORS WITHOUT
EXPLICIT REFERENCE MEASUREMENT

Efforts to combine morbidity and mortality into a
single measure without explicit preference (value) measurement have resulted in diverse formulations similar to the
Pan American Health Organization index.   The Q-index (Miller,
1970) ranks diseases affecting the American Indian population
according to potential response to intervention and days lost
due to premature death, hospitalization, and clinic visits.
The index is expressed as:

$$Q = MDP + 274 \ A/N + 91.3 \ B/N$$

where

Q   =   a numerical index for the program priority of a
        given disease

M   =   age and sex adjusted disease-specific Indian mor-
        tality rates as a ratio to the same rates for the
        U.S. population

D   =   crude disease-specific mortality rate for the target
         population

P   =   years of life lost because of premature death

274 =   100,000/365, a conversion factor to convert A to
         years/100,000 population

A   =   number of inpatient days due to the disease

N   =   target population

91.3 =   274/3, a conversion factor weighting an outpatient
         visit as loss of one-third of an inpatient day, to
         convert B to years/100,000 population

B   =   number of outpatient visits due to the disease.

The Indian Health Service used the index to establish
priorities in the early days of program budgeting; efforts
continued for a time to incorporate the index into more comprehensive planning models.

The Q-index provides a crude indicator for program
planning in the selection of disease for research and service.
Existing data are sufficient for the derivation of the index.
The index, however, omits many important health states that
deviate from well-being, rendering the index insensitive in
expressing the outcome of many health activities. For
planning, the Q-index is limited to disadvantaged groups
since it requires a reference population with lower mortality
to establish the potential vulnerability of the disease to a
program. Moreover, the weighting between mortality, inpatient days, and outpatient visits is arbitrary.

The Q-index has inspired a number of investigators to
devise new indexes following the same pattern. M. K. Chen
(1973) formulated the G-index but based it on crude disease-
specific mortality (for both the reference and the target
populations) and the difference between observed and expected
years lost from disease-specific mortality and morbidity in
the target population. More recently, M. K. Chen (1976) has
proposed a K-index based on unnecessary disability and death.
Operationally, this formulation of the index still requires
a reference group.

Chiang (1965) proposed a health index based on the expected duration in various health states for the fraction of
a year and the weights assigned to each state. The model is
expressed as:

$$H_x = 1 - \bar{N}_x \bar{T}_x - 1/2\ m_x$$

where

H_x = mean duration or average fraction of the year the individual is healthy in age group x

$\bar{N}_x$ = the average number of illnesses per person in age group x

$\bar{T}_x$ = the average duration of illness for group x as fractions of a year

m_x = the age-specific death rate for the year.

In a more recent formulation (1976), his model has taken the form:

$$H = W_1E_1 + W_2E_2 + ---- + W_sE_s + W_rE_r$$

where

H = health index

$W_1, W_2, ----, W_s$ = weights assigned to health states $1, 2, ----, s$

W_r = weight assigned to death state r

$E_1, E_2, ----, E_s$ = expected duration in health states $1, 2, ----, s$

E_r = expected duration in death state r.

$E_1, E_2, ----, E_r$ are to be derived from transition probabilities, whereas $W_1, W_2, ----, W_s$ represent the rapidity with which an individual in various health states returns to state 1, the perfect health state. These weights are to be derived from the incidence rates obtained through data collection from a sample survey of a population. Chiang's index, as developed, appears useful as a social indicator; the index, however, is less useful as an effectiveness measure in resource alloca-tion. A framework for linking the index to health services or biomedical advances has not been provided and the weights to be derived do not relate to a preference or value scale. Therefore, the operational definition of health states is yet to be completed.

Sullivan (1971) proposed a single index of mortality and morbidity that represents a valuable social indicator; it could be adapted to measure effectiveness. The index is based on the concept of "expectation of life free of dis-ability" and is computed by subtracting from the life ex-pectancy the probable duration of bed disability and in-ability to perform major activities according to cross-sectional data from the National Health Interview Survey.

With a conventional expectation of life at birth for all persons in the United States in 1965 of 70.2 years, the approximate expectation of life free of disability was 64.9 years.

Sullivan's index is perhaps one of the most advanced social indicators currently available. An increase in disability-free years could be computed as an effectiveness measure resulting from the implementation of a specific health activity or biomedical advance for a specific population. But the index still lacks sensitivity to many life changes that require a more refined set of disability levels and the determination of their relative values. While additional data on limitations in major and other activities are readily available from surveys conducted by the National Center for Health Statistics (1964), from a value standpoint it appears inappropriate to group these lesser types of disabilities with disability as severe as work loss or bed disability. Finally, the expectation of a disability-free life contains an undesirable technological lag behind the transition patterns that are already operating in the population but have not yet affected the cross-sectional distribution vector among the restricted activity levels.

In summary, mortality and morbidity indexes do produce some crude measures that can be used in monitoring total populations. For resource allocation among multiple programs, however, such indexes suffer one or more of the following deficiencies: (1) They implicitly assume that, regardless of severity, many disability illness states, even including death, are equally undesirable. (2) The classifications of disability lack sufficient discriminatory power to differentiate between many important health states. (3) No method is provided for specifying the relation between policy variables and the indexes. (4) For health planning, no systematic method has been proposed for determining values for the disability levels. (5) Except for mortality, no attention has been given to incorporating current transition patterns among disease states and health levels into the indexes.

Clinical Disability Ratings

A group of summary measures has a clinical orientation. These summary measures are mainly useful for clinical assessment and individual patient management; they are of little use as aggregate social indicators. At the same time, summary measures may be modified to serve as effectiveness measures and as a starting point for monetary benefit evaluation. These measures are usually in the form of a scale; many of these measures have a simple scoring system without an explicit value scale to express the relative desirability of individual items.

As the notion of health includes the capacity to perform the full range of daily activities, one approach to developing an effectiveness measure would be to adopt clinical
evaluation of a health state on a disability scale. In many
injury cases, particularly under the workmen's compensation
system, physicians are asked to give their evaluation of the
percentage of disability that the plaintiff suffers. The
process of disability evaluation generally follows the Guides
to the Evaluation of Permanent Impairment developed by the
American Medical Association (1971).

These percentages represent subjective physician judgments about "impairments of the whole man," after the maximum benefits of therapy have been achieved; the percentages
are used to compute the amount to be compensated for the
residual permanent disability. Although the percentages may
be used in planning models, serious questions must be raised
about the sources, validity, and comparability of the values
inserted. Most important, the ratings do not provide a
method for assessing the improvement to be expected from the
application of a treatment or activity. In fact, the ratings
exist only for those cases that have already achieved maximum therapeutic benefit and for which, given the existing
technology, no further change can be expected.

Furthermore, the permanent impairment rating scales
confound probabilities (prognoses) with preferences, preventing separate determination to compute precisely the effectiveness of specific health services to defined persons.
Moreover, because of their unstructured derivation, the subjective values incorporated in the "degree of disability" are
not scientifically reproducible and are of doubtful gen-
erality for social decision making.

Many other disability scales also exist. Karnofsky and
Burchenal (1949) proposed a comprehensive set of 10 disability
levels to which they assigned arbitrary 10-point intervals
from 0 to 100. Although the levels were not sufficiently defined operationally to serve as a sensitive general effectiveness measure, the scale possesses some degree of sensitivity
for evaluating special treatment advances, such as cancer
chemotherapy.

Wylie and White (1964) developed the "Maryland Disability Index" for measuring the effectiveness of rehabilitation activities. A patient in coma, who is unable to perform any activity, receives no points, while the patient who
can perform skillfully all specified activities receives 100
points. The disability scores corresponded well with the
usual clinical judgment on the patient's condition, and death
rates increased as the disability became more serious. The
index appropriately describes the health state in rehabilitation; the index is less useful, however, as a general effectiveness measure, since the prognoses cannot be explicitly

manipulated to quantify specific changes due to particular health services or advances.

Katz and his colleagues (1963) developed an "Index of Independence in Activities of Daily Living" for measuring the functional status of the elderly and chronically ill. Changes on the scale cannot be used as a measure of effectiveness for optimization, however, since (1) performance is graded only on an ordinal scale, (2) the applicable population and range of disabilities is very limited, and (3) important activities, such as walking, were omitted. Recently, Katz and his colleagues (1973) have proposed expansion to a more comprehensive set of activities, but retention of the ordinal characteristic of the performance scale prevents its general use for program selection under uncertainty, which is prevalent in health services and biomedical advances.*

Most recently, Reynolds and his colleagues (1974) have applied and extended the work of Bush and his associates (1973, 1972) on health state index, using four dimensions: role activity, self-care activity, movement, and mobility. Each dimension consists of several steps, with higher scores indicating, presumably, a higher health state. Scores are arbitrarily assigned to these steps, that is, 0 for the lowest step, 1 for the second lowest, and so forth. The index has been computed with the data obtained from a household survey of two economically depressed counties in Alabama. By correlating the index with a variety of factors, such as health contacts and perceived health status (in addition to other validity tests), it was found that the index conforms to the expectation. The usefulness of the index lies primarily in the area of social indicators; it is less useful in resource allocation since no explicit preference scale is used and no formal framework is developed to link health programs with the index. A prognostic element is not present in the index, although efforts are under way to take into account the transition probabilities.

Williamson and his colleagues developed a valuable effectiveness measure called "Preventable Impairment Unit Decades" (PIUD); this measure expresses the extent to which an untreated patient's impairment might be prevented or remedied by a specific health service (Williamson, 1968; Berdit and Williamson, 1973). Although no empirical method of scaling the degree of impairment was presented, this effectiveness measure represents a significant advance over most of the disability and disease rating scales inasmuch as prognoses, differential levels of disability, and durations in the levels were all explicitly recognized in the computation of effectiveness. A refined impairment scale and an

---

* But see Jones and others in this volume.

empirical method of valuing the impairment would make the
PIUD a very useful criterion for cost-effectiveness
analysis of health services and biomedical advances.

HEALTH STATUS MEASURES WITH
EXPLICIT PREFERENCE SCALES

relative desirability

So far, we have reviewed mainly those disability-
dysfunctional scales of health status that do not incorporate
explicit preference measurement in the scale. Because of recent advances and wide application of modern decision
theory's psychometric scaling methods and utility measurement
techniques, a spurt of research activities has ensued, focusing on the empirical scaling of the array of health conditions in terms of preference or, simply put, relative desirability. The preference scale thus developed can be used
as a set of weights to combine various health states into a
single composite health status index. Such an index should
be most useful for resource allocation purposes.

Many authors have recognized that health involves a
value judgment and the value needs to be made explicit via
vigorous scaling methods. In modern decision theory
(stemming from the work of von Neumann and Morgenstern (1944)),
two parameters are crucial: probabilities and preferences.
In the measurement of health effectiveness, the probabilities
are governed by the disease process interacting with the patient characteristics and the course of treatment. Preferences are intended as the guide to social values concerning
the relative desirability of different outcomes of the disease or injury, depending on medical care and the biomedical
advances used.

Forst (1973) proposed measuring the patient's utility
function for various health states by determining his values
based on major variables, such as probability of death, duration of incapacity, and reduction in wealth. Through careful consideration of several hypothetical situations, the
patient generates a utility function. Aside from the questions of validity and reliability, the procedure requires a
tedious introspection from each individual; it could not be
used efficiently for decisions involving large numbers of
patients. Some generalizations might be drawn from multiple
analyses of typical or recurrent situations, but Forst does
not deal with the problem of social utility (welfare) that
forms the basis for planning in the health field.

Barnoon and Wolfe (1972) have proposed a model that
makes a major advance in the application of statistical decision theory to measuring the effectiveness of medical
treatments. The measure is computed as the expected gain
from a given treatment expressed in utilities associated

with lifetime intervals and levels of disability. Where the therapeutic course is clear-cut, the model should be validated against medical decisions; it should be possible to adjust the parameter values so the model can be confidently applied to new and marginal cases. As with Forst's proposal, the model is constructed for individual decision making and the problems associated with its extension to public health programs and biomedical advances have not been addressed.

Because of the uncertainties, high personal stakes involved, and the availability of medical data and specialists interested in sharpening their clinical judgment, individual medical decision making offers a fertile area for effectiveness research for many years to come. By applying the results from one analysis to the next cohort of patients, any proposed treatment advances can be efficiently tested for their practicality and acceptability to both patients and professionals. The close analysis of medical decisions will naturally help the clinician perform his role to the benefit of the patient.

Unfortunately, the emphasis on individual decisions may not help, and may even contribute to, some of our major health care problems. Because of the high utility losses associated with individual decision making and the externalization of costs to third parties through insurance and government subsidies, decision theory based on individual preferences will almost certainly lead to still more hospitalization, more expensive diagnostic tests, and marginally beneficial therapeutic procedures; this is all rational from an individual point of view. The analysis of individual decisions, therefore, may simply result in diverting resources to the more elaborate and expensive treatment modules with marginal effectiveness for a selected few in academic medical centers. This will be done at the expense of a more fundamental search for prevention of diseases. For public decision making, a decision framework that deals with identified individuals with identified diseases or conditions needs to be supplemented by models that will deal with individuals as statistical persons.

Contrary to individual decision models, several authors have proposed health status measures based on the weighted sum of the numbers treated in each patient diagnostic category, with the weights for the cases to be derived from medical expert judgment. The weights could be a meaningful tool for productivity analysis, assuming that physicians' judgments represented social values in some sense. Neither author suggested a method for deriving the weights.

Torrance and his colleagues (1972) have developed a utility measure for the total effectiveness of health programs. Health state utilities are measured by the von Neumann-Morgenstern (1944) standard lottery scheme and by a

time-equivalence technique. Health states are defined by
disease treatment categories (such as kidney transplant or
sanitarium confinement) or by limitations (such as restricted
activity and confinement to an institution). Similar to the
models of Forst (1973) and Barnoon and Wolfe (1972),
Torrance has recognized the need for a utility dimension in
an effectiveness measure, but various problems deserve
further attention: (1) A more systematic and complete definition of health states, divorced from disease categories,
is required if we are to achieve the goal of comparing different health and biomedical research programs. (2) The
probabilistic nature of treatment outcomes must be explicitly
recognized and incorporated into the model. (3) Simpler,
more efficient, utility measurement techniques must be devised if we are to determine values from household interview
surveys. (4) Some theoretical justification must be provided
if we are to accept a social utility scale for the health
states derived from the measurement of individual preferences.
Torrance's model would be particularly useful for the purpose
of resource allocation; it would not be suitable for
social indicators.

     Bush and co-workers (Bush, 1973, 1972; Kaplan, 1976)
have developed a general index, based on the twin concepts
of function and prognosis, for use as a social indicator and
effectiveness measure. A detailed classification of over 40
function levels was developed based on mobility, physical
activity, and social activity. These health states apply
across all disease forms and health service/research programs. Prognoses, or the probabilities that govern the
transitions between the health states over time, are determined from medical data of expert judgment; a table that
distributes life expectancy among the different health states
is constructed. The vector of health state expectancies is
mapped into a scalar value called function years (quality-
adjusted life expectancy) using a set of social values
(health state weights) that have been empirically measured
to produce an interval scale. The expected increase in
function years for a patient type, given a defined service,
constitutes an effectiveness measure of the program or
treatment advances. This effectiveness measure incorporates
the probabilities characteristic of the disease and the
social values characteristic of the deviations from well-
being (Patrick, 1973). The index has been applied to a
probability sample of a community population; it can be
useful for evaluating advances in biomedical research.

     The Sickness Impact Profile (SIP) uses a measure of
sickness-related behavioral dysfunction consisting of approximately 190 items in 14 categories, such as social interaction, ambulation, and intellectual function (Gilson, 1975).
These items are derived from open-ended descriptions of behavioral dysfunction given by patients, health care professionals, individuals caring for patients, and the apparently

healthy. The investigators have adopted a psychometric scaling technique and equal-appearing method to construct the preference scale for these items. The SIP presents a valuable, sensitive measure of health status that can be used in the assessment of health program effectiveness. The incompleteness of SIP comes from the lack of frameworks to incorporate prognoses and to integrate cost with effectiveness for resource allocation purposes. SIP, with some modification, could also be used for social indicators.

Psychometric methods have also been widely used in one scaling of disability and diseases. Wyler and colleagues (1968) have developed a "Seriousness of Illness Rating Scale" for 126 diseases commonly seen in medical practice. "Seriousness of Illness" loosely includes such factors as prognosis, duration, threat to life, degree of disability, and degree of discomfort. A magnitude estimation method was used to obtain the rating. The result showed that dandruff and common cold occupied the lower end of the seriousness scale while cancer and leukemia were rated as the most serious diseases, more so than heart failure or heart attack. A highly significant individual concordance (Kendall's W) was found in the ranking of the diseases. Although useful as a guide for clinical judgment (the scale reflects the seriousness both of the present disability and the prognosis under stated conditions), it does not provide a way to judge the probable improvement of a person who receives a defined health service.

Most of the health status measures we have discussed fall into the category of behaviorally-based function/dysfunction status measures. On the other hand, investigators have attempted to elicit subjective feeling or assessment of personal health status (Ware, 1976). Ware has used health perception questionnaire items describing feeling states with accompanying response categories to each item, such as "definitely true" and "mostly false." Further studies are needed to make such measures useful for resource allocation and as social indicators.

Another approach in ascertaining the implicit value assumed in the concept of health involves the economic valuation of willingness to pay implied in public decision making. Rosser and Watts (1972) analyzed 500 awards made by the high courts of Great Britain to empirically determine the relative value of health states based on monetary criteria. They defined health states jointly by a set of disability levels and a set of distress levels. To standardize the scale, the state with the lowest award, "slight social disability with mild distress," was taken as the unit. On the average, the amount awarded to the state "confined to bed with severe distress" was 158 times that of the least severe state. The value for the death state cannot be readily obtained with this type of valuation. Moreover, the award represents considerations for both the seriousness of the disability and

of prognosis. Since the disability state and the prognosis
are not treated separately, each change in prognosis, even
for the same disability state, requires a new evaluation.
This approach, however, represents one of the best areas of
research for a meaningful effectiveness measure derived from
monetary evaluations.

USES OF HEALTH STATUS MEASURES
IN PUBLIC DECISION MAKING

As was said previously, health status measures may be
used (1) as social indicators, (2) as effectiveness criteria,
(3) as starting points in benefit measurement in dollar
terms for evaluating the payoffs from health services and
biomedical research, and (4) in the analysis of distribution.
We shall discuss each of these possible uses.

Social Indicators

Health status measures can be used as social indicators in various ways: (a) to summarize the current level of
physical and mental well-being with respect to health in a
community or nation, (b) to construct a time series for detecting trends or changes, and (c) to compare different population groups cross-sectionally. Health indicators thus
become an important component of social indicators for indicating the level of well-being in the nation or a community.
A trend analysis based on the time series would disclose a
pattern of shift in health status over time, indicating the
need for possible action. For example, by analyzing the data
on the national aggregate of age-adjusted death rates for all
causes for the period of 1900-75, we may show the long-term
trends that lead to a questioning of the factors accounting
for the pattern of change. Although the overall pattern
clearly exhibits a downward trend, the 1952-70 period does
not show any detectable change (Chen, M. M. and Wagner, 1978).
Cross-sectional analysis would reveal the differential distribution of health status among population groups. Some
disadvantaged groups can then be identified in the comparison. For example, infant mortality rate of the American
Indian population or the core city area may be exceedingly
high relative to some reference group. A number of authors,
in developing health status measures, have attempted to use
measures explicitly for population comparison (Miller, 1970;
Chen, M. K., 1976).

Effectiveness Criteria

Health status measures can be used as effectiveness
criteria and can be combined with measures that indicate
relative change for defined population groups. Efforts to
measure the effectiveness of health activities originate in

many disciplines, including clinical medicine, public health,
biostatistics, medical sociology, economics, operations research, and, more recently, the discipline of interdisci-
plines, health services research. For convenience, we follow
the convention of distinguishing effectiveness from benefit
measures in terms of measuring unit used: non-monetary
(effectiveness) versus monetary (benefit). Quite often cost-
effectiveness, by itself, has been used for allocative decision making, without converting benefits to dollar measures.

Various health status measures have been used as
effectiveness criteria in the evaluation of health services
and biomedical advances, including mortality, disease incidence rate, and bed-disability. Strictly speaking, health
status measures per se do not constitute an effectiveness
criterion; only the difference between health status measures
attributable to a specific service or advance can be properly
identified as an effectiveness measure. For example, if a
treatment will prolong life from 40 to 45 years, the health
output (and the effectiveness) of the treatment will be five
years, ignoring other aspects of health. When other aspects
of life are taken into account in a continuum from "minimal
health" to "optimum health," measured on an interval or ratio
scale, the overall effectiveness may be expressed as:

$$\Delta Q = Q_1 - Q_0$$

where

ΔQ =   change in health output (effectiveness)

Q_1 =   health output with the treatment

Q_0 =   health output without the treatment.

Health ceases to have any value once an individual reaches
the death state. Q_1 and Q_0, in effect, summarize health over
the time period between intervention and death. Many authors
have referred to such measures in various terms: for example,
value (or quality)-adjusted life years, effective years, productive years, and disability-free years (Chen, Bush, Patrick,
1975; Zeckhauser and Shepard, 1976). These measures, in a
sense, represent one possible operational definition of
"stock of health" as used by Grossman (1972) in his analysis
of demand for health.

In using effectiveness criteria for allocating resources, many health effectiveness measures may be used
simultaneously. For example, given the limited attention
span of most decision makers, a category of five or six
measures may be approximately used for comparing competing
health services or research projects. A set of such indicators (six health state descriptions) were tested in a recent experiment related to biomedical research and

prevention, control, and education (National Institutes of
Health, 1977).

     The need for weighting arises when there are many
measures involved and these measures give conflicting indications of effectiveness; in addition, the relative weights,
in terms of preference to be assigned to various measures,
become troublesome. On the other hand, a single measure,
derived from either adopting a dominant measure or integrating
various measures, can facilitate comparison between programs
more readily.

     A cost-effectiveness model may be used to select health
activity/target populations according to their ranking of
cost-effectiveness ratio until the budget is exhausted. Such
a procedure will not necessarily produce optimum results and
furthermore will be cumbersome to use when various constraints
(including equity consideration) are considered. A 0-1 programming method would be more appropriate (Chen and Bush,
1976). At present, the need for such refined modeling is not
obvious due to the lack of a uniform and sensitive measure of
health status change.

     For a given budget allocation to health, the cost-
effectiveness model will be adequate for optimum allocation
within health activities without the benefit of dollar
measurement. The problem becomes troublesome, however, when
health programs compete for allocation with other social programs, such as education and welfare. The insistence on a
single measure cutting across health, education, and welfare
will require us to develop a measure of "hew" as suggested by
Richardson (1972) ignoring other major functional areas of
public programs, such as defense, criminal justice, and agriculture. Of course, a uniform measure, such as monetary
unit, will enable us to compare programs not only for their
relative effectiveness but for their cost as well.

Starting Points for Benefit Measurement

     Health status measures can serve as a starting point
for benefit (in monetary terms) measurement if such a measure
is desired. The monetary representation of benefit facilitates comparisons across health indicators and the total
range of private and public services as well as between benefit and cost. The monetary representation, however, suffers
several deficiencies: (1) Definitional difficulties, both
conceptual and operational, are difficult to surmount.
(2) The resulting discrimination and reenforcement of status
quo (especially in health care) are not particularly attrac-
tive to a large segment of the population. (3) The resulting
valuation may be unacceptable to decision makers at all levels
of government as well as to private agencies with a pattern

of diffused power distribution. Whatever is the merit or de-
merit of the monetary benefit measure, it still depends on
the array of health conditions--such as mortality, morbidity,
function status measures, pain--to make the valuation. Accordingly, health indicators would serve as a starting point
for monetary benefit measurement. From a public policy point
of view, it appears to be more meaningful to begin the
analysis by expressing the payoff from health programs in
terms of health status change.

Analysis of Distribution

        Health status measures can also be meaningfully ap-
plied to the analysis of distribution. The equal access to
care is meaningless without some measures of health status.
If we view the health status as a stock concept, then the
distribution of such stock among subgroups or individuals in
the population will give us a precise measure of the distribution in terms of health. Because of the lack of acceptable comprehensive measures of health status, the distribution implications of many public programs are not clear.
Since the majority of publicly-financed health programs are
in-kind transfers of one sort or the other, their distributional impact in terms of health is not clear. Because of a
lack of viable health status measures, even the flow of federal funds to state and local governments cannot be analyzed
for the funds' distributional impact in terms of health
(Chen, M. M., 1976). The interaction of the interest groups
in political exchange often obscures the distributional
impact further.

REFERENCES

Acton, Jan Paul
    1973   Evaluating Public Programs to Save Lives: The
              Case of Heart Attacks. Santa Monica: The RAND
              Corporation, R-950-RC (January).

Ahumada, Jorge, et al.
    1965   Health Planning: Problems of Concept and
              Method. Publication No. 111. Washington, D.C.:
              Pan American Health Organization (April).

American Medical Association
Committee on Rating of Mental and Physical Impairment
    1971   Guides to the Evaluation of Permanent Impair-
              ment. Chicago: American Medical Association.

Barnoon, Shlomo and Harvey Wolfe
    1972   Measuring the Effectiveness of Medical Decis-
              ions: An Operations Research Approach.
              Springfield, Ill.: Charles C. Thomas.

Berdit, Martin and John W. Williamson
    1973   "Function limitation scale for measuring health
              outcomes." In Berg, Robert L. (ed.), Health
              Status Indexes. Chicago: Hospital Research
              Educational Trust, pp. 59-69.

Berg, Robert L., Dean S. Hallauer, and Stephen N. Berk
    1976   "Neglected aspects of the quality of life."
              Health Services Research 11(4) (Winter):452-463.

Bonnet, P. D.
    1969   Increased Production and Better Utilization.
              Report of the National Conference on Medical
              Costs, June 27-28, 1967. Washington, D.C.:
              U.S.DHEW.

Bush, James W., Milton M. Chen, and Donald L. Patrick
    1973   "Health status index in cost-effectiveness:
              Analysis of PKU program." In Berg, Robert L.
              (ed.), Health Status Indexes, Hospital Research
              and Educational Trust, Chicago, pp. 172-194.

Bush, James W., Sol Fanshel, and Milton M. Chen
    1972   "Analysis of a tuberculin testing program using
              a health status index. Socio-Economic Planning
              Sciences 6(1) (February):46-68.

Chen, Martin K.
    1976   "The K index: A proxy measure of health care
              quality." Health Services Research 11(4)
              (Winter):452-463.

Chen, Martin K.
    1973   "The G index for program priority." In Berg,
              Robert L. (ed.), Health Status Indexes, Hos-
              pital Research and Educational Trust, Chicago,
              pp. 28-34.

Chen, Milton M.
    1976   Federal Health Grants-in-aid to States:
              Rationale and Interstate Redistributional
              Effect. Paper presented at Eastern Economic
              Association meeting, Bloomsburg, Pa. (April).

Chen, Milton M. and James W. Bush
    1976   "Maximizing health system output with political
              and administrative constraints using mathe-
              matical programming." Inquiry 13(3) (Septem-
              ber):215-227.

Chen, Milton M., James W. Bush, and Donald L. Patrick
    1975   "Social indicators for health planning and
              policy analysis." Policy Sciences 6(1) (March):
              71-89.

Chen, Milton M., James W. Bush, and Joseph Zaremba
    1975   "Effectiveness measures." In Shuman, L.,
              R. Speas, and J. Young (eds.), Operations
              Research in Health Care--A Critical Analysis.
              Baltimore: The Johns Hopkins University
              Press, pp. 276-301.

Chen, Milton M. and D. P. Wagner
    1978   "Gains in mortality from biomedical research,
              1930-1975: An initial assessment." Social
              Science and Medicine (forthcoming).

Chiang, C. L.
    1976   "Making annual indexes of health." Health
              Services Research 11(4) (Winter):442-451.

    1965   "An index of health: Mathematical models."
              Vital and Health Statistics, series 2, no. 5,
              National Center for Health Statistics,
              U.S.DHEW.

Dorfman, Nancy S.
    1979   "The social value of saving a life." In
              Mushkin, Selma J. and David W. Dunlop (eds.),
              Health: What is it Worth? (this volume).

Dublin, Louis I. and A. J. Lotka
    1946   The Money Value of a Man. New York: The
              Ronald Press.

Feldstein, Martin S.
    1968   Economic Analysis for Health Service Efficiency.
               Chicago: Markham.

Forst, Brian E.
    1973   "Quantifying the patient's preferences." In
               Berg, Robert L. (ed.), Health Status Indexes,
               Hospital Research and Educational Trust,
               Chicago, pp. 209-228.

Gallup Poll
    1975   Release. Princeton, N.J. (December 2).

Gilson, Betty S., et al.
    1975   "The sickness impact profile: Development of
               an outcome measure of health care." American
               Journal of Public Health 65(12) (December):
               1304-1310.

Gordon, Gerald and G. Lawrence Fisher
    1975   The Diffusion of Medical Technology: Policy
               and Research Planning Perspectives.
               Cambridge, Mass.: Ballinger Publishing Co.,
               appendix 5A, p. 97.

Grossman, Michael
    1972   The Demand for Health. New York: National
               Bureau of Economic Research.

Kaplan, Robert M., James W. Bush, and Charles C. Berry
    1976   "Health status: Types of validity and the
               index of well-being." Health Services
               Research 11(4) (Winter):478:507.

Karnofsky, David A. and J. H. Burchenal
    1949   "The clinical evaluation of chemotherapeutic
               agents in cancer." In McLeod, Colin (ed.),
               Evaluation of Chemotherapeutic Agents.
               New York: Columbia University Press,
               pp. 191-205.

Katz, Sidney, et al.
    1973   "Measuring the health status of populations."
               In Berg, Robert L. (ed.), Health Status
               Indexes. Chicago: Hospital Research and
               Educational Trust, pp. 39-52.

    1963   "Studies of illness in the aged." JAMA 185(12)
               (September 21):914-919.

Miller, J. E.
    1970   "An indicator to aid management in assigning
               program priorities." Public Health Reports
               85(8) (August):725-731.

Mishan, E. J.
    1971   "Evaluation of life and limb: A theoretical
              approach." Journal of Political Economy
              79(4) (July/August):687.

Moriyama, Iwao M.
    1968   "Problems in the measurement of health status."
              In Sheldon, E. B. and W. Moore (eds.),
              Indicators of Social Change: Concepts and
              Measurement. New York: Russell Sage,
              pp. 573-600.

Mushkin, Selma J.
    1962   "Health as an investment." Journal of
              Political Economy 70 (October):129-157.

National Center for Health Statistics
U.S. Department of Health, Education, and Welfare
    1977   "Current estimates from the health interview
              survey, United States--1975." Vital and Health
              Statistics, series 10, no. 115, Rockville, Md.
              (March), p. 19.

    1964   "Health survey procedure: Concepts, question-
              naire development, and definitions in the
              health interview survey." Vital and Health
              Statistics, series 1, no. 2, Rockville, Md.
              (May).

National Institutes of Health, Division of Lung Diseases
U.S. Department of Health, Education, and Welfare
    1977   Respiratory Disease Task Force Report on Pre-
              vention, Control, and Education, U.S.DHEW pub.
              (NIH) 77-1248 (March).

Nunnally, J. C.
    1967   Psychometric Theory. New York: McGraw-Hill.

Parsons, Talcott
    1958   "Definitions of health and illness in light of
              American values and social structure." In
              Jaco, E. Gartley (ed.), Patients, Physicians,
              and Illness, pp. 165-187.

Patrick, Donald L., James W. Bush, and Milton M. Chen
    1973   "Toward an operational definition of health."
              Journal of Health and Social Behavior 14(1)
              (March):6-23.

Reynolds, W. Jeff, William A. Rushing, and David L. Miles
    1974   "The validation of a function status index."
              Journal of Health and Social Behavior 15(4)
              (December):271-288.

Rice, Dorothy P. and Barbara S. Cooper
     1967   "The economic value of human life." American
               Journal of Public Health 57(110 (November):
               1954-1966.

Richardson, Elliot L.
     1972   "The inescapable necessity of choice."
               Los Angeles Times, section 5, p. 6 (February
               20).

Rosser, Rachel M. and Vincent C. Watts
     1972   "The measurement of hospital output."
               International Journal of Epidemiology 1(4)
               (Winter):361-368.

Schelling, T. C.
     1968   "The life you save may be your own." In
               Chase, Samuel B. (ed.), Problems in Public
               Expenditure Analysis. Washington, D.C.: The
               Brookings Institution, pp. 127-162.

Sullivan, Daniel F.
     1971   "A single index of mortality and morbidity."
               HSMHA Health Reports 86(4) (April):347-354.

Thurston, L. L.
     1959   The Measurement of Value. Chicago: University
               of Chicago Press.

Torrance, George W., W. H. Thomas, and D. L. Sackett
     1972   "A utility maximization model for evaluation of
               health care programs." Health Services
               Research 7(2) (Summer):118-133.

U.S. Office of Management and Budget
     1973   Social Indicators. Washington, D.C.

von Neumann, J. and O. Morgenstern
     1944   Theory of Games and Economic Behavior. Prince-
               ton, N.J.: Princeton University Press.

Ware, John E.
     1976   "Scales for measuring general health per-
               ceptions." Health Services Research 11(4)
               (Winter):396-415.

Weisbrod, B. A.
     1961   "The valuation of human capital." Journal of
               Political Economy 69 (October):425.

Williamson, John W.
     1968   Prognostic Epidemiology: Concept, Process, and
               Product. Baltimore: The Johns Hopkins School
               of Hygiene and Public Health, Dept. of Medical
               Care and Hospitals.

Wyler, Allen R., M. Masuda, and T. H. Holmes
    1968   "The seriousness of illness rating scale."
              Journal of Psychosomatic Research 11:363-374.

Wylie, Charles M. and Betty K. White
    1964   "A measure of disability." Archives of
              Environmental Health 8:834-839.

Zeckhauser, Richard and Donald Shepard
    1976   "Where now for saving lives?" Law and
              Contemporary Problems (Summer).

2 An Approach to the Assessment of Long-Term Care

Ellen W. Jones
Barbara J. McNitt
Paul M. Densen

Progress in developing methods for assessing the quality of medical care is dependent on (1) the completeness of information on the natural history of disease and (2) the relationship between the processes of medical care and patient outcomes (Brook, 1973; Donabedian, 1966; Katz, 1972; Shapiro, 1967; Gonnella, 1975). With regard to long-term care, such information depends upon the development of a standard terminology for describing the health status of chronically ill patients at different points in time or at different stages of disability. More than 20 years ago, the Commission on Chronic Illness in the United States recognized this requirement and recommended "the adoption and widespread use of comparable terminology... [as] essential steps toward improving the usefulness and meaning of data collected and analyzed for various purposes by health organizations and by persons who investigate needs and resources for care of long-term illness" (Commission on Chronic Illness, 1956). In the years since the Commission's report, many classifications of long-term care patients have been proposed (Ryder, 1971; Akpom, 1973; Bruett, 1969), but none has gained widespread acceptance in the sense of being incorporated systematically into service programs generally. The research project reported in this paper used the classifications in the Patient Classification for Long-Term Care: User's Manual (Jones, 1974) as the basis for developing a patient-assessment procedure which could be implemented in long-term care facilities and which would provide information for planning and evaluating patient-care, as well as for program review.

In order to develop such a patient-assessment procedure, it was decided that the assessment system would have to (1) provide information on patients which could be used for decisions about the type and place of care appropriate to their needs and (2) be sensitive to changes over time in the conditions of patients; thus, the outcomes of patients in different types of care programs could be evaluated. The developed procedure was tested by assessing patients in

Long Island Chronic Disease Hospital and in seven nursing
homes providing both skilled and intermediate levels of care.*
Specific aims of the project at Long Island Hospital were to
assist the hospital staff in assessing needs of patients, including determination of levels of care, and to reassess patients at a later date in order to measure the effects of the
hospital's program changes on the patient population. In the
nursing home study, the aims were to assess all newly admitted
patients and reassess the same patients at periodic intervals
thereafter until their discharge, up to two years after admission. Data from these assessments and reassessments in the
project report exemplify the utility of the assessment system
for placement and care planning, for quantifying changes in
patient status, and for study of patient outcomes.

METHODS

        Sources of information about patients included in the
study were the medical and administrative records of the pro-
vider facilities and interview responses from personnel who
were in a position to observe patients regularly; these latter
included licensed nurses, aides, social-work personnel, and
medical specialists. Since the sources were multiple and
varied from setting to setting, an assessment-abstract form
was developed for recording the information. The form was
designed to organize information in a way that would be useful to both a care planner and reviewer. For example, the
columnar arrangement for checking a patient's classification
with respect to specific items of information at four different times shows, at a glance, the direction of change in
the patient's status. In addition to the patient's medical
and functioning status, as well as socio-demographic characteristics, as defined in the Patient Classification for
Long-Term Care: User's Manual, the form includes information
on services performed for the patient, on the patient's
transfers away from and into the facility, and on the frequency of social visits made to the patient, according to the
relationship of the visitor to the patient. In selecting and
defining these additional items of information, the concepts
used in the development of items in the Patient Classification
were adhered to; for example, the service items were defined

---

*   Long Island Chronic Disease Hospital is located in Boston
    Harbor. It is a part of the Boston City Department of
    Health and Hospitals. The seven nursing homes and their
    locations in Massachusetts are as follows: Dexter House,
    Malden; D'Youville Manor, Lowell; Elm Hill, Roxbury;
    Franvale, South Braintree; Mary Immaculate, Lawrence;
    Normandy House, Melrose; Prospect Street, Cambridge. Five
    homes are proprietary and two are non-profit.

as services actually performed or actions taken (rather than proposed actions), and were expressed in objective terminology.*

For personnel in the participating facilities, project staff conducted orientation sessions on the use of the abstract form for patient assessment. Procedures for collecting information differed slightly between the chronic disease hospital and the seven nursing homes. In the hospital, sociodemographic information was abstracted from records by project personnel; medical information was recorded by the hospital's full-time clinician; functioning-status information was recorded by hospital nursing staff. The three parts were put together and discussed in team conferences organized for the purpose. In the nursing homes, at the beginning of the study, project staff obtained and recorded information from all sources (by copying from the medical records or interviewing the appropriate nursing home personnel). During the project, however, members of nursing home staffs became increasingly active in the assessment process and began to implement the procedure within their ongoing service programs. In this changeover, project staff continued to review the assessment information with nursing home personnel to insure that standard definitions were being adhered to. A test of reliability of the data collection procedure by project staff was carried out in one nursing home. As a result of the test, some errors in classification due to differences in interpretation of definitions were detected and the coding of the study data was corrected accordingly.

The assessment-abstract forms were duplicated so that one set could be retained by the facility and the other could be used for data processing. In Long Island Hospital and in several of the nursing homes, the forms were incorporated in the patient's medical record. Personnel in the homes began to find the form information useful to them in a variety of ways and reported these uses to the project staff. An important part of the process of developing the patient-assessment procedure was a series of meetings between project staff and personnel from all participating facilities. At these meetings, the results and implications of periodic data analysis were discussed together. At intervals, the project staffs were also able to discuss the progress of the study with an advisory committee of experts in the long-term care field and with a larger group of participants in three nursing home conferences (Harvard Center, 1974, 1973, 1972), including members of the four university groups who had collaborated in the development of the Patient Classification for Long-Term Care.

---

* Two training manuals have been produced which were built on the study procedures and experience (Falcone, 1976; McNitt, 1976).

APPLICATION OF THE PATIENT CLASSIFICATION TO PROGRAM
EVALUATION IN LONG ISLAND CHRONIC DISEASE HOSPITAL

In 1972, a cooperative study had been started at Long
Island Hospital as a result of the clinical director's estimation that between 40 and 50 percent of the hospital's pat-
tients might be appropriately cared for in other and less
costly locations. At that time, an assessment of the needs
of patients, based on their physical and social functioning
as well as their medical status, showed that indeed 53.2 percent were appropriately located, but that, with the exception
of 2.4 percent judged to need psychiatric hospital care, the
remaining 44.4 percent could have their needs met by facilities providing less intensive levels of care. In 1975, on
the basis of the individual assessments and these findings,
the hospital staff undertook specific activities to improve
their program for patient care, including the following:

(1)   discharge planning whenever possible for
        patients judged to be inappropriately
        located;

(2)   use of patient-assessment procedure in
        preadmission screening;

(3)   use of patient-assessment procedure in
        utilization review; and

(4)   implementation of specific rehabilitation
        techniques to improve the functioning
        status of patients throughout the hospital.

On February 1, 1975, a second survey of the hospital
population was carried out for all inpatients. Of the 279
patients assessed,* 158 patients had been assessed in the
survey in 1972.

Results of activities in the first three categories
above, (1) discharge planning, (2) preadmission screening,
and (3) utilization review, are reflected in the fact that
the percentage of patients judged to be appropriately
placed in the chronic disease hospital increased from 53.2
in 1972 to 67.4 in 1975.

It was not feasible to transfer all patients who could
be theoretically transferred elsewhere. Patients in Long
Island Hospital are unlike patients in nursing homes or the
general population in certain characteristics: 64 percent
were males compared with 27 percent in a national nursing-
home sample (Public Health Service, 1975); twice as many

---

* Seventeen other patients were discharged or died before
  their assessments were scheduled.

were single (never married) as in the national sample; about
two-thirds had been in the hospital for more than two years;
and the two most frequently reported diagnoses were neurological disorders (43.0 percent) and alcoholism (42.6 percent).
However, 29 patients were transferred to nursing homes and
seven were transferred to other long-term care facilities out
of the group of 295 assessed in 1972.

Effects of the rehabilitation programs instituted by
the hospital were seen in the comparison of functioning status
items for the 158 patients who were assessed in the two surveys, for example:

	Percent in category in	
	1972	1975
Confined to chair or bed	48.1%	7.0%
Wheels without assistance	4.4	9.5
Wheels with help of another person	1.9	36.1

In addition to this increase in mobility of patients in a two-
and-a-half-year period, there was improvement in the functioning status of activities of daily living (ADL), such as
transferring (in the sense of moving about), bathing, and
eating, and even a small increase in the number of patients
toileting themselves. There was also improvement in the
orientation status of patients. Among the 158 assessed in
both surveys, the percentage who were disoriented as to time,
place, and person decreased from 31.6 in 1972 to 5.7 in 1975.
One explanation for this decrease is that an active reality/
remotivation program in which all staff participated was instituted by the hospital in the time between the two surveys.
However, change in functioning status went in the opposite
direction--that is, toward a lower percentage performing in-
dependently--in the activity of dressing, and more than half
the number of patients at both surveys were not dressed.

In 1975, increasing numbers of impairments were noted
in this group of 158 patients. While some change for the
worse, such as deterioration in vision or hearing, might be
accepted as an unavoidable concomitant of aging in a population with multiple chronic conditions, the increase in joint
motion impairments was a cause for concern. This was called
to the attention of the Physical Therapy Department in particular and to medical and nursing staffs for evaluation of
their responsibilities in this connection.

In summary, the systematic use of patient assessment at
Long Island Hospital has (1) pointed out program areas in need
of attention and (2) demonstrated the effectiveness of staff
efforts to improve the functioning status of patients in their
care.

THE ASSESSMENT OF CARE IN SEVEN NURSING HOMES

        The primary purpose of the study of nursing homes was
to develop a method of looking at issues of quality-of-care on
patient-status information, as defined in the Patient Classification. The data were obtained from periodic assessments of
patients admitted to the seven nursing homes in the period
February 1, 1973 to November 30, 1974. Initial assessments of
patients were done within the second week of the patient's
residence in the home; reassessments were done at intervals of
six weeks, three months, six months, one year, 18 months, and
two years after admission.

        Of the 1,745 patients admitted to the nursing homes
during the study intake period, 211 (12.1 percent) were discharged before they could have an initial assessment. About
70 percent of this group with very short stays either died in
the nursing home (79 patients) or were discharged back to the
acute-care hospital (68 patients). Further follow-up of those
discharged to hospitals revealed that about half of these died
in the hospital. The very high early mortality among these
211 patients raises questions about the appropriateness of the
nursing home placement in the first place, the transfer back
to the hospital, or both. The effect of regulatory and fiscal
reimbursement policies on such transfers of patients needs
examination.

        Patients remaining in the homes and having an initial
assessment numbered 1,534. Of these, 902 (58.8 percent) remained in the homes and were reassessed at six weeks; 582
(37.9 percent) were present for a three-months reassessment.
Numbers present for reassessment at each subsequent point in
time were the following:*

              Initial assessment   1,534
              6-weeks reassessment   902
              3-months reassessment   647
              6-months reassessment   425
             12-months reassessment   205
             18-months reassessment   112
             24-months reassessment   14

In addition to the assessments done on the regular schedule,
520 were done at the time of discharge or readmission of a
patient, making a total of 5,359 patient assessments in the
nursing home study.

_____

*   It should be noted that the decrease in numbers available
    for reassessments after three months was the result not
    only of discharges, but also of foreshortened periods of
    observation for patients admitted late in the study.

Demographic characteristics of the patient population were generally comparable with those observed in the national survey (Long-Term Facility Study, 1975): 24.6 percent were 85 years of age or older, and a total of 47.0 percent were 80 or older; females outnumbered males by more than two to one and only 24.5 percent had a living spouse, although 60.9 percent had one or more living children. Almost all (96.8 percent) of the patients in these seven nursing homes were white and for 79.0 percent, their former residence was in the same town as the nursing home or a neighboring town.

The most frequently reported medical diagnosis among patients in the study was one or more of the specifically defined heart conditions: angina, myocardial infarction, cardiac arrhythmia, or congestive heart failure. These conditions ranked first for patients admitted at all levels of care; however, there were differences between levels of care in the ranking of other medical conditions, as shown in table 1.

Table 1. Five Most Common Diagnoses by Patients' Level of Care on Admission.

Level I (formerly Extended Care Facility, ECF)	Level II	Level III (Intermediate Care Facility, ICF)
1. Heart disease 2. Hip fracture 3. Stroke 4. Diabetes 5. Malignancy	1. Heart disease 2. Diabetes 3. Stroke 4. Malignancy 5. Arthritis	1. Heart disease 2. Diabetes 3. Arthritis 4. Neurologic disorders 5. Hypertension

All of the information collected in the assessment process is used in planning care of patients--medical diagnoses, personal characteristics, physical impairments, and tests and measurements indicating fragility or the need for special follow-up attention. But the observed performance of patients with respect to the ADL is the basis for much of the nursing care plan and also indicates the amount of nursing care required. Similarly, the degree of dependence in function determines, to a large measure, the level of care or type of program assigned to a patient. Systematic assessment of all patients admitted to the nursing homes, as in Long Island Hospital, focused attention on specific areas of function in which care was needed; for example, the improvement of ambulation in a patient requiring assistance in walking or the encouragement of a patient to feed himself.

Data from the study showed that a sizable proportion
of patients admitted to the homes were in need of a great deal
of nursing care. In order to summarize the detailed data on
functioning status items, each patient was classified according to the "Katz Index of the Activities of Daily Living," a
classification that has been validated as "a measure of
primary sociobiological functions" in several types of care
settings and with many different groups of patients (Katz,
1976). The index is a scale on which patients are graded
from independence to dependence (A through G) in six ADL
activities: transferring, bathing, dressing, toileting,
eating/feeding, and continence. The percentages of patients
admitted to the nursing homes in the two most dependent categories (F and G, dependent in five or six of the six functions) were 57.0 for Level I, 69.9 for Level II, and 31.8 for
Level III. The distributions of patients by ADL categories
varied among the nursing homes in the study even when the
level of care was held constant. The range in percentages of
Level II patients classified F or G was 47.4 to 79.6, and the
range for Level III was 22.2-51.5. This variation within
levels of care raises questions about reimbursement formulae
based solely on level-of-care criteria.

As one approach to the assessment of appropriateness of
care, data from the study were used to show how information
about services provided to patients could be related to information about patient status. For example, at the time of
initial assessment, 97.9 percent of the patients with a
diagnosis of hypertension had a blood pressure recorded;
monitoring was continued for patients with this diagnosis,
with 99.3 percent having a blood pressure recorded at the
six-weeks reassessment date. On the other hand, among patients with diuretics prescribed, only 25.0 percent had a
weight recorded at initial assessment, and there was no increase in this percentage at the time of the six-weeks reassessment. The data in this format do not permit conclusions
about effectiveness of services, but they illustrate a line
of questioning that may be pursued in a nursing home's self-
evaluation or in surveillance of care programs generally.

Different approaches to issues of quality through
measurement of change--made possible by sequential patient
assessments employing standard terminology--were exemplified
as follows:

(1)   change in specific items used on the assessment-
      abstract form;

(2)   change in incidence or prevalence of a specific
      condition;

(3)   change in the functioning status profile of a
      patient population (outcomes);

(4)   changes in the functioning status of individual
       patients and the direction or nature of these
       changes (outcomes); and

(5)   (a) calculation of the probabilities of change
       associated with certain characteristics of pa-
       tients at the time of first observation and
       (b) the application of this method to managerial
       and epidemiological questions.

An example of the need for number (1) was given above.
Only 25 percent of patients with diuretics prescribed had
their weight recorded in the initial assessment. For an example of number (2), change in incidence or prevalence of
a specific condition, data on decubiti were presented. At
the time of admission to nursing homes, 17.1 percent of all
patients had one or more decubiti. However, of those who
remained in the homes for six-weeks reassessment, 37.1 percent had their decubiti successfully treated while, during
the same time period, only 4.4 percent of the patients without decubiti on admission developed them. Number (3), changes
in profiles of patient populations, were illustrated by the
classification of functioning status of patients who were
present in the nursing homes for initial assessment and six-
weeks and three-months reassessments. Although changes in
this patient group were small, the changes were, for the most
part, in a positive direction. At least it could be said
that function in the basic ADL was being maintained.
Number (4), functioning status changes of individual patients (outcomes), were shown for patients in different ADL
categories at the time of initial assessment. For example,
of 481 patients classified as G (receiving assistance with
all six ADL functions), 23 percent died within six weeks of
admission to the homes; of 301 surviving the six-weeks
period, 71 percent remained in the dependent category, but
29 percent had improved in functioning status to some degree. Study of the data for patients in all categories led
to two general conclusions. One was that the ADL status of
patients at initial assessment is highly predictive of the
patient's type of discharge within the ensuing six-weeks
period; the percentages of patients dying in the homes before the six-weeks date can be seen in table 2. The second
general conclusion was that among patients remaining in the
nursing homes for six weeks, change in functioning status
was a common occurrence.

At the three-months reassessment period, the picture
of change becomes very complex. For example, some patients
who improved in the earlier periods, initial assessment and
six-weeks reassessment, relapsed in the later; some who
worsened at first, subsequently recovered their initial
functioning status; others delayed any change until the
later period. Nevertheless, it was evident that patterns
of change could be described quantitatively. Given large
enough numbers to start with, data of this type could be

Table 2.   Percentages of Patients Dying in Nursing Homes.

ADL categories	Number of patients in each category	Percent dying in nursing homes within six weeks
A	161	1.2%
B	53	1.9
C	93	1.1
D	72	4.2
E	325	4.9
F	349	10.6
G	481	22.7

used to describe expected patient outcome. Observed outcomes in different settings, with different treatment
modalities, could then be compared.

The last approach to analysis of changing status of
patients, number (5), was the application of modified life-
table methods of calculation of probabilities of survival,
death,* or other change within specified time intervals. As
shown by the data in table 3, the ADL status of patients at
initial assessment was highly predictive of survival or death
not only over a six-weeks period, as mentioned above, but
over a span of one year or more. Of those in the categories
A through E, 74-77 percent survived one year and the two-year
survival for the combined group was 65 percent (not shown in
the table); for those in the F category, 50 percent survived
two years, and for those classified G, only 28 percent survived two years. Probabilities of survival differed for patients under and over 80 years of age and for patients with a
diagnosis of cancer. Prognosis of two-year survival was very
low for cancer patients with F or G status at time of initial
assessment.

The methodology of number (5) could also be used to
examine the probabilities of such changes as movement from one
ADL category to another, return to preadmission functioning
status, transfer to acute care hospitals, and discharge to
lesser levels of care. Thus, this methodology is a powerful
tool for comparing outcomes of patients in different settings.

----

*   Facts of death were ascertained by checking the death
    certificate files of the Massachusetts Department of
    Public Health. Thus, the data include all deaths in
    the study population irrespective of the place of
    death within the state.

Table 3. Probabilities of Surviving to Specified Time Periods after Admission to Nursing Homes, for Patients in Selected Categories at Initial Assessment.

Category	Number of patients in category	Probability of surviving after admission					
		One month	Two months	Three months	Six months	One year	Two years
Patients with initial assessment, total	1,534	.854	.792	.754	.681	.602	.501
Age:							
Under 80 years	813	.870	.814	.773	.695	.638	.562
80 years or over	721	.836	.767	.732	.664	.560	.425
ADL status:[+]							
A	161	.950	.944	.918	.847	.741	.599[f]
B	53	.943	.925	.867	.806	.747	.747[f]
C	93	.914	.892	.869	.806	.762	.711[f]
D	72	.912	.870	.855	.825	.762	.556[f]
E	325	.923	.892	.865	.812	.770	.685[f]
F	349	.854	.786	.737	.651	.558	.503[f]
G	481	.744	.633	.586	.498	.401	.275[f]
Number of medically defined conditions:							
None	145	.883	.819	.797	.773	.658	.589[f]
One	550	.862	.795	.761	.701	.627	.572[f]
Two	529	.843	.780	.740	.657	.583	.451[f]
Three or more	310	.845	.796	.744	.643	.564	.391[f]
Diagnosis of cancer (CA):							
All patients with CA	260	.746	.625	.536	.397	.303	.238[f]
A or B status	35	.829	.800	.655	.525	.427[f]	.284[f]
C, D, or E	70	.757	.685	.625	.415	.294[f]	.294[f]
F or G	155	.723	.558	.468	.360	.275	.193[f]

+ ADL = activities of daily living: bathing, dressing, toileting, transferring, continence, and feeding. A = no assistance with any of the activities, B = assistance with one, C with two, D with three, E with four, F with five, and G = assistance with all six activities.

f Fewer than 10 person months of observation in final month of period.

It also provides the opportunity to assess the impact of
policy decisions on changes in patient status and costs of
care over time. For instance, in this study of nursing home
lengths of stay, it was evident that the probability of remaining in the homes was a function of the payment mechanism
as well as of the characteristics of patients. Only about
one-fourth of the Level I patients (24.2 percent) remained
as long as three months after admission, and very few remained one year. Of Level II patients, 50 percent remained
three months and 26.3 percent remained one year or longer.
The longest stays were averaged by Level III patients; 63.3
percent were in the homes for three months and 36.7 percent
stayed one year or more. If the present policies of payment
for long-term care were to be changed, one could then observe
the resulting changes in the lengths of stay as calculated
above.

SUMMARY AND CONCLUSIONS

        The development and use of a patient-assessment system,
based on the Patient Classification for Long-Term Care, has
shown that widespread use of the common language incorporated
in the system is feasible and practical. Data obtained in
the development project, An Approach to the Assessment of
Long-Term Care, were used to show that health status of
chronically ill and aged individuals is measurable and that
changes in status are also quantifiable. Specific examples
were presented of how the data might be used to approach
issues of quality of care, both from the individual-patient
standpoint, as in current utilization review procedures, or
from the group standpoint, as in the determination of norms
of patient care. Analysis of change in patient status was
shown to be a potent tool for comparing outcomes of patients
in different settings, that is, in different treatment
modalities. Based on this experience, a number of next
steps are seen as important:

        ● Agreement must be reached among regulatory
          agencies at both state and federal levels
          about the content and structure of the
          patient-oriented information that long-term
          care facilities are required to report.
          This would reduce the time and cost now
          associated with the reporting of overlapping
          data items on a multiplicity of forms. Once
          such agreement is reached, technical aspects
          of reporting need further development; for
          example, efficient and economic methods of
          abstracting information from individual pa-
          tient records for use in manual and electronic
          data-processing systems.

- Training and orientation activities in patient
  assessment, coordinated at state, regional, and
  federal levels, should be continued and expanded.

- The patient assessment process should be applied
  in longitudinal studies of population groups for
  analysis of two types of questions: (1) Which
  characteristics of patients are associated with
  use of long-term care resources? (2) What relationship is there between types of service
  (specific processes of care) and patient outcomes? Data from such longitudinal studies
  are needed for evaluation of existing alternative modes of care for the aged and
  chronically ill and for the identification
  and development of new forms of service
  programs.

- Much more work needs to be done to determine
  the feasibility of linking reimbursements for
  long-term care to performance criteria expressed in terms of patient outcomes. It is
  now theoretically possible, since the characteristics and outcomes of patients can be
  described in the standard terminology of the
  patient assessment system, to experiment with
  reimbursement mechanisms which offer incentives
  of different types and to analyze the relative
  costs and effectiveness of different reimbursement formulae and methods of payment.

Acknowledgments.

     Research for this paper was done under Research
Grant HS-01162, National Center for Health Services Research,
Health Resources Administration, U.S.DHEW.

REFERENCES

Akpom, C. A., S. Katz, and P. M. Densen
    1973   "Methods of classifying disability and severity
             of illness in ambulatory care." Medical Care
             11:125-131. (Supplement.)

Brook, R. H. and F. A. Appel
    1973   "Quality of care assessment: Choosing a method
             for peer review." New England Journal of
             Medicine 288:25, 1323-1329.

Bruett, T. L. and R. P. Overs
    1969   "A critical review of 12 ADL scales."
             Physical Therapy 49:857-862.

Commission on Chronic Illness
    1956   Chronic Illness in the United States, Vol. II.
             Care of the Long-Term Patient. Cambridge,
             Mass. Published for the Commonwealth Fund by
             Harvard University Press.

Donabedian, A. D.
    1966   "Evaluating the quality of medical care."
             Milbank Memorial Fund Quarterly 44:166-206.
             (Supplement.)

Falcone, A. R. and S. M. Bright
    1976   Patient Assessment: A Training Manual for Use
             of Patient Classification in Long-Term Care.
             Prepared by the Harvard Center for Community
             Health and Medical Care for the Division of
             Long-Term Care, Health Resources Administra-
             tion, Public Health Service and the Depart-
             ment of Health, Education, and Welfare (June).

Gonnella, J. S. and M. J. Goran
    1975   "Quality of patient care - a measurement of
             change: The staging concept." Medical Care
             13:6, 467-473.

Harvard Center for Community Health and Medical Care
    1974   Summary of Proceedings: Third Invitational
             Conference on Nursing Home Care. Boston,
             Mass. (May 30).

    1973   Summary of Proceedings: Second Nursing
             Home Conference. Cambridge, Mass.
             (December 6).

    1972   Conference Highlights. Nursing Home Care:
             Problems Perceived by Providers, Standard
             Setting Agencies and Fiscal Agencies.
             Cambridge, Mass. (November 28-29).

Jones, E. W., B. J. McNitt, and E. M. McKnight
    1974   Patient Classification for Long-Term Care:
              User's Manual, U.S.DHEW Publication No.
              HRA 75-3107, Health Resources Administration,
              Bureau of Health Services Research and
              Evaluation, U.S.DHEW.

Katz, S. and C. A. Akpom
    1976   "A measure of primary sociobiological
              functions." International Journal of Health
              Services 6:493-507.

Katz, S., A. B. Ford, T. D. Downs, M. Adams, and D. I. Rusby
    1972   Effects of Continued Care: A Study of Chronic
              Illness in the Home. U.S.DHEW Publication No.
              (HSM) 73-3010, Health Services and Mental
              Health Administration, National Center for
              Health Services Research and Development,
              U.S.DHEW.

McNitt, B. J. and P. C. Brown
    1976   Guide for Completing Patient Appraisal and Care
              Evaluation (PACE) Instrument. Prepared by
              Harvard Center for Community Health and Medical
              Care for the Office of Long-Term Care, Depart-
              ment of Health, Education, and Welfare (July).

Public Health Service, Office of Nursing Home Affairs
U.S. Department of Health, Education, and Welfare
    1975   Long-Term Care Facility Improvement Study.
              Introductory Report (July).

Ryder, C. F., W. F. Elkin, and D. Doten
    1971   "Patient assessment - An essential tool in
              placement and planning care." HSMHA Health
              Reports 86:10, 923-932.

Shapiro, S.
    1967   "End result measurements of quality of medical
              care." Milbank Memorial Fund Quarterly 45:2,
              part 1, 7-30.

Valuing Health and Health Benefits

3 The Social Value of Saving a Life
Nancy S. Dorfman

The expanding role of government in fields such as health and environment has intensified the need for a measure of how much society is willing to spend to save a human life. Without such a measure, we have no way of knowing whether the public is being asked to invest too much or too little in medical research, air pollution abatement, nuclear plant safety, and similar efforts. Too much would mean that we are spending more than the public is willing to pay for the marginal benefits it receives in return. Too little would imply that the public is willing to pay the price of still greater lifesaving activities in return for the expected rewards.

The lifesaving efforts this paper is about concern not the life of a named individual, who can be identified ex ante, but, in the probability distribution, the life of an unspecified victim that will be lost if the government fails to act. Even if we knew what society was willing to pay for the life of such a person, we would be a long way from commanding all of the information needed to make optimal decisions about lifesaving activities. We have much to learn about how many lives, or life-years, will be saved by various programs. But I want to focus on a narrow but important aspect of the problem. Assume that all possible programs for saving the lives of anonymous persons can be arrayed with price tags in order of increasing cost per life saved. We have, in other words, a supply curve. Where along that supply curve should we stop investing further resources? The problem is to determine the public's demand function for saving a life. For present purposes, we will assume that the demand price is constant within the relevant range of lives saved.

HOW MUCH TO SAVE A LIFE

To simplify the problem further, consider it in the context of a society made up of exactly n persons. The question, then, is how many dollars would all n persons

together be willing to contribute to a program that promised
to eliminate the premature death of one additional person in \
the population in a given year and restore that person's life
expectancy to normal for his age (the life to be saved is not
specific to any subgroup in the population and individuals
have no control over their own exposure to the particular
form of risk). At the time the investment is made, every
member of the population is guaranteed a reduction in the
risk of premature death during the coming year amounting to
$1/n$. If $n = 1,000$, a person who previously faced a $5/1,000$
chance of dying next year will find it reduced to $4/1,000$ as
a consequence of the public expenditure.

Public Good

        The benefit produced is what economists call a "public
good." No one can be excluded from its consumption. Hence,
if it is available to one, it is available to all. Consumption by one person furthermore does not interfere with
its consumption by another. To be sure, in the end the death
of only one person will be prevented, but at the time the investment decision is made, everyone is offered an equal reduction in risk. Unlike private goods, such as home fire ex-
tinguishers or physical checkups, each of which we can assume
is worth to consumers what they pay for it, the value of a
public good is measured by adding up the amounts that everyone who benefits from it is willing to pay for what each re-
gards as his share. We need to know the sum of what each of
the n persons in the community is willing to pay for a program that will reduce the risk of an individual's own death
along with that of every other member of the group by $1/n$.
This sum will probably differ from what society would be
willing to pay to save a particular life, and it will differ
from what an individual would be willing to pay to save a
particular life, including his own.

WHAT THE AVERAGE PERSON WILL PAY

        Depending on their incomes, risk preferences, ages,
and other factors, different people will be willing to pay
different amounts for the reduced risk of death in the population. We cannot, then, generalize from what members of
an unrepresentative sample of people are willing to pay and
arrive at a value of the public good to society as a whole.
Let us assume, therefore, that we can identify a person in
the population who is average in terms of characteristics
that determine willingness to pay. The amount he is willing
to pay for a reduction in the risk of death for everyone in
the population of $1/n$ multiplied by n gives us the amount
society as a whole would be willing to pay to prevent a
single death.

The Benefits Expected

The amount this average person will pay for
in question will naturally depend on the benefits he
expects to enjoy as a consequence. What are these b
likely to include? Mishan (1971) and Schelling (196.., in
separate articles, have suggested three. The first and most
obvious comes from the reduced risk of the person's own
death, for which we would expect the average person to pay a
price we will call p_1. Second, the average person will consider that he benefits from the reduced risk of the death of
various others in the community, among family, friends, and
even among persons he does not know or know of. We will call
the price the average person would pay for this benefit p_2.
Third, the average person will gain or lose "financially,"
as Mishan calls it, from the prevention of a death, depending on whether the person whose life is saved (if it is not
his own) is expected to produce more or less than he consumes
over the remainder of his life. The expected value of the
financial gain or loss to the average person from preventing
a random death in the population can be estimated. It constitutes the one part of the risk of death that is insurable.
Let us call its value to the average person p_3.

There may be other components of individual demand for
a reduction in the death rate; for example, some who are relatively well off may be willing to contribute to saving the
lives of others who are not well off out of a sense of moral
obligation. But the three we have mentioned probably constitute the major benefits for which individuals will pay a
price. The average person would be willing to pay the sum
of $p_1 + p_2 + p_3$ for the lifesaving activity. Let us call
this sum L. Society as a whole would be willing to pay nL
for the same activity; nL is the social value of saving a
life in the present context.

HOW TO QUANTIFY nL

Now nL is difficult to quantify. No attempts I know
of have been successful. Several different approximations
tend to be used when a number is needed. I have no substi-
tutes to propose. I want, in the remainder of this paper,
to examine some of the implications of the conventional
measures to see how well they approximate what we want to
measure, namely, nL.

Human Capital Valuation

The most commonly used measures are one or the other
of two variants of human capital valuation. The first values
a life saved according to the present value of future earnings of the average person in the group at risk, and the

second, according to his future savings. Let E, for earnings,
stand for the first, and E minus C, for earnings minus consumption, stand for the second.

Sidestepping the problems these measures present when
it comes to valuing lives of those who will not, in the
future, be in the labor force, note that the human capital
approach equates the value of saving a life with the value
of goods and services that would be lost to society if the
life were not saved. A human life is treated just as any
other capital asset. A life and a bulldozer with similar
earning capacity are interchangeable. The two human capital
measures differ in that, according to the larger (E), the
consumption of the person in question is of value, while,
according to the smaller (E-C), consumption is merely the
cost of keeping the person alive in order to produce savings.
The smaller of the two, E-C, can fairly be said to tell us
the absolute minimum that society would be willing to pay
to save a life. Society will definitely benefit to the extent of E-C and should be willing to pay as much as its expected value (although it should be noted that E-C may turn
out to be negative). Saving "as much" is a bit like determining that a work of art is worth at least the canvas it
is painted on; few of us would pay an appraiser for that information. Notice that E-C corresponds to np_3, the financial
rewards that all n members of the population can anticipate
from the saving of a life. What does this tell us about the
larger human capital valuation, E? If

$$n(p_1+p_2+p_3) = E, \text{ and}$$

$$np_3 = E-C,$$

$$n(p_1+p_2) = C, \text{ and}$$

$$p_1+p_2 = C/n.$$

This says that the average person would be willing to pay
C/n for the non-financial benefits that he perceives from
reducing the risk of death in the population by 1/n.

Consumption-related Valuation

I have looked for ways to justify this implication of
the human capital approach. How might we explain finding
that the value of all the benefits a person anticipates from
a given percentage reduction in the risk of his own death,
as well as the death of all others in the population, is
equal to the present value of his future consumption times
the percentage reduction in risk?

The two explanations that have any appeal at all fail
on close inspection. The first explanation that comes to
mind is that a person may value his own life according to

the present value of his future consumption, C, and therefore, be willing to pay C/n to avoid a 1/n risk of losing his
life. One trouble with this line of reasoning is that it
leaves nothing for p_2, the value to the average person of the
reduced risk of death to all others in the population. I
conjecture that p_2 may be very much larger than p_1. I suspect that a typical person in a family of say, four, who
would pay $10 to reduce the risk of his own death by 1/n
would happily pay an additional $30 to extend the same in-
surance to the other three members of the family if the opportunity presented itself.

     The other problem I find with this explanation is that
I do not think it likely that persons equate the value of
their own lives with the value of their consumption. I am
not even sure the two are positively correlated across the
population, except insofar as both the amount one can afford
to pay to save a life and the amount one consumes are positively related to income or wealth.

     This brings us to a second possible explanation for
the human capital approach. A person's willingness to pay
to reduce the risk of death must be based on ability to pay.
A person can afford to pay no more to prevent the certain
death of anyone than the present value of his own lifetime
earnings (plus any additional assets on hand or expected in
the future). Is it not reasonable to assume, therefore, that
E is the amount a person would pay to prevent his own certain
death and E/n what he would pay to reduce the risk of death
by 1/n? Alas, a person cannot afford to pay E for anything
but his own death because such a commitment would leave
nothing to consume for the rest of life. At most, a person
can pay E minus the cost of the consumption that would make
life preferable to death. On these grounds, E is too high a
figure. But looked at another way, E is too low, for although a person cannot afford to pay as much as E to prevent
a 100 percent chance of dying, he can afford to pay a good
deal more than E/1,000 to prevent a 1/1,000 chance of dying.
This suggests that L may be much higher than E/n and nL
greater than E. It seems to me that we are left without any
very good idea of how society's willingness to pay for preventing a death is related to lifetime earnings or
consumption.

     Measures of human capital were not invented to assess
the value of life. They serve a useful purpose in helping
to assess the country's capacity to produce marketable goods
and services, that is, gross national product (GNP). The
value of capital embodied in the future earnings of the average person measures the loss in GNP that can be averted by
saving such a life, on the assumption that the lost production would not be replaced through immigration or an increase
in births. It would be merely a happy coincidence if this
turned out to approximate what society is willing to pay for

the reduced risks associated with an activity that will save
a life.

Compensation Valuation

Other approaches have been suggested, or actually
tried, for measuring willingness to pay for a reduced risk of
death.   One alternative is based on the compensation that
persons employed in hazardous jobs demand in return for accepting identifiable risks.   For small changes in risk exposure, the compensation demanded to undertake it will be
roughly the same as what one would pay to avoid it.   Any
concrete data that help illuminate the problem must be wel-
comed.   But in interpreting studies of actual risk compensation, we should bear in mind that the data probably capture
p_1 without regard to p_2 or p_3, unless the risk taker in-
ternalizes the loss to which his death would subject others.

Another serious question concerning such data is
whether individuals who accept hazardous positions come close
to representing the average person in terms of the amount of
compensation they demand.   It is a reasonable conjecture that
such persons are less risk-averse than the average, or that
their marginal utility of money is higher.   To the extent
that either their incomes or their aversion to risk are less
than average for the population, the compensation they receive will understate what the typical person would be willing to spend to reduce the risk of his own death; the compensation may not at all reflect the interest of others in
preventing their own death.

Political Valuation

Another approach that has been proposed is the political one.   Let the legislature decide; or observe what political decision makers seem to regard as the value of saving
lives in contexts other than hazardous jobs.   Limited evidence suggests that there is little consistency in the
amounts that policy makers actually do direct toward marginal
reductions in mortality rates via different means, such as
highway safety, public health, and medical research.
Furthermore, it is often difficult to calculate the real
social cost of existing policies as distinct from what the
government spends.   What is the full social cost, for example, of achieving a reduction in deaths by enforcing reductions in highway speed limits?   And besides, to abandon
the task of policy makers is to relinquish responsibility
for aiding in the making of rational economic choices.
Finally, how are we to know whether the amount of resources
devoted to highway safety reflects a judgment of the value
society places on saving lives or the value legislators
place on the goodwill of the construction industry?

An alternative to observing how policy makers appear to value lives is to determine what it actually costs, by the least costly means, to prevent a death in the population. This will provide a measure of the maximum value to society of the saving of a life by any other means at the present margin. It will provide no clue as to whether we should move up or down the supply curve.

Response to Questionnaire

As a last resort, there is always the questionnaire. Economists tend to eschew this approach, largely because they believe that it is almost impossible to get a valid answer to a hypothetical question. Their preference is to observe what people do rather than what they say they would do. In view of the abysmal lack of data on which to base an evaluation of benefits in the present instance, however, a well-designed sample survey might shed light on the issue. Several economists have come out in favor of an attempt, and some have given it a try. Although it cannot be expected to produce a definitive answer, it might provide a useful guide in interpreting estimates arrived at by other means. As far as I am aware, no such effort has taken steps to assure that the survey sample was representative of the population in terms of the characteristics that influence willingness to pay. Because willingness to pay is bound to vary with income, age, family size, risk averseness, and other factors, careful selection of the survey sample is essential. There are, in addition, the well-known problems associated with obtaining honest answers concerning expenditures on public goods. It would be a mistake to understate the difficulties that will have to be overcome before respondents are able to evaluate their own attitudes with respect to lifesaving, much less articulate them accurately and honestly.

CONCLUSION

I believe that we are presently a long way from being able to estimate, within a reasonable range, how much society, as a whole, wants to contribute to the saving of a life, or any number of life-years, of an anonymous person. Until we have a sounder basis for doing so, I would like to recommend that we refrain from placing a dollar sign on lives saved. I am in favor of calling a life a life, with whatever additional descriptive information seems appropriate. In the meantime, without monetizing lives, there is much that needs to be done to advance the ability of decision makers to make rational choices. These choices will assure that the resources allocated to measures for saving lives are directed where they will do the most good.

REFERENCES

Mishan, E. J.
     1971   "Evaluation of life and limb: A theoretical
                approach." Journal of Political Economy
                (July/August):687-705.

Schelling, Thomas C.
     1968   "The life you save may be your own."
                In Chase, Samuel B. (ed.), Public Expenditure
                Analysis. Washington, D.C.: The Brookings
                Institution.

4 Social Valuation of Life- and Health-Saving Activities by the Demand-Revealing Process

Edward H. Clarke

A fundamental problem of making public choices has been the lack of a mechanism for making social valuations that directly reflect individual preferences. As a consequence, there has been a long history of efforts to measure benefits indirectly. The difficulties and the drawbacks of the various approaches are well known.

The demand-revealing process provides a way of solving two fundamental problems of making social choices based on individual values by removing the individual's incentive to hide these values and by developing a formal communication procedure among consumers that results in non-strategic, consistent patterns of social choice. A systematic treatment of the incentives necessary to remove the natural tendency of individuals to hide their true values was theoretically employed by Clarke (1971) in the context of a theoretical analysis of alternative methods for pricing public goods. Thus, the approach embodied in the demand-revealing process as initially defined by Clarke largely overcomes the "free rider" problem set forth by Samuelson (1954) and more fundamental problems of making collective decisions based on individual values, which are embodied in the Arrow Theorem (Arrow, 1963).

This paper considers the potential application of demand-revealing procedures to health resource allocation and extends the theory to a range of public-goods problems, such as dealing with externalities in the consumption of health care. The paper also derives a new willingness-to-pay criterion that can be applied to public choices about life- and health-saving activities generally, and to health research decisions in particular.

The demand-revealing process would permit each person to state his willingness to pay for these activities—presumably the amount that would compensate him for increased risk of death or decline in functional health status.

69

This is the "compensating variation" first set forth by
Mishan (1971). Although choices would be made according to
the traditional criterion that equates aggregate willingness
to pay with cost, each person would be required to pay an
amount equal to the net benefits sacrificed by others as a
result of taking that person's preferences into account. In
contrast to the "compensating variation," which measures net
benefits sacrificed by each individual at the margin, this
reflects the net benefits sacrificed by all others for changes
that result from taking the individual's preferences into
account.

     Application of this new willingness-to-pay criterion
for arriving at optimal choices by direct revelation of preferences would supplement indirect approaches for measuring
benefits. Further, this new criterion would involve individuals in making tradeoffs among a range of life- and health-
saving activities, including the defensive activities of
individuals, as well as those outside their control and
within the purview of curative or preventive health services.

     In a world of reasonably well-informed individuals,
who can easily perceive risks, direct revelation could be
rather easily integrated with indirect approaches for arriving at the optimum individual and social allocation of
resources. The true world of uncertainty and imperfect
information, however, presents real difficulties (Arrow,
1965a). These difficulties may largely explain the lack of
individual participation in important group or collective
decision-making processes--which remains a problem for the
demand-revealing process as well. Addressing this problem
requires determining how information flows and networks can
be efficiently organized so as to help determine individual
preference and shape public choices about life- and health-
saving activities. At the same time, the means by which
individual values can be reflected in social choices must
be retained.

     The first section of the paper illustrates the appli-
cation of the new willingness-to-pay criterion under rather
simple assumptions, with gradual introduction of more
realistic ones, such as uncertainty and imperfect information. In this context, the application of the willingness-
to-pay criterion to group decision making is illustrated, and
the results are compared with present approaches to economic
and social valuation.

     The second section considers the problem of motivating
individual citizens to devote time and effort to determining
and communicating preferences for life- and health-saving
activities. The potential complementarity between indirect
approaches (e.g., looking at revealed preferences in the
market) and direct approaches (e.g., asking individuals about
their willingness to pay) is considered. The aim is to use

both approaches to help individuals make educated and internally consistent choices, both public and private, that
will lead toward individual and social optima. The provision of information, itself a public good, and the feedback of
information to and from a sample of individual citizens, is
posed as a way to address this motivational problem. Further,
an analysis is conducted of how individual preference information can be incorporated into the demand revelations of
groups, thereby utilizing the present reality and structure
of our political system. The intent is to strike a balance
between reliance on representatives, issue-specializing
bureaucrats, and group providers of health care to perform
informational and social choice functions while retaining
optimum room for taking individual values into account.

     The paper concludes by considering the possibility of
experimental applications with the new criterion in sampling
individual preferences, oriented initially toward group
choices closest to the individual. The results of a series
of such experiments might provide the basis for broader application to the social valuation of governmentally-provided
life- and health-saving activities.

ILLUSTRATING THE NEW WILLINGNESS-TO-PAY CRITERION

     Setting aside uncertainty and imperfect information
and making assumptions that all persons have the same general
health experience, the simplest form of the new willingness-
to-pay criterion can be described in the context of determining the optimal level of provision of a public good.
For a "pure" public good--biomedical research and innocula-
tions against communicable disease being reasonably good
examples--it is necessary to determine an optimal amount that
will equate the aggregate willingness to pay with the cost
of provision. This result is achieved by charging each individual the net cost to others, as measured by individuals'
aggregate willingness to pay and the cost of provision to
them. This is distinct from changes in the level of provision that result from taking an individual's own willingness
to pay into account. As indicated below, this charge solves
the "free rider" problem of public goods.

     In figure 1, assume that AD represents society's ag-
gregate willingness to pay for expenditures on biomedical research and that the line at $1/unit represents the social cost
schedule for purchasing different quantities of such research;
the efficient level of expenditures on research by society is
thus defined as the quantity Q_E. The problem heretofore has
been determining individual willingness to pay in a way that
would lead to honest statements of preferences. For example,
if cost-sharing for biomedical research expenditures is based
on stated willingness to pay, then the individual is better
off to underrepresent "true" willingness to pay for these expenditures. On the other hand, if cost-sharing is separated

Figure 1.   Equilibrium and a Clarke Tax for Expenditure
            on a Public Good.

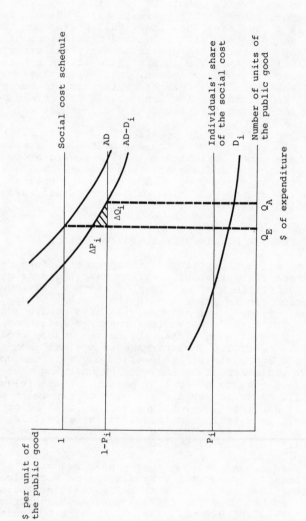

Source: Derived from Tideman, T. N., Introduction to Public
          Choice (Spring supplement, 1977), and Tideman, T. N.
          and G. Tullock, "A new and superior process for
          making social choices," Journal of Political Economy
          84(6) (December 1976):1153.

from the stated willingness to pay, given the present tax
system, then one has an incentive to overrepresent the "true"
value of biomedical expenditures.

The demand-revealing process solves this fundamental
problem, regardless of what cost-sharing rule is employed.
Assume that each individual (i) is assigned a share of costs
equal to P_i, in figure 1, and asked to indicate his willingness to pay for alternative quantities of this public good
and thus defining the individual's demand for his good, D_i.
For each individual, two calculations would be made:
(a) a determination of the social outcome that would be
chosen by all other persons if the one person abstains (indicated by the quantity Q_A in figure 1) and (b) the amount
that others would have to be compensated so that they would
be indifferent between this quantity, Q_A, and the amount that
is actually selected, Q_E, as a result of taking i's preferences into account. In figure 1, the net benefits sacrificed
by all others (e.g., benefits of future reductions in risk
of mortality or morbidity less their share of expenditure) is
the shaded area. The individual is now taxed that amount in
addition to his contribution for the social quantity chosen,
equal to $P_i(Q_E)$. By similar reasoning, the same optimal
quantity and the contribution from every other individual can
be determined. Elsewhere, it has been shown that this tax
payment motivates honest revelation of individual willingness
to pay (Clarke, 1971; Tideman and Tullock, 1976a).

In order to keep the incentives correct, any amounts
collected in excess of the cost of provision must be wasted.
For this reason, the approach seems strange, although in
cases of large numbers of participants, the taxes would be
very small. It is projected (Tideman and Tullock, 1976b)
that "if the citizens of the United States were voting on
the annual federal budget, the [upper limit] of the grand
total of all the Clarke taxes charged would be in the
neighborhood of $2,000 or about one-thousandth of a penny per
person." Voting on health research would, of course, lead to
a proportionately smaller upper limit. And if the initial
allocation of shares had reflected true preferences, the excess would disappear, assuming that each individual's willingness to pay at the margin were equal to each individual's
cost share.

The new willingness-to-pay criterion could, of course,
be applied to any public good or externality in the allocation of resources to health. Although it is controversial,
in part because of lack of an acceptable criterion for income
distribution, consider the application to determining an optimal level of health care subsidies. Pauly (1971) has shown
that this problem can be considered in the context of externalities in the consumption of health care, where the consumption of each individual is taken as a separate public
good. Given the aggregate willingness to pay of those who

wish to redistribute income to others who suffer large medical
expenses in relation to their income, the optimum quantity
for each person is defined by vertically adding the aggregate
willingness to pay of the former to the individual demand
curves of the latter.

In a world where individuals were reasonably knowledge-
able about risks, the demand-revealing process could be used
to determine an optimal pattern of insurance subsidies that
would take into account externalities in consumption for insurance against these risks. The insurance subsidies would
vary according to ways in which the society's aggregate willingness to pay varies with respect to different illnesses.
For example, communicable diseases might receive higher subsidies than some forms of psychiatric care. The rub, of
course, in such an approach comes when genuine uncertainty,
as opposed to simple risk, arises in the context of
widespread imperfections in information. As Arrow has observed, information then becomes an "elusive" commodity, which
may explain many of the special characteristics of medical
care markets designed to compensate for its imperfect market-
ability (Arrow, 1965a). Transactions costs, on both the
buyer and seller side, can reinforce a tendency toward non-
market forms of allocation, as can increasing returns in both
the provision of information and other aspects of the provision of health care (Arrow, 1965b).

These aspects of health care are often suggested as a
rationale for collective provision, including group provision
of health care and insurance. Here the individual sacrifices
some elements of personal choice to enjoy the efficiency of
group insurance and provision and to reduce information and
transaction costs. The problem is twofold: (a) How to determine optimal group provision as opposed to illnesses that
can be separately insured for by the individuals? (b) How
to allocate resources paid for by the group among various
types of interventions? The efficient use of co-insurance,
deductibles, and user charges represents one set of allocation mechanisms. But there is a problem about how to determine the optimal pattern of resource allocation that will
permit individual preferences to be taken into account, particularly in determining preferences for extra market allocations of health care resources.

Lipscomb's paper (1979) in this volume addresses
this issue and suggests two potential approaches. The first
approach is a (full pay) tax and transfer mechanism designed
to ameliorate such behavior, which depends, in part, upon
countervailing forces in a constrained optimization process
where the modules are "competing" with each other for resources and, in part, upon philanthropic motivations. The
second is a variant of the demand-revealing process, which
addresses the strategy problem more directly but generates
deficits and, in some sense, is inefficient.

Discrete Case Illustration

The application of the new willingness-to-pay criterion for determining group preferences for extra-market allocations can best be illustrated by abstracting from the
income-redistributive aspect of health care discussed earlier.
For illustrative purposes, assume the population has been
asked to efficiently allocate resources amongst a number of
health-promoting and medical care activities that dif-
ferentially impact on the health status of various groups or
modules of the population, defined according to income and
risk of disease. Using traditional benefit-cost techniques,
an initial resource allocation solution for an assumed health
expenditure budget across 20 groups in the population is presented in table 1, as initial solution A. In this analysis,
the 20 groups have been further collapsed into three modules
that similarly perceive the benefits derived by the initial
allocation solution across the health-promoting activities.
Finally, it is assumed that the costs are shared equally
among the various modules, each of which has an equal aggregate income, such that while per capita or household incomes
in each module are equal, they are not equal between modules.

The two alternative case.--The relevant question at
this point is to determine whether the initial solution is
preferred by all modules such that they would not be willing
to pay the net costs to others to alter that solution. For
purposes of illustration, assume that module M_1 is the only
one dissatisfied with the initial solution of health programs
and expenditures. The representative of M_1 proposes alternative B that, for purposes of illustration, includes more
funds for biomedical research (since the individuals in this
module presumably suffer more from presently non-curable
diseases). The representative of each module is then asked
to state the group's willingness to pay for each alternative,
assuming that the cost of each alternative will be shared
equally among the groups. The result is shown in table 1.
The value of alternative B to module 1 is $20 million, and
the four groups comprising module 2 each value alternative
B at $4 million, or $16 million total. The "low risk" groups,
on the other hand, comprising module 3, prefer solution A
and would be willing to pay $2 million each, or a total of
$30 million, to retain solution A.

The more efficient allocation, however, is B because
the net benefits of $36 million to the five groups of people
in the higher risk groups in the population, those represented
by modules 1 and 2, are in excess of the net benefits of $30
million to the other 15 lower risk group people. This efficient allocation could be attained through honest revelation
of preferences if each module were charged the difference in
net benefits between the two alternatives, calculated without
the module's vote--if its vote changes the outcome. In this
case, M_1 would pay a tax of $14 million, which represents the

Table 1.   Two Alternative Health Expenditure Allocation
           Solutions.

Number of groups per module	Alternative Modules	Initial solution A	Alternative B	Tax
1	1 $= M_1$	0	$20m	$14m
4	2-5 $= M_2$	0	16m($4m per group)	0
15	6-20 $= M_3$	$30m($2m ea.)	0	0
	Total net benefits	$30m	$36m	$14m

Total without indicated net benefits

For module 1:	2 + 3	30	16
2:	1 + 3	30	20
3:	1 + 2	0	36

difference between the net benefits accruing to the other two
modules for the solution A that would have been picked if
module 1's preferences had not changed the outcome so that
alternative B is actually chosen.   Thus, the tax calculation
for module 1 = $30 - $16 = $14 million.   If module 2, which
is comprised of four groups, consisted of only one group,
it too would have paid a tax of $10 million, the difference
between $30 and $20 million.   However, since each group in
module 2 paid only $4 million, that amount by any one group
would not have altered the solution decision so that they
would not be required to pay the tax.   Finally, module 3
did not change the outcome of the demand-revealing process
away from alternative B and thus would not be required to
pay a tax.

     The three alternative case.--The results reached here
are easily generalized.   Any other group could presumably
offer other alternatives and the alternatives might also
extend to other types of interventions (e.g., for pollution
control that could complement or substitute for expenditures
on health services).   In table 2, for example, lower risk
groups are assumed to offer a third alternative that em-
phasizes the control of toxic substances through regulation.
Additional expenditures over alternative B include some re-
allocation of health services expenditures to bring about a
more optimal balance between health services and pollution
control.

Table 2. Three Alternative Health Expenditure Allocation Solutions.

Number of groups per module	Alternative Modules	Initial solution A	Alternative B	C	Tax
1	1 = M_1	0	$20m	$30m	0
3	2-4 = M_2	0	12m(4m)	9m(3m)	0
1	5 - M_3	0	10m	5m	0
8	6-13 = M_4	16m(2m)	8m	0	0
7	14-20 = M_5	21m(3m)	0	28m(4m)	0
	Net benefits	$37m	$50m	$71m	0

Total without indicated values

For module				
1: 2 + 3 + 4 + 5	37	30	41
2: 1 + 3 + 4 + 5	37	38	62
3: 1 + 2 + 4 + 5	37	40	66
4: 1 + 2 + 3 + 5	21	42	62
5: 1 + 2 + 3 + 4	16	50	43

It is interesting to observe first that this example illustrates the potential for "cycling" or inconsistent patterns of social choice that lie at the heart of the Arrow Theorem. If we were to use some conventional voting process, such as majority voting, to make choices among any two paired alternatives that somehow get on the agenda, the result would be a "cycle." If, for example, we compare A with B, 15 groups (M_6 through M_{15}) would favor A while five groups (M_1 through M_5) would favor B. Alternative A would thus be preferred to alternative B by a margin of 3 to 1. Similarly, if we compare preferences for alternative B as opposed to C, the former would be favored by a margin of 3 to 2. But if we then compare alternative C with alternative A, alternative C would be preferred by the same 3 to 2 margin.

We avoid the Arrow problem through demand revelation by letting the groups communicate the intensity of their preferences which they will do honestly. Thus, as Tideman and Tullock (1976) observe, we get around the Arrow problem by not meeting Arrow's assumptions. Heretofore, no way has

been devised for getting around the problem without giving
rise to strategy in communicating the intensity of
preferences.

Table 3 also illustrates the result that the magnitude
of any excess taxes will decline as the number of individual
participants or groups in the decision increases. In fact,
no excess taxes arise in the context of the stated preferences
in table 3, although M_1 comes close to paying a small amount.
The reason that no module or group pays a tax for alternative
C is because (as can be seen in the first row of part b of
table 3) alternative C would have been picked as the preferred alternative by the other four modules, excluding
module 1. In the case of module 5 (see last row in the lower
part of table 2), while the other modules would have picked
alternative B rather than C, so that a tax of $7 million
(the difference between $50 million and $43 million) would
be warranted since it is comprised of seven groups, with the
value of alternative C to each group only equal to $4 million,
that amount would not have altered the solution decision
from C to B.

In this example, low risk groups in module 5 (groups
14-20) put high values on pollution control, but relatively
low values on more health services; high risk groups, such
as the one comprising module 1, put high values on both
pollution control and health services. This interaction tends
to alleviate the type of situation illustrated by table 1,
where conflict over the health services budget led to rather
substantial excess taxes for M_1.

APPLICATION OF THE CRITERION

What is the feasibility of implementing a new
willingness-to-pay criterion incorporating demand-revealing
procedures? The question of feasibility is largely one of
information. Conventional political and bureaucratic
decision-making processes also require information that is
not easily obtained from individual citizens. Political
theory suggests that, given any degree of knowledge about
benefits, majority voting will lead to efficient outcomes
only in very special circumstances that are unlikely to be
satisfied in a realistic setting.

The informational problem exists for the demand-
revealing process as well. When the number of individuals
increases, each has a diminishing incentive to participate.
The problem is compounded when an individual's own tastes
are unknown and can be discovered only at a real cost in
resources. How can citizens rely on others to perform
information and social choice functions while retaining
means by which their own values can be reflected in these
choices? This problem has been addressed elsewhere in

Table 3. Evaluation of Discrete Alternatives by
          Population Groupings.

a. Two Alternatives

Number of groups per module	Alternative Modules	Initial solution A	Alternative B	Tax
1	M_1	0	$20m	$14m
4	M_{2-5}	0	16m($4m ea.)	0
15	M_{6-20}	$30m($2m ea.)	0	0
		$30m	$36m	$14m

b. Three Alternatives

Number of groups per module	Alternative Modules	Initial solution A	Alternative B	C	Tax
1	M_1	0	$20m	$30m	0
3	M_{2-4}	0	12m(4m)	9m(3m)	0
1	M_5	0	10m	5m	0
8	M_{6-13}	$16m(2m)	8m	9	0
7	M_{14-20}	21m(3m)	0	28m(4m)	0
		$37m	$50m	$71m	0

Voting by majority rule (cycles)

A preferred to B - 3 to 1
B preferred to C - 3 to 2
C preferred to A - 3 to 2.

looking at the possible application of the process to making
environmental quality choices--for example, among water
quality goals and pollution abatement projects for individual
areas or jurisdictions in a given water or airshed (Clarke,
1977a). Here, the more difficult problem of its application
to the evaluation of public and private life- and health-
saving activities is considered.

Private activities are important because the acts of
individuals in their own life- and health-saving activities,
and the process by which they make rational and consistent
choices between private and public activities, can be an
essential element of the social valuational process. In this
regard, the usefulness of thinking about the potential complementarity between efforts to measure benefits indirectly
(e.g., revealed preferences for the value of life by the defensive life-saving activities of individuals) and efforts to
ask individuals directly how much they would be willing to
pay for life-saving activities is presented. The evaluation
of private activities, ranging between the more obvious (e.g.,
smoking, diet, use of seat belts, or health-screening procedures) to the more subtle (e.g., purchase of insurance
annuities, arranging of bequests), can also be an important
way to motivate individuals to think about the value of
public interventions. These interventions include (a) better
access to response programs (e.g., faster delivery to special
care units for heart attacks) at the community level,
(b) strategies for allocating public health resources among
various disease or treatment categories at both the community and national levels, and (c) allocation of insurance
subsidies, biomedical research dollars, and choices about
environmental health regulatory and research strategies at
the national level.

If decision making could be made efficient by properly
addressing the information problem, individuals might be
motivated to invest time and effort in trying to effect in-
ternally-consistent resource allocations among discrete life-
and health-saving activities. Private and public expenditures on health services alone are approximately $140 billion
annually, or more than $2,000 for each family, not including
costs resulting from the regulation of environmental hazards
or those resulting from precautions voluntarily taken by, or
imposed on, individuals (e.g., use of seat belts or air bags).
It is possible that individuals would be interested in ways
of better arranging both group and individual insurance contracts so that they are more in accord with individuals'
willingness to pay for protection against risks. In the
context of considering their own individual or household
evaluations, people might be motivated to generate much useful information about external benefits in consumption, particularly in determining a more optimal allocation of subsidies among various disease or treatment programs.

Families might also be motivated to think more systematically about consumption/savings patterns, including not only the purchase of life and health insurance, but also the purchase of annuities and the arranging of bequests. These consumption/savings patterns (over the life cycle) can also be taken into account, along with defensive life-saving activities, in determining implied valuations of willingness to pay. These valuations can be used, in turn, to help make resource-allocation decisions.

In addition to obtaining information about what house-holds actually do and how they might change their individual behavior based on more information, it would be useful to group them for purposes of both medical evaluation and pref-erence revelation. For both purposes, the groups should be relatively homogeneous with respect to present and likely future health states. As suggested by Lipscomb (1979), in-dividuals might be assigned to various risk classes on the basis of characteristics (e.g., weight, age, sex, medical history) that have been linked with various health states and probabilities of survival. It is possible that house-holds or individuals within each category would be interested in obtaining information about various private activities that could improve functional health status (e.g., reduction in smoking, sanitary conditions within the home for those at risk to certain diseases) or increase the probability of sur-vival (e.g., use of seat belts or secondary control methods, such as the use of better screening and recordkeeping for those at risk to certain diseases). Education and train-ing activities aimed at populations subject to different types of risk could be conducted in conjunction with attempts to gauge each population's willingness to pay for public goods.

Experimental Application

A group of citizens in one or more communities might be asked to participate in a preference revelation experiment for the group provision of health services. This experiment would include a process of evaluating private and public life- and health-saving activities affecting the group. They could then better arrange their private activities and, in turn, the group provision of health services in a more optimal way. The process would help determine an appropriate balance be-tween private and group access to health services. For ex-ample, should access to very expensive technologies or treat-ments be made available to the group, or should individual members merely be informed of the availability of appropriate catastrophic insurance?

The main objective of the proposed experiment is to de-termine an optimal pattern of individual and group activities, including the scale of group provision and the allocation of resources to group activities, based on the revealed

preferences of the enrolled group population. The demand-
revealing experiment would first find an appropriate way to
subclass the population into "modules" for purposes of both
medical evaluation and the assessment of preferences. For
each module, a set of strategies for health status improvement could be defined by experts. Perhaps the experts might
represent individual modules rather than using "medical
Delphis."

An objective is to determine preferences for information, education, and training strategies aimed at prevention.
This provides a key link with individual life- and health-
saving activities in trying to improve health status by relying on strategies within the control of the individual or
household. It would also help effect educated and internally-
consistent choices about individual strategies, and more informed choices about group provision (e.g., education and
training) relating to these activities. Techniques of
traditional cost-benefit analysis or health resource allocation could determine an "initial solution" for a presumed
optimal set of strategies for each module, allocating costs
to each according to perceived benefits. Group representatives would then be permitted to change the allocation by the
approach illustrated earlier.

The effects of the initial round of information, education, and training could then be evaluated to see what
changes in individual and household defensive activities
occur. Part of this evaluation could include a predictive
model describing how similarly situated individuals and households in each module behave and the value they implicitly
place on life- and health-saving activities. In turn, modular
representatives could be further educated about the results of
the evaluation and members encouraged to think about a more
optimal pattern of individual activities based on observed
inconsistencies in their own behavior and the activities of
similarly situated individuals. Their response or adjustment
patterns would further modify the implicit values, as well as
suggest redefinition of "similarly situated individuals." A
determination of individual willingness to pay could be made
for both (a) information provision designed to assist in
better private choices and (b) the allocation of resources to
both health-promoting activities and "curative" medical
treatments.

The public choice problem is to make effective tradeoffs between the proposed strategies. As suggested earlier,
there is the problem of choosing between interventions that
will be available for all in the groups versus those that
will be available to only those that have appropriate insurance. A good example would be kidney disease or ESRD
facilities that might cost up to $50,000 per patient per
year. Such a choice involves individuals in the evaluation
of very complex probabilistic alternatives. Lipscomb's

paper (1979) discusses the types of probabilistic information
that might be presented individuals, recognizing the difficulties of obtaining willingness-to-pay-expressions for
changes in the probability of health (also see Fischer's
paper, this volume).

In spite of the difficulties, individuals in each
module may devote some time to determine their willingness to
pay for reduced probabilities of mortality or morbidity if
they were compensated (because of the value of this information to others) and if this activity produced value to them
(e.g., the improved design of individual life and health insurance contracts). The difficulties could be improved if
individuals were provided "starting points" that reflected
willingness to pay values implied by their own behavior and
the behavior of similarly situated individuals.

To reduce the costs of decision, the representative of
each module might rely on an optimal sample of its members to
determine how to modify willingness-to-pay starting points
so as to better reflect group preferences. Appropriate
weighting in the samples might be given to individuals who
tend to produce high standard errors in the predictive model
(e.g., those whose willingness to pay is very uncertain because of inconsistent patterns of defensive behavior or consumption). The representatives would make decisions on
project proposals or plans advanced by cost-benefit analysts
or health resource planners using the willingness-to-pay
criterion suggested earlier. Given the allocation of group
health resources, additional information provision would
assist in the readjustment of individual strategies, such as
insurance for illnesses not covered by group provision.

One such experiment would facilitate and reduce the
costs of implementing other ones. In particular, the information gathered from members of one group health plan
could be used to allocate costs among members of another
group plan without motivating strategic misstatements of
preferences. The information would also enable (a) more
precise initial willingness-to-pay starting points and
(b) help groups determine the ways in which their preferences
are likely to differ from these starting points (e.g., the
standard errors in the predictive model may indicate areas
where further sampling would provide more precise estimates
of preference).

Broader Application

A number of such experiments could be conducted to determine their reliability, and could be used to bring to
value public activities that fall outside the scope of group
insurance and provision, such as (a) government or voluntary
provision of information about health and safety precautions,

and biomedical research, (b) the provision of health services
and medical insurance subsidies, and their allocation among
different types of medical interventions, as well as among
income groups, and (c) the shaping of environmental health
control and research strategies. The example in table 2 illustrated the application of demand-revealing procedures for
choosing between health services and environmental strategies.
The major difference between this example and the evaluation
of group health resource budgets is the problem of valuing
non-group inclusive benefits. Yet, if experimentation with
procedures designed to encourage improved individual and
group choices could be initiated, a stock of information
relevant for valuing broader strategies could be developed.
Individuals who had performed well in previous experiments,
properly validated and replicated, could become "surrogate"
decision makers in these broader settings.

     The sampling of individual preferences within rel-
atively homogeneous groups might eventually become a routine
complement to government cost-benefit techniques in making
decisions. Presumably, the sampling would also be subject
to usual political safeguards. The executive branch and the
Congress could always override the result arrived at by
applying the new criterion if either wished to do so. In
many cases, however, use of the willingness-to-pay criterion
defined via the demand-revealing process would not only be
fairer and more efficient, but would avoid the Faustian
bargains that cannot be addressed by cost-benefit analysis
and are often explicitly avoided by legislatures (Kneese,
1973). Of further importance, the process permits the expression of diverse preferences or differing values on the
avoidance of risks. Also, it enables the expression of different values placed on life-saving and health-promoting
activities, given precautions that take into account differences in the capacity to pay, since it is premised on individuals' stated willingness to pay rather than the perceptions of bureaucrats and politicians. Finally, by per-
mitting different valuations placed on life-saving and
health-promoting activities, it provides greater decision-
making flexibility than is presently possible when
traditional benefit-cost analysis is used and where the
"value of life" is considered to be the same for all members
of the population.

Health Research Decisions

     The problems in applying a demand-revealing approach
can be illustrated in the context of the allocation of resources to biomedical research. As indicated earlier, biomedical research comes very close to being a "pure" public
good, but it is also one which presents difficult obstacles
in obtaining information on individual preferences. The
dollars allocated to biomedical research are also not large

--only about $40 per family in fiscal year 1978 of federal government expenditures, and slightly over $60 if we include all health research expenditures.

In this context, it would be difficult to motivate individual citizens to make informed choices about the allocation of health research dollars. Even the most educated, informed, and vitally interested citizen could receive only a few additional dollars' worth of satisfaction utiles (most of which would presumably reflect his preferences for the welfare of future generations), even if he could dictate the allocation and level of support of all health research.

The series of experiments described earlier in this section, however, can provide a range of consumer willingness-to-pay valuations that reflect differences in socioeconomic and risk characteristics, motivated by the consumer surplus arising out of changes in thousands of dollars per family in health care expenditures and other costs of life- and health-saving activities, public and private. These valuations could be taken into account in making health research allocations at virtually no incremental expenditure whatsoever and use them to value the medical and scientific community's evaluations of the likelihood of life-saving and health status improvement from changes in health research resource allocations.

With very little incremental expenditure, representatives of various groups, homogeneous with respect to social, economic, and health status, could communicate group preferences by interpreting the willingness to pay of their group and evaluating the differing evaluations of probabilities from medical, scientific, and other groups. Such an approach might provide useful information where there are particularly important social choices, such as expenditures on biomedical versus environmental health research. The paper by Schulze and others (1979) in this volume provides an indication of the potential gains from better resource allocation decisions. Further inconsistent decisions could be avoided by using information obtained from the process defined above.

The final, and more costly, step is likely the sampling of individual preferences about health research decisions. As in early examples, sampling could be used to reduce high estimation errors deriving from those with very uncertain individual willingness to pay for life- and health-saving activities. Those who have participated in previous experiments and who would also reduce their own uncertainty from participation might add useful information that would be worth the cost--both to them and those making decisions about research.

Despite the potential efficacy of the results, bureaucrats and politicians may rebel at the thought of such experimentation aimed at providing better measures of social

valuation for any government activity. The surrogate
decision makers would be better educated and better informed
than the citizenry in general, even though they would presumably reflect the same socioeconomic characteristics.
Further, the opportunity to use information to better arrange
private activities suggests different social optima for the
surrogates as opposed to otherwise similarly situated citizens. Despite the many ways, including errors in estimation,
in which the aggregate willingness to pay of the surrogates
would depart from true aggregate social willingness to pay,
the perceived differences would often suggest the desired
direction of social policy; for example, increased investment
in information, education, and training for the general
citizenry according to the guidance provided by participants
in the experiment. The implementation of such a process
would be gradual and would allow for feedback from the experience of individual citizens involved in the process of
making public choices about life-saving and health-promoting
activities.

     Biomedical research may seem distant and remote from
most citizens. Thus, their participation in its decision
process may seem irrelevant. However, citizens may contribute more to both the political economy and the long-run
interests of future generations than those bureaucrats and
politicians presently entrusted with this responsibility.
An actual subsidized experiment, oriented initially toward
life- and health-saving choices by individuals and groups,
and designed so as to elicit information about individual
willingness to pay for publicly-provided goods and services,
may be the only way to determine if individuals can be
motivated to think about complex uncertainties that affect
their lives and those of future generations.

CONCLUSION

     In discussing the possible practical relevance of the
new willingness-to-pay criterion to the social valuation of
life- and health-saving activities, the focus has been on the
simplest form of application to supplement existing institu-
tions. There are, of course, a range of objections that
could be raised about any such application--ethical and
theoretical, as well as practical. These problems have recently been explored in a special issue of Public Choice
devoted to demand revelation (see Clarke, 1977b). This
paper, however, has set aside many of these problems with the
primary aim of showing how demand-revealing procedures could
complement existing decision-making approaches.

     In particular, the complementarity with cost-benefit
analysis has been highlighted, including the reliance on
indirect valuation and the improvements that could be made
with experiments that incorporate direct revelation of

preferences. Such experiments could also be a by-product of information provision aimed at improved individual life- and health-saving choices. By providing a better way to link the valuation tools of economics with those of politics, demand-revealing experiments in preference-revelation could lead to better public choices involving human life and health.

REFERENCES

Acton, Jan Paul
     1973   Evaluating Public Programs to Save Lives.
             Santa Monica: The RAND Corporation.

Arrow, Kenneth J.
     1965a   "Uncertainty and welfare economics of medical
             care." American Economic Review (March).

     1965b   "Reply." American Economic Review (March).

     1963   Social Choice and Individual Values (Second
             Edition). New Haven: Yale University Press.

Blomquist, G.
     1976   "Value of life: Implications of automobile
             seat belt use." Ph.D. dissertation, University
             of Chicago.

Blomquist, G. and G. Tolley
     1977   "The value of life as influenced by bequest,
             insurance annuities, and age." Paper presented
             at Conference on Environmental Benefit Estima-
             tion, University of Chicago (June).

Bowen, H.
     1943   "The interpretation of voting in the allocation
             of economic resources." Quarterly Journal of
             Economics (November).

Burger, E.
     1974   "Protecting the nation's health." A New
             Perspective on the Health of Canadians: A
             Working Document. Canadian Ministry of Health,
             Ottawa.

Carey, J.
     1970   "Factors in determining the level of biomedical
             research support." Address to Council of
             Academic Societies, Chicago (February).

Clarke, Edward H.
     1977a   "Social valuation of environmental quality by
             the demand-revealing process." Paper presented
             at Conference on Environmental Benefit Estima-
             tion, University of Chicago (June).

     1977b   "Some aspects of the demand-revealing process."
             Public Choice (Special Spring Supplement).

Clarke, Edward H.
    1971   "Multipart pricing of public goods." Public
            Choice (Fall).

Downs, A.
    1957   An Economic Theory of Democracy. New York:
            Harper and Row.

Good, J.
    1977   "Justice in voting by demand revelation."
            Public Choice (Special Spring Supplement).

Green, J. and J. J. Laffont
    1977   "Imperfect personal information and the demand-
            revealing process: A sampling approach. Public
            Choice (Special Spring Supplement).

Hinich, M. J.
    1975   "A rationalization for consumer support for food
            regulation." Virginia Polytechnical Institute
            (January) (Mimeographed.).

Kneese, Allen
    1973   "Benefit-cost analysis and unscheduled events in
            the nuclear fuel cycle." Resources (September).

Kneese, Allen and William Schulze
    1977   "Environment, health, and economics - The case
            of cancer." American Economic Review 67:1.

Lipscomb, Joseph
    1979   "The willingness-to-pay criterion and public
            program evaluation in health." In Mushkin,
            Selma J. and David W. Dunlop (eds.), Health:
            What is it Worth? (this volume).

Mishan, E. J.
    1971   "Evaluation of life and limb: A theoretical
            approach." Journal of Political Economy
            (July/August).

Pauly, M.
    1971a   Medical Care at Public Expense. New York:
            Praeger.

    1971b   Medical Care at Public Expense. Chapter 3.

Samuelson, Paul
    1954   "The pure theory of public expenditure."
            Revue of Economics and Statistics 36:387-389.

Starr, P.
    1976   "The undelivered health system." Public
            Interest (Winter), p. 82.

Tideman, T. N. and G. Tullock
    1976a   "A new and superior process for making social
            choices." Journal of Political Economy
            (December).

    1976b   "A new and superior process for making social
            choices." Journal of Political Economy
            (December), p. 1158.

Tullock, G.
    1977   "The demand-revealing process as a welfare
            criterion." Public Choice (Special Spring
            Supplement).

5 The Willingness-to-Pay Criterion and Public Program Evaluation in Health

Joseph Lipscomb

The purpose of this paper is to introduce a resource planning model for determining the efficient allocation of inputs among competing medical care programs that would, on average, lead to maximum improvement in population health status. The primary focus of the model will be on how individual preferences for alternative program outcomes can be channeled directly into the decision-making process. Thus, what at first might sound suspiciously like a centralized scheme strengthening the bureaucrat's grip on policy will, in fact, be an algorithm structured to be responsive to the collective preferences of the public. This raises the crucial question of precisely how public preferences should be reflected in medical care allocation decisions; much of this paper is devoted to examining this question from a theoretical perspective.

The conceptual framework for the allocation model itself has its foundation in Bush (1973, 1970); Chen (1977, 1975); Torrance (1973, 1972); and Lipscomb (forthcoming; 1975). In their scheme, health status is defined in terms of expected population movement through non-disease-specific function levels. These levels, which are the defined states of health to be used in the allocation model, are assigned relative value weights on the basis of sampled population preferences, which are aggregated in some fashion. Diseases of interest are divided into clinical stages; each stage is associated with a corresponding function level and is assigned the relative value weight given that level by the population. The effectiveness of a particular health program for the target population is gauged by its impact on the expected health state occupancy pattern relative to the status quo pattern that would be expected to result were the program not instituted. It is through the application of these relative value weights to the derived health state occupancy patterns that individual preferences influence allocation decisions.

91

The first section of the paper deals with the substitution of a willingness-to-pay mechanism for this relative
value weight-voting scheme. There are a number of potential
advantages to this method. It is shown that under one set of
assumptions, a willingness-to-pay approach can lead to Pareto
optimal allocations that reflect eleemosynary considerations,
including traditional philanthropic contributions. Under certain other assumptions, the usual motives for individuals to
understate their true preferences for outcomes is eliminated.
While such willingness-to-pay votes would doubtlessly be a
function of the prevailing income distribution, there are
rational means for guaranteeing minimum medical care benefit
packages to selected population subgroups.

In this paper, the objective function will be given a
statistical (semi-Markovian) interpretation, which establishes
a direct and natural correspondence between model parameters
and the traditional epidemiologic components of disease prevalence. The constraint set will be structured for the allocation of physical resources rather than a budget. The result is that the potential specificity of resource allocation
recommendations is increased, albeit at the expense of requiring much data which would link the medical care process
(treatment) to outcome. In general, experimental data of this
type have not been available for large population groups.
Health program impact information has usually been obtained
either through adaptation of certain epidemiologic models from
the clinical medicine literature (Torrance, 1973, 1972) or by
the aggregation of expert medical opinion (Bush, 1972).

However, recent developments in federal health care
regulation have established mechanisms with the potential for
continuous collection of data, linking treatment to outcome
for all demographic groups of the U.S. population. In 1972,
Congress mandated the development of a nationwide network of
Professional Standards Review Organizations (PSROs), whose
principal responsibility is to monitor the quality and cost
of hospital care for Medicare and Medicaid patients (U.S.
DHEW, 1974). The current focus of most PSROs appears to be
on traditional parameters of inpatient care appropriateness,
such as diagnostic-specific length of stay. However, there
is the potential for PSROs to selectively embark on a more
detailed examination of the relationships between health programs and health function levels for different demographic
categories of patients (in outpatient as well as inpatient
settings).

It is assumed that health care--or any commodity that
is the focus of such an allocation model--is a "merit" good
(see Musgrave, 1959; Pauly, 1972). That is, because of consumer ignorance, perceived income inequities, or other
factors, the good, in the absence of public intervention,
would be underconsumed by certain segments of the population.
As a result, a formal service planning mechanism is required

of the public sector. In special settings (such as an American Indian reservation) where there is not a significant organized market for modern medical care, an allocation model,
such as the one presented here, could become the principal
external mechanism for determining the mix of services received by the population. In the more general case where a
market does exist but is decreed inadequate by the public
sector, the model could be viewed as providing allocative
guidelines for supplementing the medical care consumed by
specific population groups. Under this conceptualization,
the status quo value of the health status index is precisely
that which arises in the presumed absence of extra-market
intervention. The public's perception that this status quo
value is unacceptable becomes the normative basis for intervention in a market or non-market context.

     This paper deals neither with how such a public per-
ception of health care inadequacy emerges nor with how these
perceptions are translated organizationally into a public will
to act. The paper also does not confront a central issue that
should be made endogenous in all discussions of merit good
provision: How does society come to know whether, and to what
extent, it is "underconsuming" a good or service? The basic
approach taken here and by Acton (1973) is not to ask the
population if they would rather have more of service X or Y;
to pursue this course of inquiry in medical care is often to
assume that the responding consumer has unbiased, low-variance
estimates of the relationship between the adoption of X or Y
and resultant changes in his own function status. Given the
complex nature of medical technology and the slow rate of information transfer from providers to consumers, it is not
evident that the typical consumer is in a rational position
to deal directly with this choice between X and Y, per se.
The strategy advocated here is to elicit consumer preferences
for health program outcomes, delineated in terms of levels of
human physical and social function. Then one uses the allocation model to explore the relationships between (a) the
medical care processes (programs) required, on average, to
produce the desired outcomes, (b) the resources required for
these processes, (c) the opportunity costs of these resources,
and (d) the value society places on these expected health outcomes, that is, whether the value is sufficient to pay the opportunity costs of these resources. If society does value
these health outcomes sufficiently, it proceeds to provide the
programs in the most efficient manner possible. If the opportunity costs cannot be voluntarily covered, then society
may choose not to provide the programs--in essence, they are
declared not to be merit goods.

     In the next section, the new allocation model is pre-
sented with the traditional relative value weight-voting
scheme. In the following sections, criticisms are addressed
to this formulation. Thereafter, willingness-to-pay schemes
are introduced. A concluding section summarizes the results.

AN OPTIMIZATION MODEL FOR
RESOURCE ALLOCATION TO HEALTH

The purpose of this section is to present and discuss
in some detail the allocation model that will be used subsequently in the development of a willingness-to-pay approach
to health program determination.*

Structural Features

The health status-oriented models of Bush (1973, 1972,
1970), Chen (1977, 1975), and Torrance (1973, 1972) share certain important structural features that will be embodied in
the model proposed here. In particular, these cost-
effectiveness models have certain features:

They explicitly take account, in the allocation decision process, of individual consumer preferences for alternative states of health. These expressions of preference have
so far taken the form of utility weights based ultimately on
consumer statements concerning their choices among alternative functional states of nature. Yet, as will be demonstrated subsequently, the structure of these models can
also permit program priorities to be set on the basis of
individual statements of willingness to pay for program
outcomes. Furthermore, a consumer can be held account-
able for these preference statements because they can
become the basis for raising the tax bill to reflect the
proposed programs.

They allocate a given budget to maximize the improvement in a population's health status over time. Setting the
allocation model in a willingness-to-pay context is important,
for it makes program evaluation goal-directed. Health status
indexes have been introduced in the literature a number of
times, but only a few of these are readily adaptable for use
in mathematical programming analysis (see Lipscomb, 1977). As
will be seen later in the paper, there is an additional advantage to using a constrained optimization model in a
willingness-to-pay context, in that, the appropriate levels
and distributions of taxes and expenditures can be determined
simultaneously.

The allocation model under discussion is intended
specifically for the allocation of human and physical resources among competing health programs. Accordingly, in

---

* Much of this section and the Appendix has been adapted from
  Lipscomb (forthcoming) where these issues of model specification and parameter estimation are pursued in more
  depth.

addition to the general properties noted above, some additional requirements will be imposed:

     As with the models of Chen (1975) and Bush (1973), a
delineation of the target population into modules is required,
such that each is relatively homogeneous with respect to
transitions among disease states and durations of stay in
stages. Since one is dealing now with specific diseases, a
module might be ideally defined as a subpopulation whose members are at approximately the same risk to a particular
disease. Individuals would be assigned to risk levels on the
basis of certain predisposing characteristics (for example,
weight, age, sex) that have been previously linked with the
severity of the disease.

     It may be particularly true with acute diseases, such
as infant gastroenteritis and respiratory infections, that
prevalence patterns are seasonal. Since changes in expected
prevalence within a module directly influence the optimal set
of intervention strategies and their associated resource requirements, the model should account for possible cyclical
variations in epidemiologic parameters.

     Because the model is intended to relate inputs to out-
puts (in the form of health outcomes), it must incorporate
information on the processes of medical care. These processes must be linked simultaneously with the structure of
care (the distribution of available inputs) and the outcome
of care. Information is required on (a) the types of resources potentially able to meet the health needs of a target
population, (b) the effective availability of each resource,
(c) alternative intervention strategies at each clinically
defined stage of each disease at which programs might be
directed, (d) the amount of each resource required to undertake each alternative intervention strategy, and (e) the expected impact of each strategy on the health status of each
subpopulation, that is, module in the target population.

     The resource drain from non-intervention must be ex-
plicitly accounted for. Thus, for a given module, one might
have choices among interventions a, b, or c or no intervention
at all. But not intervening at all does represent an intervention in one important sense: These module members are
likely to consume health care resources over time, and this
may have the effect of shrinking the resource pool that sup-
ports the "active" interventions a, b, and c.

Semi-Markovian Properties

     Unlike the formulation of Torrance (1973, 1972), the
allocation model will have an explicit stochastic structure.
Departing from the models of Bush (1972) and Chen (1975),

this structure will be semi-Markovian rather than pure
Markovian in thrust. The motivation for this departure is
that a pattern of disease prevalence typically involves not
only transitions among states, but stays of <u>variable duration</u>
in each state. Because (in contrast to a pure Markovian
model) a semi-Markovian model treats these durations as
random variables, it is a natural framework for epidemiological analysis. However, there have been comparatively few
applications of these concepts to health services delivery
problems. (For an excellent exception, see Kao (1972).) The
statistical framework to be used in this analysis may be
introduced as follows:

We let p_{ij} be the probability that a semi-Markovian
process which entered state i on its last transition will
enter j on its next transition;

$$p_{ij} \geq 0 \text{ and } \sum_{j=1}^{N} p_{ij} = 1, \text{ for } i, j=1,\ldots,N,$$

where N is the number of states in the model. (These
transition probabilities are, in fact, those of the Markovian
process that is "imbedded" in the more general semi-Markovian
formulation. One way to conceptualize a semi-Markovian
process is to imagine that after the process enters state i, it
determines its next state j according to the p_{ij}. Then,
conditional on the choice of j, the process holds in i for a
time τ_{ij}. These holding times are positive, integer-valued
random variables with densities $h_{ij}(s) = P(\tau_{ij} = s)$, for s
= 1,2... and for all i and j. It is assumed that all holding
time means

$$\bar{\tau}_{ij} = \sum_{s=1}^{\infty} s \, h_{ij}(s)$$

are finite and that each holding time is at least one time
unit in length, so that $h_{ij}(0) = 0$. In applications, one can
assign this fundamental time unit any desired value.

One key assumption of the semi-Markovian (and pure
Markovian) model should be noted, namely, that each transition probability and holding time distribution is a function
solely of i, the current state of occupancy. In actual applications, this "memoryless" characteristic of the process
may be too strong an assumption. There are practical rem-
edies, but these will not be discussed here (see Chen, 1975;
Lipscomb (forthcoming)).

The principal epidemiological result that emerges from
this framework is that the expected value of the prevalence
of a health state j over a time period t--call it $\overline{pp}_{j}(t)$--
can be expressed succinctly as a function of <u>all</u>
transition probabilities and holding time distributions.

This result is derived in the Appendix. It implies that for any period t, one can forecast period prevalence by first obtaining estimates of all transition probabilities and holding time distributions and then employing the general expression for $\overline{pp}_j(t)$ given in the Appendix.* These transition probabilities and holding time distributions will give rise to a particular pattern of prevalence over time that can, of course, be determined by direct observation ex post. In principle, a health care program alters outcomes (prevalence patterns) by inducing changes in the P_{ij} and $h_{ij}(\cdot)$. But one need not obtain separate estimates of these underlying semi-Markovian parameters in order to forecast the impact of selected programs on health outcomes; a regression model for accomplishing this purpose has been developed by the author (Lipscomb, forthcoming).

In the allocation model to be described, period prevalence will be defined over an interval of length t whose starting point is assumed to be randomly selected (see the Appendix). The model is structured as a mathematical program whose optimal solution permits calculation of the amount of each limited resource needed in each population module for each treatment strategy. The objective function is maximized, subject to the constraints (1) that total available resources not be exceeded by requirements, (2) that each module member may be treated by one, and only one, disease strategy, and (3) that all diseases are treatable in all states, for all population modules: maximize

$$\Delta H(t) = \left[\sum_{d=1}^{D} \sum_{m=1}^{M} \sum_{i=0}^{S_d} \sum_{j=1}^{N} U_j \; (\overline{pp}_{jm}^{d_o}(t) - \overline{pp}_{jm}^{d_i}(t)) \right] P_m^{d_i} X_m^{d_i},$$

subject to $\displaystyle\sum_{d=1}^{D} \sum_{m=1}^{M} \sum_{i=0}^{S_d} A_{mp}^{d_i}(t) \, X_m^{d_i} \leq R_p(t)$, for p=1, ..., Q;

$$\sum_{i=0}^{S_d} X_m^{d_i} = 1, \text{ for m=1, ..., M}$$

$$d=1, \ldots, D; \text{ and}$$

$$X_m^{d_i} \geq 0, \text{ for i=0, ..., S}$$

$$d-1, \ldots, D,$$

$$m=1, \ldots, M$$

---

* It can also be shown (see Lipscomb, 1977) that within this semi-Markovian framework, the expected prevalence of state j can be expressed as the product of the expected incidence of j and the expected duration-of-stay per entry.

where

U_j = the consumer-provided preference, or utility, weight for health state j

$\overline{pp}_{jm}^{d_i}(t)$ = the expected time a typical member of module m will spend in the stage of disease d associated with health state j during the time interval t, given that intervention strategy i against disease d is implemented

$\overline{pp}_{jm}^{d_o}(t)$ = the special case of $\overline{pp}_{jm}^{d_i}(t)$ when no special intervention strategy (i=0) is implemented and the status quo is assumed to exist within module m with respect to disease d over t

t = the time duration over which the strategies are being evaluated

$P_m^{d_i}$ = the size of the population at risk to disease d in module m which can <u>potentially</u> be affected by intervention strategy i

$A_{mp}^{d_i}(t)$ = the total amount of resource p required to treat the expected prevalency of disease d, in its entirety, with strategy i in module m over t

$R_p(t)$ = total amount of p available over t

$X_m^{d_i}$ = that fraction of the population of module m, potentially treatable under strategy i against disease d, which should in fact be treated via that strategy if the optimal allocation of resources is to result

N = the number of health states

S_d = the number of intervention strategies against disease d subject to allocative decisions

M = the number of population modules

D = the number of diseases in the decision problem

Q = the number of resources subject to allocation decisions.

The objective function, $\Delta H(t)$, is interpreted as expected improvement in the health status of all modules of the
target population over a time period of length t. To see
this, note first that the expression within the inner parentheses represents the expected change in the total time of
occupancy of state j over t for a typical individual in
module m, who is subject to strategy i against disease d instead of the status quo. The model is a one-period construct,
and the time interval may be set at any value. However, it
is desirable to choose t such that observed prevalence rates
for the health states under consideration are reasonably
stable, so as to approximately meet the model's stationary
requirement.

Solution of the model also requires that a duration-
of-stay value be assigned to the terminal, that is, "trapping" health state. Yet there is nothing in semi-Markovian
theory to suggest the proper termination times for trapping
states. Death is the ultimate trapping state, and one is
forced to employ exogenous assumptions in choosing the
associated mean duration-of-stay parameter value. If the
optimization interval t is sufficiently long, the problem is
readily resolved by defining a Standard Life to be some arbitrary large value, say 100 years. Then, (1) sample individuals are "dropped" from the optimization analysis once they
reach this age or (2) are assigned to the death state for a
period equal to the difference between the Standard Life value
and the actual expected age of death. This procedure has
been employed by Bush (1972). It can be shown (Lipscomb,
1977) that optimal resource allocations are invariant to a
choice of the Standard Life length, so long as it exceeds
the greatest life expectancy in the target population. For
simplicity, it is assumed that an individual can occupy
one, and only one, disease state at any moment. More complicated models allowing multiple stage occupancy may be
developed, but these would not serve a purpose here.

The Uj serve to weight each alternative state (stage)
occupancy according to its relative social utility. Since
the objective function is structured to represent a minimiza-
tion of value-weighted disability, the Uj are better thought
of here as disutility weights whose numerical values are inversely related to state desirability. Therefore, the expression within square brackets can be defined as the expected change in health status for an individual in module m
who receives treatment strategy i. Multiplying this number
by

$$P_m^{d_i}$$

yields the total expected change in health status if strategy
i against disease d is administered to the entire population
assumed to be at risk to d in module m. In solving the
mathematical program, one is trying to determine that set

of values,

$$X_m^{d_i},$$

on the closed interval $[0,1]$, each of which represents
the fraction of a population at risk that should receive
a certain treatment strategy. It should be noted that
while the model is specified here as a linear program,
one can convert it to a dichotomous (0-1) integer program
by simply restricting the

$$X_m^{d_i}$$

to lie on an endpoint of $[0,1]$. Under this specification,
a treatment strategy--if it were administered within a
module at all--would be made available to the entire at-
risk population in the module. This permits acknowledg-
ment of the arguments made by Chen and Bush (1977) and
Torrance (1973) that fractional funding of modules may
be administratively and politically infeasible.

     Turning now to the constraint set, first consider
the Q-inequality resource constraints. Each

$$A_{mp}^{d_i}(t)$$

represents the total amount of resource p needed to admin-
ister strategy d_i to the entire population assumed to be at
risk to d in module m. It is computed as the product of
the amount of resource p needed for that purpose _per_
individual and

$$P_m^{d_i},$$

the _total_ population at-risk in the module. Once the
mathematical program is solved, the set of products

$$A_{mp}^{d_i}(t) \quad X_m^{d_i}$$

can be easily computed separately. From a policy standpoint,
these are the key results; each

$$A_{mp}^{d_i}(t) \quad X_m^{d_i}$$

represents the optimal amount of resource p to be devoted to
treatment of disease d via strategy i in module m.

     The second section of the constraint set consists of
the M·D equality constraints of the general form

$$\sum_{i=0}^{S_d} X_m^{d_i} = 1.$$

As mentioned above, the constraints require that, for each
disease, each module member be subject to one, and only one,
strategy. Under the dichotomous integer programming formulation, each module will be allocated exactly one strategy for
each disease.

Overall, the model may be viewed as a large production
function, which indicates the maximum amount of output--
defined here as expected improvement in total population
health status--obtainable from a given vector of inputs.
However, since this production function is structured basically as a linear program, there is a concomitant assumption
that the care rendered with inputs explicitly in the constraint set is subject to constant returns-to-scale. This
requirement may seem unduly restrictive, but several steps
can be taken to weaken its practical impact: (1) For any
particular application, one must determine the nature of
the short-run within which production is proceeding. The
constraint set for that application should include only the
factors assumed to be variable. To be sure, the cost of
fixed factors can also be calculated and should in fact be
for long-run planning purposes. (2) If it is believed that
these variable factors do not combine in a manner consistent
with the constant returns assumption throughout the relevant
output range, the range can be divided into regions such that
over each region, the assumption is more reasonable. The

$$A_{mp}^{d_i}(t)$$

production coefficients could then be adjusted as needed
to reflect the particular input proportion characteristics
relevant to each output region. (3) From a modeling viewpoint, one can "unfix" fixed factors and calculate the
maximum obtainable output from all relevant short-run con-
figurations of medical care structure. This also implies
that the optimal long-run input configuration for the
system can be calculated. Of course, the ability of a decision maker to move to that optimum may be limited by an
external funding constraint, or perhaps even by an absolute
shortage of one or more productive factors. Because these
considerations are assumed for now to be external to the
system decision maker, they are not brought explicitly into
the allocation model.

INDIVIDUAL PREFERENCES FOR SOCIAL GOODS

        The utility weights employed by Bush, Chen, Torrance,
and the author possess at least two major limitations as
guideposts for health resources allocation:

        (1) The first limitation of the utility weight ap-
proach is that while the weights may represent an individual's relative preferences for the health states themselves,* they do not indicate the individual's relative
preferences between health per se and other goods and services. Consequently, they cannot be used as the final criteria in determining how a government allocates its (tax-
derived) resources among public goods, one of which is health
care. (This is also pointed out by Fischer (1977).) It is
in somewhat this same vein that Acton (1973) criticizes the
use of human capital or "livelihood" measures as a basis for
resource allocation. He writes: "The major objection to a
livelihood evaluation is that it does not clearly correspond
to the amounts the decision maker or members of the community
would want to pay for a particular project." When an individual (truthfully) states what he is willing to pay for a
health program, he is explicitly evaluating the expected
(total) benefit of that program relative to the expected
benefits that could be derived from the most preferred alternative use of those funds. It is a sobering realization
that there is nothing in the utility weights themselves to
indicate how much of a society's resources should be devoted
to health nor whether any resources at all should be budgeted
to health. Consequently, the allocation model discussed
above and Bush and Torrance's allocation model presuppose
that society has decreed its optimal total allocation of
health care resources to the modules under consideration.
The only question left--though it is a difficult and important one--is the optimal distribution of those health care
resources among the modules.

        (2) A second limitation of the utility weight approach
(as it has been developed thus far) is that a consumer is
permitted only a partial expression of the intensity of his
preference among health state alternatives. It is true in
this paradigm that the voting consumer can express preference
intensity by assigning to each state, in effect, any desired
real number from the closed interval on which the utility
weights are scaled, for example, [0,1]. It is also true--
most explicitly in the Bush approach to weight construction

----

*   It is, in fact, not a trivial problem to demonstrate that
    a given set of utility weights elicited from individuals
    represents a valid summarization of their preferences for
    states. For an excellent discussion of the validation
    issue, see Kaplan (1976).

--that the voting individual is to express ethical
(society-minded) rather than personal preferences for the
states (see Harsanyi, 1956).

Under these limitations, it is perfectly possible for
two individuals, A and B, to have assigned identical sets of
interval-scale rankings to states and yet for A to feel much
more intensely about the outcomes on either end of the preference continuum. A's deep involvement may stem from concern about his own health status, the family's, or the
health and well-being of the community. Conversely, individual B may feel much less concern for the health status
of anyone; but (assuming he was willing to endure the preference survey in the first place) his set of utility weights
will count just as much as A's in the aggregation of votes
that follows. Admittedly, any voting scheme that establishes
upper and lower numerical bounds on preference expression is
subject to this same commentary. When the upper and lower
bounds are the same for all individuals, the scheme is effectively "one man-one vote." It is precisely this egali-
tarian concept that is embodied in the utility weights of
Bush and others.

This policy can be rationally defended if at least one
of the following conditions is assumed:

(1)   All individuals have identical utility
      functions, which include health status
      as an argument.

(2)   There is little a priori information on
      the distribution of preference intensity
      for health status across the population;
      appealing to the Principle of Insufficient
      Reason, the policy maker acts as though
      each individual regarded health identically.

(3)   It is agreed that the distribution of in-
      come is so unsatisfactory that statements
      of preference that might be influenced by
      this distribution are not acceptable for
      social policy formation.

(4)   Questions of economic efficiency aside,
      society agrees a priori that social
      justice requires one man-one vote schemes
      for all balloting (but this does not pre-
      clude private, legally sanctioned action
      to influence the outcome).

Few would concur that (1) is reasonable. A satisfactory analysis of (4) is beyond the scope of this paper;
clearly, if one accepts this principle, much of the im-
mediately proceeding discussion becomes irrelevant--but

so does any voting scheme that might be structured to permit
direct expressions of altruism to influence the outcome.
It could be claimed that alternative (2) is not unreasonable;
even though consumers do register preference intensity for
health status with their dollar votes in the market place,
it can be persuasively argued that these "votes" are biased
by consumer ignorance, supply constraints that muffle the
expression of effective demand, and an unjust income distribution. Given all this "noise" in the market place
"ballot box," a more defensible strategy for gathering information on the demand for health for social policy purposes might be simply to assign each consumer the same effective supply of utility weights and let the voting proceed
through such devices as consumer surveys. But it is precisely through such carefully planned surveys that additional
information could be obtained on preference intensity for
health--information that would distinguish between the de-
sires of individuals A and B by requiring each to state how
much income he is willing to forego to obtain program outcomes. In its most basic form, the "willingness-to-pay"
approach to program determination consists of the following
procedure:

        (1) To determine from each member of a population how
much he is willing to contribute toward the provision of alternative quantities of a public good. From this information, each individual's demand curve for the public good is
derived. It is not required that each polled individual be
a direct beneficiary of the good. Each individual's response
reflects jointly his desire to see the good provided both for
himself and for all other individuals who might benefit. The
response of the philanthropic individual will clearly reflect
his differential valuation of the health of various subgroups
within his community. For example, willingness to pay $100
for a certain program could imply that the philanthropist
believes that the direct benefits received by him are worth
$50, that those accruing to his family are worth (to him)
$45, and that those to be derived by the community at large
are worth (to him) $5.

        (2) To sum all of the individual expressions of worth
to obtain a level aggregate willingness to pay for each alternative quantity of the public good. When ordered, these
levels yield the aggregate demand curve for the good.

        (3) To provide that quantity of the good given by the
intersection of the aggregate demand and supply curves; to
tax each individual an amount equal to his stated willingness
to pay for the number of units of the good to be provided.
These tax contributions, while not covering administration
expenses, will cover the total cost of the quantity of the
good provided and, in fact, yield a producer's surplus if
aggregate supply is not perfectly elastic. Given the downward slope of each individual demand curve, each contributor

will enjoy a consumer surplus in the standard sense. Assuming that the prices of all inputs and other outputs remain
unaffected, provision of the good meets the Pareto criterion
for the improvement of the collective welfare.

The willingness-to-pay approach to cost-benefit
analysis has been endorsed by Mishan (1971) as the only
method consistent with Pareto optimality. It is the corner-
stone of Pauly's (1972) suggested policy for the efficient
provision of medical care. Acton (1973) has provided an example of how this methodology can be used to determine a community's demand for alternative life-saving programs, such as
those intended to reduce heart attack mortality.

Health care resource allocations, based on interval
scale, health-state utility weights, alone, can make no similar claim to Pareto optimality. These weights indicate
nothing about the relative value of health versus non-health
goods and services to the individual; consequently, they cannot reflect the total opportunity cost of health care provision. Under a willingness-to-pay approach, a society's legal
currency is automatically the instrument for the commensura-
tion of values and the aggregation of preferences. Citizens
can be polled on their willingness to pay for each type of
public good; in principle, the aggregate demand for each good
could be derived and thus their optimal quantities determined.

The crucial issue for legitimizing this method is
whether society should regard the individual's set of "dollar
votes" for the various public goods as a valid expression of
his relative preferences for those goods. There are two
potential problems with this approach:

(1) It can be argued that the acceptability of willingness to pay as a criterion for allocation is directly related to the social acceptability of the prevailing income
distribution. It is reasonable to posit that the individual's
stated demand for a public good is, like the demand for goods
in general, a function of his income. It follows that a significant redistribution of income could result in a significant alteration in the volume and composition of public goods
demanded. Chen, Bush, and Zaremba (1975) also argue the following in this regard:

Analytically, this proposal [willingness to pay]
suffers from all the defects of using actual expenditures as a surrogate for the effectiveness
of health activities. Furthermore, unless the
assumption that [there is] an equal distribution
of income is valid, "the willingness to pay"
criterion results in reinforcement of the status
quo, i.e., unequal access to health care.

    This criticism is overstated for two reasons:
First, the socially preferred income distribution need
not be an equal income distribution; this would be
the case, in general, only if all individuals possessed an
identical utility function for money. More importantly,
there is a basic distinction between willingness-to-pay
expressions for a public good and those expenditures actually
made on the good (if any) in the market place. Expenditures
represent the effective demand for health care, reflecting
the complex interactions among (a) the consumer's willingness
to pay (his true demand) for health outcomes, (b) the consumer's knowledge of the relevant market variables (for
example, price and quality of care) and of the technical relationship between health care and outcomes, and (c) the
existing supply of health care. Expenditures will have a
(perhaps undesirable) status quo orientation because they are
partially predicated on (b) and (c). A properly formulated
willingness-to-pay scheme need not be encumbered with these
distorting complications. It must be acknowledged that to
the extent that (i) the distribution of income is socially
unacceptable and (ii) the income elasticity of willingness-
to-pay statements is non-zero, assumption (c) above becomes
salient and the utility weight approach becomes a more at-
tractive alternative. But given (i) and (ii), there is the
alternative--discussed in the next section--of using
willingness-to-pay information as the primary demand-side
determinant of public health expenditures, while guaranteeing
economically disadvantaged modules certain minimum benefit
packages.

    (2) Another major criticism of the willingness-to-pay
approach, as it has been traditionally conceptualized, is that
there is always the opportunity and often the motive for a
strategic understatement of true preferences. For instance,
assume an individual believes (a) that he and numerous others
highly value a prospective health care program, (b) that most
or all fellow citizens will state their true willingness to
pay for the program, (c) that his own true willingness to pay
--while no small sum to him--would be but an insignificant
proportion of the total amount stated, (d) that all pledges
will be collected in taxes if the good is provided, and (e)
that all citizens have equal access to the program, if provided. The individual may then be led to underrepresent how
much the program is worth to him. Acton (1973) has briefly
raised this possibility and makes the distinction between
"manifest" (actual) and "latent" (true) willingness to pay.
His conclusion on the issue is that, "Manifest preferences
are probably a much better guide to latent preferences than
any of the alternatives that do not consider preferences at
all." However, one of the alternatives that Acton does not
appear to consider is the use of interval-scale utility
weights in the manner of Bush, Torrance, and the author
(Lipscomb, forthcoming). Because these weights are not explicitly linked to tax schemes to pay for the "fixed" resources being allocated, the motive for a systematic

underrepresentation of preferences is not apparent. (On the
other hand, there might be occasions where an individual believes a strategic redistribution of utility weight "votes"
among states might favorably affect an allocation solution.
This issue of strategic "point" voting is largely unexplored.)
The question remains whether the willingness-to-pay criterion
can be implemented in a context that reduces undesirable
strategic behavior.

Acton's (1973) analysis of alternative means of reducing heart attack mortality represents the one major effort
to adapt and implement the willingness-to-pay approach for
the evaluation of health care programs. His analysis focused
on two states of health, death and non-death, and individuals
were asked, essentially, how much they would be willing to
pay, or advise others to pay, for certain reductions in the
probability of dying from a heart attack.

WILLINGNESS TO PAY AND THE OPTIMAL
ALLOCATION OF HEALTH RESOURCES

One of the principal features of the willingness-to-
pay allocation model developed below is that the optimal distributions of expenditures and taxes are determined simultaneously. (As will be shown, the notion of optimality here
is predicated on, among other things, a preference for a
benefit theory of taxation, modified wherever deemed necessary to compensate for unacceptable differences in ability
to pay. Throughout the early discussion on benefit determination, it is assumed that people do express their true
preferences for health outcomes.

The context of the willingness-to-pay allocation
model problem is much the same as that for the resource
allocation model. There exists a target population at
risk to a number of diseases. There are alternative strategies for preventing or treating each disease, every strategy
being characterized by minimum standards of care, reflected
in the associated resource requirements coefficients (the
$A^{d}_{mpi}(t)$). There is (for the moment) a fixed vector of resources assumed to be exogenously given. Each
strategy has an expected medical outcome, expressed in terms
of a time-flow pattern of health state occupancy for each
member of the target population. The population itself is
divided into modules, each of which is thought to be relatively homogeneous with respect to both the expected outcome
and the resource requirements of any set of intervention
strategies. The major distinction between the allocation
model and the willingness-to-pay allocation model is that
population expressions of willingness to pay for interventions
replace the interval-scale utility weights, U_j. These
willingness-to-pay statements are presumed to be elicited on
behalf of each module from a "contributing" population that

may be, but need not be, identical with the target population. This leads to the objective function variations of
interest.

Objective Function I

In this formulation, willingness-to-pay expressions
play a comparable structural role to the utility weights in
the basic model. With respect to any module m, the contributing population is defined as:

$$C = C_m + C_{m'} + C_{m''}$$

where

C_m =   set of individuals <u>in module m</u> who may be asked
             to contribute to the provision of one or more
             intervention strategies in m

$C_{m'}$ =   set of individuals in the target population <u>not</u>
             in module m who may be asked to contribute to
             one or more intervention strategies <u>in m</u>

$C_{m''}$ =   set of individuals <u>not</u> in the target population
             who may be asked to contribute to one or more
             intervention strategies <u>in module m.</u>

Next, let

k^w_{jm} =   the maximum amount that person $k \varepsilon C_m$ is willing to
             pay to convert 24 hours of state j occupancy into
             24 hours of optimal (good health) state occupancy
             for himself (24 hours is set as the fundamental
             semi-Markovian time unit here)

w_{jmk} =   the maximum amount that person $k \varepsilon C_m$ is willing to
             pay to convert 24 hours of state j occupancy into
             24 hours of optimal (good health) state occupancy
             for one other person within module m

w_{jmg} =   the maximum amount that person $g \varepsilon C_{m'}$ is willing
             to pay to convert 24 hours of state j occupancy
             into 24 hours of optimal (good health) state
             occupancy for one person within module m

w_{jmh} =   the maximum amount that person $h \varepsilon C_{m''}$ is willing
             to pay to convert 24 hours of state j occupancy
             into 24 hours of good health person in module m.

It follows that

$$W_{jm} = \sum_{k=1}^{C_m} \left({}_k w_{jm} + w_{jmk} \right) + \sum_{g=1}^{C_m'} w_{jmg} + \sum_{h=1}^{C_m''} w_{jmh} = w_{jm} + w_{jm'}$$

$$+ w_{jm''}.$$

This is the maximum amount the contributing population is willing to pay to convert 24 hours of state j to 24 hours of good health within module m.

Each w represents the maximum amount person k in module m would prefer to pay rather than spend 24 hours in health state j. Whenever k is confronted with the opportunity of paying ${}_k w_{jm}$ for such an improvement, he will benefit by doing so. That is, there is some ${}_k w_{jm}^I$ which makes k indifferent between payment and the function status improvement, and it is always the case that

$$_k w_{jm}^I - {}_k w_{jm} = \varepsilon \geq o.$$

In practice, of course, ε should be only as large as the smallest unit of relevant currency, for example, one cent. Thus, in general, while a consumer surplus exists on each day of function status improvement "purchased" by any member of the contributing population on behalf of any member of the target population, the magnitude of the consumer surplus is not likely to be significant.

Applying these constructs, willingness-to-pay Objective Function I of the basic model becomes the following:

$$B^1(t) = \sum_{d=1}^{D} \sum_{m=1}^{M} \sum_{i=0}^{S_d} \left[\sum_{j=1}^{N} W_{jm} (\overline{pp}_{jm}^{d_o}(t) - \overline{pp}_{jm}^{d_i}(t)) \right] P_m^{d_i} X_m^{d_i}.$$

When this expression is maximized, subject to the original resource constraints, an optimal set of intervention strategies is determined. Corresponding to this optimal solution, there is an expected total benefit accruing to the contributing population because of programs in module m; this benefit is defined on the basis of the willingness-to-pay expressions themselves. Let $\{X_m^{d_i}\}$ be the optimal solution vector. Then the total expected benefit associated with module m is:

$$\overline{B}_m^1(t) = \sum_{d=1}^{D} \sum_{i=0}^{S_d} \left[\sum_{j=1}^{N} W_{jm} (\overline{pp}_{jm}^{d_o}(t) - \overline{pp}_{jm}^{d_i}(t)) \right] P_m^{d_i} \hat{X}_m^{d_i}.$$

There are several aspects of this form of the model to note:

(1) Given the simple and isolated manner in which
the elements of W_{jm} are elicited from individuals, the possibility of diminishing marginal utility in the occupancy of
particular health states is not reflected in the W_{jm} and
therefore does not influence the allocation solution. Thus,
demand curves for states are implicitly assumed to be infinitely elastic, and the usual notion of consumer surplus
does not enter the analysis.

(2) The relatively "minor" consumer surplus that
arises because of the difference between $_kw_{jm}$ and $_kw_{jm}^I$
will not be treated as significant quantitatively.
The role it does play is to insure that the utility-
maximizing person k values the change from j to good health
more than he does $_kw_{jm}$. This, in turn, means that any action
k might take--such as not revealing his true preferences--
would cause him not to receive program benefits, resulting
in an expected loss in welfare.

(3) The period t is sufficiently short so that discounting program benefits to present value is not a practical
concern.

(4) The individual willingness-to-pay expressions,
w_{jmr}, are assumed to be characterized by linear additivity of
the following sort: (a) the amount that r would be willing
to pay to convert Q days of state j to Q days of good health
for a person in m is $Q.w_{jmr}$, (b) the amount that r would be
willing to pay to convert a day of state j to a day of state
j' is $(w_{jmr} - w_{j'mr})$, (c) the amount r would be willing to
pay to convert Q days of j to Q' days of j' in m is given by
$(Q.w_{jmr} - Q'.w_{j'mr})$. This latter expression may be positive,
negative, or zero. The linear additivity assumption is
admittedly stringent, but it is precisely this assumption that has been adopted by Chen and Bush (1977),
Torrance (1973), and the author (Lipscomb, 1977) in allocation models that employ the linear scale utility weights.

One of the fundamental characteristics of the
willingness-to-pay expressions, w_{jmr}, is that they represent
evaluations of health states that are presumed to be attain-
able with certainty; this arises essentially from the
straightforward manner in which the w_{jmr} are elicited. It is
also the case that the interval-scale utility weights employed
by Bush (1972), Torrance (1972), and the author are designed
to reflect the relative value of these states irrespective of
their probability of occurrence to individuals. Torrance
(1973) has gone to considerable lengths to insure that his
utility weights are untainted by prognoses. Bush and his
associates have sought to develop a single set of function
states and associated utility weights that can be applied
directly in the evaluation of different health programs with
diverse prognostic characteristics.

But the question can be raised, why should not the probability of a state--or at least the individual's perception of that probability--be regarded as a possible attribute of the state itself? Health status may indeed be a matter of preference and prognosis, but it is not clear why prognosis should be left unrelated to preference. As a counterexample, consider the usually undisputed designation of death as the lowest function level. The problem with death, it might be argued, is not so much the pain and anguish involved, but that the prognosis is poor. For models that do employ interval scale utility weights, one important but difficult extension would be the development of weights that incorporate the influence on consumers of perceived probabilities of state occupancy.

It might even be argued that any program which alters these perceived probabilities favorably has improved the person's health status even if the objective, etiologically-based probabilities are not, in fact, altered. This is all, admittedly, speculative at this point. But, in principle, the theories of conjoint and functional measurement, as described by Luce and Tukey (1964) and Anderson (1970), would be used to develop such utility weights. The key innovation would be designating the perceived probability of the state as an attribute of the state, so that the functional inter-action of this attribute with others (for example, physical dysfunction and social dependence) could be analyzed. Under this research strategy, it need not be assumed that prognosis and preferences for the other attributes (that is, preference for the "state" as it has been traditionally defined) are in-dependent; the assertion can be tested directly.

The most salient practical reason for considering a more probabilistic assessment of state utility is that it should enhance the likelihood of obtaining realistic evalua-tions for states that are extremely undesirable, such as death. When the alternatives to death presented in a utility assessment session are primarily long-term chronic conditions --which, if the conditions attained, would have substantial impacts on the entire function history of the individual-- persons can be led to deal with the issue of (relative) dis-utility of death. Torrance (1972) has presented preliminary evidence to support this.

However, when the alternatives to death are acute dis-ease stages of short expected durations, it is difficult to conceive of how these states and death could be simply arrayed by the individual along an interval scale in terms of relative disutility. In his willingness-to-pay evaluation of heart attack programs, Acton (1973) recognized these diffi-culties and instead asked individuals what they were willing to pay to achieve certain reductions in the probability of heart attack. His analysis proceeded by relating these willingness-to-pay expressions to the costs of alternative

programs for obtaining these probability reductions. As
Acton acknowledges, it is not a trivial matter to obtain
willingness-to-pay expressions for changes of probability
in health. In so proceeding, one can, in principle, arrive
at willingness-to-pay valuations that summarily reflect the
complex interaction of prognosis and preferences for the
usual (non-probabilistic) attributes of each state. As a
practical matter, the individual's willingness to evaluate
death in relation to other alternatives is enhanced because
it is more realistic, and less threatening, to deal with
projected changes in the probability of death than its occurrence with certainty.

      In view of these considerations, an alternative ob-
jective function form will be proposed.

Objective Function II

      Acton's model required only that the individual make
willingness-to-pay assessments regarding changes in the probability of occupying a single state, death. To integrate
this approach into the allocation model here requires, in
principle, that the breadth of the willingness-to-pay elici-
tation process be greatly expanded. For now, given the
status quo, there are N-1 non-fatal transient states of
health--each with an associated expected prevalency over
period of length t--plus the trapping state death, which
occurs with some probability. This probability and the
other expected prevalencies are a function of all transition
probabilities and holding time distributions. There will be
also a different set of expected prevalencies over t corresponding to each intervention strategy d_i, and these will
be module-specific as well.

      What is proposed is that each person in the contribu-
ting population be presented, in a concise format, (1) the
expected prevalencies of the N-1 states and the death probability in module m over period t, given intervention strategy d_i and (2) the corresponding pattern of parameter estimates for module m over t, given d_o, the status quo. The
person would be told to assume in all cases that death--if it
does occur during t--happens at the midpoint of the interval.

      It would be emphasized to the individual that informa-
tion on the likely health status within module m after
period t is not available and that, if he must speculate on
this, the speculations should be guided by a criterion of
"reasonableness." For example, it is probably not reasonable
to assume that a typical member of module m will suffer sudden
death just after the end of t; nor is it reasonable to assume
that this typical member of m will be in a good health state
throughout his life expectancy. Clearly, as the length of
the intervention interval, t, increases, the amount of

function time unaccounted for in the model--namely, the difference between the expected age of death and the end of interval t--approaches zero; as this occurs, the impact of an
uncertain future on the contributing individual's willingness-
to-pay statements is reduced.

Thus, let $v_{mr}^{d_i}(t)$ be the maximum amount that individual
r is willing to pay for intervention strategy d_i per person
in module m, rather than have the module receive the status
quo "intervention," d_o. (Again, this amount is assumed to be
less than the payment which would just make r indifferent between purchasing the intervention and not doing so.) Clearly,
$v_{mr}^{d_o}(t) = 0$. Then, for the contributing population as a whole,
one may define

$$\sum_{k=1}^{C_m} {}_k v_m^{d_i}(t) + v_{mk}^{d_i}(t) + \sum_{g=1}^{C_{m'}} v_{mg}^{d_i}(t) + \sum_{h=1}^{C_{m''}} v_{mh}^{d_i}(t) =$$

$$v_m^{d_i}(t) + v_{m'}^{d_i}(t) + v_{m''}^{d_i}(t) = V_m^{d_i}(t),$$

the total maximum amount that would be paid for intervention
strategy d_i, where ${}_k v_m^{d_i}(t)$ represents person k's willingness
to pay for d_i on behalf of himself.

Objective Function II may be expressed simply as:

$$B^2(t) = \sum_{d=1}^{D} \sum_{m=1}^{M} \sum_{i=0}^{S_d} v_m^{d_i}(t) \; P_m^{d_i} X_m^{d_i},$$

which is maximized subject to the usual resource constraints.

The basic distinction between the two objective functions lies in the divergent nature of the willingness-to-pay
expressions. The w_{jmr} of Objective Function I are probably
easier to elicit and, once obtained, are generally applicable
regardless of the number and range of diseases in the model.
Determining the $v_{mr}^{d_i}(t)$ would doubtlessly involve considerable
administrative problems; of more fundamental concern is the
suggestion in Fischer's analysis (1977) that most individuals
are not capable of validly processing the quantity and complexity of information embedded in the "simple" alternatives,
d_i and d_o. However, a regression scheme to overcome some of
these difficulties will be introduced in the next section as
part of a more basic discussion of how individual willingness-
to-pay responses are obtained.

These concerns aside, willingness-to-pay expressions
of the form $v_{mr}^{d_i}(t)$ do have the advantage of allowing the

consumer to render preference judgments which do not <u>assume</u>
the independence of prognoses and traditionally conceived
state preferences. Nor does this "episodal" approach to
willingness-to-pay evaluation require one to assume operationally that the disutility of a set of health state occupancies over an interval t is the simple, direct sum of the
disutilities of the state occupancies comprising that pattern.
(It should be noted, however, that $v^d_{mr}i(t)$ is assumed to be invariant to the sequence of state occupancies.)

Tax Schemes

        The focus shifts now to a more difficult issue: Can a
mix of taxes and expenditures be specified so that
willingness-to-pay voters are induced to express their true
preferences while, at the same time, a set of intervention
strategies is determined that is Pareto efficient? These
questions have been of central concern to economists for some
time. However, by stating the tax-expenditure problem in a
multi-output, multi-input mathematical programming framework,
some new insights emerge. The answer to the general question
posed above appears to be negative. But first, an approach
is introduced that, under appropriate assumptions, can be regarded as Pareto efficient--though preference understatement
remains a possibility. Next, a tax scheme that bears some re-
semblance to Clarke's "demand-revealing process" (Clarke,
1971) is proposed; it appears to eliminate the incentive to
misstate willingness-to-pay votes. However, there is a strong
likelihood under this scheme that some individuals not in the
target population will have to be taxed at no apparent benefit to themselves in order to support the intervention strategies adopted for the target group.

        There are then three issues of economic efficiency:

    (1)   Will individuals reveal their true preferences
          for health outcomes?

    (2)   Will individuals in the target population get
          (at least) what they pay for in terms of health
          outcomes?

    (3)   Does the implementation of the allocation de-
          cisions that are optimal for the target popu-
          lation leave the rest of society in no worse
          a position?

        In examining these issues under the two following tax
schemes (full pay and demand-revealing plan), it will also be
desirable to distinguish between two assumptions regarding
the supplies of inputs. The first assumption is that the
amount of each input is fixed and exogenously given to the
target population. The second, more complicated and more

theoretically interesting, assumption is that inputs for the
intervention strategies must be purchased from a budget formed
by aggregating all willingness-to-pay responses. If society
wishes to augment this budget, that is a separate decision
based on equity considerations. A final assumption imposed
for the remainder of the discussion is that the basic resource
allocation model will be restricted to be a dichotomous integer program. According to this condition, the entire module
receives either health strategy d_i or the status quo, that is
$x_m^{d}i = 0,1$ in all cases. This not only acknowledges the
political and administrative difficulty in funding module
programs on a fractional basis, but facilitates the development of the tax-expenditure model below.

Full pay tax scheme.--In the full pay tax scheme, each
module member--and thus each module--is taxed by the full
amount of the solicited willingness-to-pay expression. For
this scheme, there are three efficiency issues that must be
considered.

The first efficiency issue is whether individuals will
be motivated to express their true preferences. From the
public finance literature, it is clear there are rational reasons not to expect this, especially if the number of
willingness-to-pay voters is sufficiently large that each believes his own actions will have a negligible impact on the
outcome of the vote. Unfortunately, this conclusion will
finally prevail in the discussion below--but with some interesting qualifications.

To the extent that members of module m believe they
are competing fiercely with other modules for the limited
supply of resources in the constraint set, they will have a
special incentive to boost their w_{jmr} (or $v_{mr}^{d}i(t)$) to levels
sufficiently high to secure as many module-m variables in the
optimal solution as possible.* On the other hand, any individual in m who is convinced that the full panoply of
intervention strategies will be awarded to m via the optimization model, regardless of his willingness-to-pay pledges,
will have an incentive to understate his willingness to pay.

---

* Underlying this result is the fact that the rational individual k' is not indifferent between the alternatives of
expressing his true willingness to pay to avoid j, say
w_{jmk}, and obtaining the optimal state. By construction, he
would rather forego the money and attain the latter. It
follows that each member of module m would like to have as
many module-m variables as possible in the optimal solution to the mathematical program--even if doing so required
that each, in fact, pay taxes equivalent to his true willingness to pay. Of course, if a strategic understatement
of willingness to pay could be successfully made, then all
the better.

Obviously, no individual in m will be rationally motivated to
overstate willingness to pay, for his non-Paretian day-of-
reckoning will arrive at tax time.

Conversely, individuals in module m' (different from
m) will have an incentive to depress the value of W_{jm} (or
$v_{m}^{d}i(t)$) by reducing their philanthropic contributions, if it
is felt that resource allocations in module m will ipso facto
reduce the volume of interventions allocated to m'. To the
extent that one or more key resources are scarce, this will
be a rational perception. Optimal allocations are crucially
dependent on the ratio of module objective function coefficients; willingness-to-pay voting behavior that keeps contributions to module m at relatively low levels will increase
the likelihood that interventions will be allocated relatively
away from m and toward m', ceteris paribus. Thus, each
$g_\varepsilon C_m$ may have a rational motive to understate willingness to
pay.

Presumably, contributing individuals not in the target
population are philanthropically motivated in the first place.
Strategic considerations that might be relevant to the behavior of module members should not affect those $C_m"$ individuals. An incentive for the understatement of willingness to
pay arises here only to the extent that some $h_\varepsilon C_m"$ believes
that a module m is already certain to attain objective function coefficients large enough to insure the desired allocations. In this case, he will feel that his true willingness-
to-pay offerings are unneeded by m. However, to the extent
that his willingness-to-pay offerings are motivated more by
the joy of giving than a perception of what the gift buys,
the individual willingness-to-pay pledges will tend to be unbiased by strategic considerations.

Assuming the above is not valid, however, a way of
achieving honest willingness-to-pay statements would be to
elicit information in such a manner that the link between the
voter's response and his subsequent total tax bill becomes
less clear to him. The willingness-to-pay data obtained for
Objective Function I might meet this test, it can be argued.
The consumer there is asked his willingness to pay for a
change from one day of health state j to one day of optimal
function. There is no stated linkage between these
sequentially-sought w_{jmr} and any specific intervention
strategy (d_i) on which these weights will subsequently place
a social value. Nevertheless, the thoughtful consumer--
depending on how well he is informed--may perceive the implications of his willingness-to-pay pledges, may feel that
module competition for resources will not be that fierce, and
may therefore understate willingness to pay.

A somewhat more complicated alternative approach would
be to sample the willingness-to-pay sentiments of individuals
not in the target population, then use this information to

predict what target population members <u>ought</u> to be willing to
pay for outcomes. Taxes would be levied accordingly. One can
envision the following type of willingness-to-pay elicitation/
analysis, assuming now that Objective Function II has been
chosen. This scheme also illustrates how one might proceed
to overcome some of the psychological difficulties (noted in
the last section) of obtaining meaningful individual responses
to the complex, "episodal" alternatives considered in Objective Function II:

     - Develop a number of real (or hypothetical) health
program outcome alternatives, each consisting of (a) the expected prevalencies of a <u>very few</u> health states and (b) the
probability of dying over t. In constructing this set of alternatives, provide for considerable variation in the length
of t itself, the expected prevalencies and death probability,
and the state-composition of the alternatives.

     - Submit these alternatives to a large sample popula-
tion, recording each individual's income, wealth, and other
demographic characteristics. If there are numerous program
outcome alternatives, each individual would be asked to respond to only a selected subset.

     - Use this information in a statistical analysis in
which individual willingness-to-pay expressions are regressed
against their associated program outcome alternatives and the
income, wealth, and demographic composition of the respondent.

     - Finally, use (a) the estimated regression, (b) knowl-
edge of the expected prevalencies and death probabilities associated with the relevant d_i and d_o, and (c) information on
the target population's characteristics to predict
willingness-to-pay expressions for each module member for
Objective Function II.

     Clearly, if the target population is then taxed accord-
ing to these predictions, one must expect some welfare loss
(and some gain) because the predictions themselves are probabilistic. However, it should be possible to develop confidence intervals so that the policy maker could, for instance, be 95 percent confident (statistically) that an individual's true willingness to pay lies within a particular
interval. The welfare implications of this approach deserve
closer study, but it does seem possible that in this way one
could obtain raw willingness-to-pay responses that would be
unprejudiced by strategic considerations.

     The second efficiency issue is whether the target pop-
ulation receive its money's worth in terms of health outcomes. For convenience, this discussion will proceed assuming Objective Function I.

From the standpoint of the individual module member in the target population, it can be claimed that the full pay tax program is Pareto-efficient ex ante. Each person makes willingness-to-pay statements about the worth of health states achieved--or avoided--with certainty for a specified period of time (one day). Each person is taxed on the basis of these willingness-to-pay statements and the <u>expected</u> prevalencies of each of the health states over the allocation period, given the intervention strategies adopted. However, once the programs are underway, these expected state prevalencies will likely not be exactly realized because of the stochastic nature of disease processes. The health outcomes which, in fact, materialize in module m over a given t will usually be worth either more, or less, to individual r rather than his tax payment based on expected values. That is

$$
B^{-1}_{mr}(t) = \sum_{d=1}^{D} \sum_{i=0}^{S_d} \left[\sum_{j=1}^{N} w_{jmr} \left(\overline{pp}^{d_o}_{jm}(t) - \overline{pp}^{d_i}_{jm} \right) \right] P^{d_i}_m \hat{X}^{d_i}_m \neq
$$

$$
\sum_{d=1}^{D} \sum_{i=0}^{S_d} \left[\sum_{j=0}^{N} w_{jmr} \left(\hat{pp}^{d_o}_{jm}(t) - \hat{pp}^{d_i}_{jm}(t) \right) \right] P^{d_i}_m \hat{X}^{d_i}_m = \hat{B}^1_{mr}(t),
$$

where the period prevalence rates in the latter expression represent actual observations over t. If

$$
\hat{B}^1_{mr}(t) > \overline{B}^1_{mr}(t),
$$

individual r literally receives a "consumer surplus" equal to the difference between the two expressions. Otherwise, however, tax costs exceed realized program benefits for r, and the Paretian criterion is not met ex post.

At this point, one can choose from among several perspectives:

- Ex ante Paretian efficiency is the more relevant, or more reasonable and practical, criterion for the evaluation of social programs from the module member's perspective.

- Ex post Paretian efficiency--as defined above in simple terms--is the more relevant evaluative criterion from the module member's perspective. The willingness-to-pay Full Pay allocation-tax scheme may fail this test during a given period t and therefore not be socially efficient.

- If one introduces the possibility of compensation, there are conditions under which this willingness-to-pay allocation-tax plan may be made efficient ex post for each period of length t. Define $\hat{B}_{mr}(t)_k - \overline{B}_{mr}(t) \equiv N\hat{B}_{mr}(t)_k$, the

net realized benefit to individual r of programs in module m
implemented in the kth period of length t. This difference
need not be positive. Recall that C represents the total
number of people in the contributing population. Then, for
module m, if

$$\hat{NB}_m(t)_k = \sum_{r=1}^{C} \hat{NB}_{mr}(t)_k \geq 0,$$

there exists an overall tax and transfer policy that will
leave all C individuals in a Pareto-optimal position at the
end of the kth allocation period (relative to the beginning
of that period). Generalizing, the program of "optimal" intervention strategies in this k^{th} period can be regarded as
Pareto-efficient overall if

$$\hat{NB}(t)_k = \sum_{m=1}^{M} \hat{NB}_m(t)_k \geq 0$$

and if the contributing population proceeds to secure the
necessary transfers. In the absence of an actual compensation provision, the total health plan may be regarded, from
the health consumer's standpoint, as potentially Pareto
efficient in the sense of Hicks and Kaldor. The administrative costs of tax and transfer policies are ignored throughout, and it has been assumed that the provision of interventions does not result in unintended externalities in production and consumption. Also ruled out are undesirable
price effects, especially on factors of production, which may
be used for health and non-health goods and services.

It should be made clear that underlying this discussion is the assumption that the "original position" of all
module members is the status quo strategy. Thus, members of
modules that are omitted, all or in part, from the optimal
solution are presumed to be in no worse position than they
would have been if the entire merit good issue had never been
raised.

The third efficiency issue is whether the optimal set
of programs impose any unwelcome costs on that part of society
which does not voluntarily contribute toward the health of
the target population. Recall that the earlier efficiency
discussion was entirely from the perspective of the individual's voluntarily contributing to the target population (including, of course, members of that population).
It was implicit that the amounts of all inputs were somewhat exogenously given.

However, it is possible to specify a fundamental linkage between the objective function under Full Pay and the
right-hand-side resource availability parameters,

$R_p(t)$, p=1, ..., Q—a linkage that is not possible when the objective function is founded upon interval-scale utility weights. The connection exists because the contributing population can be taxed in accordance with its willingness-to-pay expressions, and the aggregate of these taxes can be designated as the budget constraint on the purchase of allocable resources. One can reformulate the optimization goal as the following:

> Maximize expected health status improvement,
> subject to the constraint that the value of
> the resources employed in the process not ex-
> ceed the aggregate value to the contributing
> population of the expected health status im-
> provement implied in that optimal solution.

The purpose of such a specification is not merely to insure that whatever health strategy is implemented break even in an accounting sense. Its purpose is, rather, that the factors of production that might be used for intervention strategies have alternative uses in society; these opportunity costs are reflected, to a great extent, in the unit prices of the production factors.

Upon this basis, the complete Full Pay willingness-to-pay model may be specified, employing Objective Function I for simplicity. The analysis can be developed most compactly if it is assumed that all resources are variable. The first problem encountered, and the most vexing, is this: the total tax contribution that each individual r is asked to make on behalf of each module m is predicated on the government's already knowing the optimal solution set,

$$\{\hat{X}_m^{d_i}\}$$

which cannot be calculated without assumed values for the elements in the resource vector. Yet the aim is to determine permissible resource vectors on the basis of the willingness-to-pay tax contributions. The problem then is to penetrate this apparent circularity.

It should be recalled that the allocation model has the form of a dichotomous integer program. Thus, if there are S_d possible intervention alternatives for disease d, D diseases, and M modules, there are

$$Y = \prod_{d=1}^{D} S_d^M$$

distinct decision variable vectors from which an optimal solution must be chosen, given particular values for the

constraint set. This follows because each module will receive one, and only one, disease-specific intervention under
this integer programming specification. The yth decision
variable vector is denoted as

$$\{X_m^{\wedge d_i}\}y, \quad y = 1, \ldots, Y.$$

From here the analysis proceeds in several steps:

- Let $\bar{B}_{mr}^1(t,y)$ be the maximum amount individual r is
willing to contribute for module m for strategies implied by
solution vector

$$\{X_m^{\wedge d_i}\}y$$

over period t. Then the corresponding total volume of
willingness-to-pay tax contributions over period t, given this
solution vector, is

$$\sum_{m=1}^{M} \sum_{r=1}^{C} \bar{B}_{mr}^1(t,y) = \bar{B}^1(t,y).$$

This is also equal to the value of Objective Function I with
$\{X_m^{\wedge d_i}\}Y$.

- Let c_p be the unit price of input p, assumed not to
vary with its use over period t. Form the budget constraint,

$$\sum_{p=1}^{Q} c_p R_p(t) \leq \bar{B}^1(t,y)$$

and let $(R_p(t))_e^Y$ be the eth resource vector that satisfies
this constraint, where $e = 1,2\ldots.$

- Insert, in turn, each resource vector, $(R_p(t))_e^Y$, into
the resource allocation model and determine in
each case whether

$$\{X_m^{\wedge d_i}\}Y$$

is feasible. Designate the subset of resource vectors that
permit feasibility as

$$(R_p(t))_{e'}^Y.$$

Denote the least-cost element of the subset as $(R_p(t))_{e''}^Y$.

- Repeat this process for each of the Y possible decision variable vectors. Denote the subset feasible vectors

as

$$\{\{X_m^{d_i}\}^{y'}\},$$

where $y'=1, \ldots, Y'$ and $Y' \leq Y$. The optimal set of intervention strategies will be regarded as the set

$$\{\hat{X}_m^{d_i}\}^{y''},$$

which is the vector-element of

$$\{\{\hat{X}_m^{d_i}\}^{y'}\}$$

that yields the largest value of $\bar{B}^1(t,y)$.

- Implement this optimal solution with resource vector

$$(R_p(t))_{e''}^{y''},$$

the least-cost vector for producing that set of intervention strategies. If

$$\overset{1}{\bar{D}}(t,y'')_{e''} \equiv \overset{1}{\bar{B}}(t,y'') - \sum_{p=1}^{Q} c_p R_p(t)_{e''}^{y''} > 0,$$

redistribute this sum to the contributing population by an agreed upon rule.

Of course, without further restrictions there may be no decision variable vector that is feasible under this regime. In such a case, the government may make a separate decision to supplement the target population's health budget on the basis of equity or other criteria. For instance, if the population were low-income, it is quite possible that the sum of their willingness-to-pay expressions would not alone constitute a budget large enough to support many--if any--intervention strategies. In the special case where all resources are fixed and require remuneration at the usual rates,

$$\overset{1}{\bar{D}}(t,y) \gtrless 0 \text{ for } y=1, \ldots, (Y).$$

That is, each of the y solution vectors, including y", may or may not have an associated willingness-to-pay great enough to cover the given, mandated resource cost. If

$$\overset{1}{\bar{D}}(t,y'') > 0,$$

the excess tax payment can be refunded to the contributing population in some fashion.

Each feasible solution represents, by construction, an allocation that meets the Paretian criterion, subject to the difficulties of interpretation raised earlier in this section. Each module m in a feasible solution will be receiving expected health program benefits equal to the willingness-to-pay tax contributions made on behalf of m. To the extent that contributions on behalf of m exceed the cost of the resources required to implement all strategies in m, other modules in the optimal solution may, in a sense, be receiving a bonus. This is because the excess contributions for m flow into the overall budget constraint,

$$\overline{B}^1(t,y),$$

and thereby establish the possibility that the necessary resources may be provided to some other modules, so that the total value of health benefits exceeds the total willingness-to-pay for those modules.

The optimality rule suggested for this particular version of the model--that is, adopt the largest Pareto-efficient

$$\overline{B}^1(t,y),$$

may not actually maximize consumer surplus, although from the earlier discussion (under Objective Function I) it is clear, by construction, that surplus is not a quantitatively significant element in this analysis. However, the above optimality criterion leans in the direction of maximizing the number of modules receiving program benefits. This, in turn, increases the likelihood that some modules are receiving bonus program benefits whose real resource cost exceeds the modules' willingness to pay, since all modules are taxed on the basis of willingness to pay.

In claiming Pareto efficiency here, several critical assumptions have been made. The possibility of preference misrepresentation has been ignored. Price effects that may disturb other markets are assumed to be negligible. Finally, module members assigned the status quo intervention for one or more diseases are assumed to be no worse off over t--in an expected value sense--than they would be were no health service interventions contemplated for anyone. (Of course, this does not imply that these module members would not have preferred the interventions to the status quo assignment. The status quo designation only implies that they remain in their "original position"--again, in an expected value sense--over the interval t.)

Demand-revealing tax scheme.--A second tax-expenditure plan focuses on the problem of inducing individuals to reveal their true willingness to pay. It may be viewed as an attempt to extend Clarke's demand-revealing process (Clarke,

1978, 1971) to the present context, where there are multiple
public outputs and inputs to be allocated simultaneously.
Like Clarke's proposal, this demand-revealing plan seeks to
establish a voting structure in which each module member cannot improve his welfare by misrepresenting his true preferences. Also, as in Clarke's proposal, this tax scheme is
developed so that the individual's willingness-to-pay statement is not the basis for computing his tax bill for services
received. One consequence of this is that the total willingness to pay by the target population may be insufficient to
cover the resource costs of the programs provided. In such
cases, society may view the deficit as the price it must,
and may wish to, pay in order to obtain valid information
on the demand for health care. Of course, this information
is valid only to the extent that the validity of individual
(true) willingness-to-pay expressions is accepted for social
decision-making purposes.

     The logic of the demand-revealing tax scheme appears
much more clear when Objective Function II is used, so it
will be adopted throughout the following discussion. It will
also be convenient to treat the population module as the basic
unit for voting analysis from this point on. In practical
terms, this requires either (a) that each individual be
formally regarded as a module or (b) that each module have a
designated decision maker/leader who uses the members'
willingness-to-pay expressions as a basis for his willingness-
to-pay bids in the module-level competition and who also taxes
his constituency on the basis of their stated willingness to
pay. The simpler viewpoint conceptually is (a); the only
difficulty with it is the operational one that the resulting dichotomous integer program becomes large and perhaps not
easily soluble by currently available methods.

     In contrast, paradigm (b) would require a type of two-
stage demand-revealing process. The first state, involving
an inter-module competition for resources, will be introduced shortly. To insure that each module leader has valid
willingness-to-pay information with which to make his bids,
module members must be taxed for services received, based
on the demand-revealing procedure described by Clarke (1971)
and Tideman and Tullock (1976). For ease of exposition,
case (a) will be assumed, and individuals will be considered
to be bidding for resources.

     The procedure of the demand-revealing tax scheme is
as follows:

     - Elicit from each individual m, $v_m^{d_i}(t)$, his willing-
ness to pay for attaining, over period t, the expected health
outcomes associated with strategy d_i rather than those expected with the status quo, d_o. Do this for all diseases
and intervention strategies. (For the remainder of the

discussion, the time-interval notation will be suppressed for
simplicity.)

  - In a manner similar to that adopted for the Full Pay
plan, use these willingness-to-pay expressions to determine
that solution set,

$$\{\hat{x}_m^{d_i}\}y'' \; ,$$

that results in the maximum obtainable $\bar{B}^2(t,y)$. Recall that
the least-cost input vector for achieving this solution set,

$$(R_p(t))_{e''}^{y''},$$

is to be selected. Assuming that these variable inputs may
be treated as infinitely divisible, it follows that all resource constraints will be binding in the optimum case (even
for the dichotomous integer program assumed here). There may
be an associated willingness-to-pay surplus to be
redistributed.

  - Tax each individual only for the active (non-status
quo) interventions assigned to him in the optimal solution.
His tax does not equal the amount of his willingness-to-pay
expression. Instead, a more complicated procedure is
adopted: for each $X_m^{d_i}$ in the optimal solution, tax individual
m an amount,

$$_\tau v_m^{d_i} \; ,$$

equal to that value of the objective function coefficient of

$$X_m^{d_i}$$

required to just maintain $X_m^{d_i}$ in the optimal solution, given
that all other objective function coefficients and all other
elements of

$$\{X_m^{d_i}\}\, y''$$

are held fixed at their original values. The tax

$$_\tau v_m^{d_i}$$

will be less than m's actual willingness-to-pay expression,

$$v_m^{d_i} \; ,$$

whenever there is an aggregate willingness-to-pay surplus associated with the optimal solution.

The claim is made that under these conditions, $_uv_m^{d_i}$
will be m's true willingness to pay for intervention
strategy d_i. To see this, first consider the disincentives
to understate willingness to pay here. If m made the strategic understatement,

$$_uv_m^{d_i},$$

there are two possibilities, ceteris paribus. Either his $x_m^{d_i}$
would remain in the optimal solution, so that he would pay
the same tax as if he had stated $v_m^{d_i}$, or else $_uv_m^{d_i}$ would
have sufficiently low value to remove $x_m^{d_i}$ from the optimal
solution. In the first case, m is no worse off than if he had
expressed his true willingness to pay. In the latter case,
he is in an inferior position since he will not have the opportunity to purchase d_i at a price,

$$_\tau v_m^{d_i},$$

which is less than or equal to his true valuation, $v_m^{d_i}$.

We next consider the incentive structure for overstatement of willingness to pay; by definition of the overstatement,

$$_ov_m^{d_i} > v_m^{d_i}.$$

Again there are two pertinent cases for m to consider. If

$$v_m^{d_i} > {}_\tau v_m^{d_i}$$

--so that the true expression of willingness to pay is sufficient to put $x_m^{d_i}$ in the optimal solution anyway--then the
overstatement,

$$_ov_m^{d_i},$$

and the true willingness-to-pay expression yield the same
outcome. If

$$v_m^{d_i} < {}_\tau v_m^{d_i} < {}_ov_m^{d_i},$$

then $x_m^{d_i}$ is contained in the solution set, but at a cost to m
since he will now be taxed an amount greater than what d_i
is truly worth to him. By overstating willingness to pay, m
can be made no better off but possibly worse off than if he
had rendered $v_m^{d_i}$. The overall conclusion of this analysis
is that he will rationally express his true willingness to
pay.

One possible problem with this scheme is that m's tax,
$_\tau v_m^{d_i}$, is restricted only in that it will be no greater than

his true willingness to pay. Since the budget from which the
inputs are purchased is based on the $v_m^{d_i}$, there may be cases
in which the total tax take from the contributing population
falls significantly short of the actual resource cost incurred. Clearly, in order to make up this deficit, a tax
cost, of unspecified magnitude, is imposed on society as a
whole. Since the mechanics of this demand-revealing tax-
expenditure plan are complex, especially for large populations, the probable magnitude of such a tax burden could best
be explored through computer simulation analysis, employing
a wide range of values for the relevant parameters.

For the demand-revealing tax scheme, the second efficiency issue must be considered: Does the target population receive their money's worth in terms of health outcomes? All of the conclusions reached above regarding ex
ante and ex post Pareto efficiency hold a fortiori here,
since each individual is taxed in an amount less than or
equal to his true willingness to pay. His tax would be
set equal to his true willingness to pay only when $D(t,y")$
= 0; in this case, implementing the optimal solution

$$\{X_m^{d_i}\}Y",$$

requires in principle an aggregate expenditure equal to the
sum of all willingness-to-pay expressions. If

$$_\tau v_m^{d_i}(t) < v_m^{d_i}(t)$$

for only one individual m, the associated aggregate willingness-to-pay amount is then inadequate ceteris paribus to support even the least cost resource vector,

$$(R_p(t))_{e"}^{Y"},$$

required to implement $\{X_m^{d_i}\}Y"$.

The third efficiency issue must also be discussed:
Does the optimal set of programs impose any unwelcome costs
on that part of society which does not <u>voluntarily</u> contribute
toward the health of the target population? Let

$$_\tau V(t)^Y = \sum_{m=1}^{M} \sum_{d=1}^{D} \sum_{i=0}^{S_d} {}_\tau v_m^{d_i}(t)^Y$$

be the aggregate tax revenue corresponding to the feasible
solution

$$\{X_m^{d_i}\}Y.$$

Define $F^2(t.y) \equiv \sum_{p=1}^{0} c_p R_p(t)_{e"}^{Y} - {}_\tau V(t)^Y$

as the deficit generated by the

$$\{\hat{X}_m^{d_i}\}^y.$$

From previous discussion, it should be clear that

$$F^2(t,y'') \geq 0.$$

In particular,

$$F^2(t,y'') = 0$$

if, and only if

$$\overline{D}^2(t,y'') = 0.$$

That is, if the sum of all willingness-to-pay expressions results in an optimal solution

$$\{\hat{X}_m^{d_i}\}$$

such that the associated least-cost vector $(R_p(t))_{e''}^{y''}$ could be just barely financed by that willingness-to-pay sum, then each m would be taxed an amount just equal to his stated willingness to pay. Otherwise his tax is less than his stated willingness to pay, and the aggregate result is a deficit that must be financed by society. The size and distributional implications of this deficit require further study.

Income Distribution

Perhaps the most frequent criticism of willingness-to-pay allocative procedures is that they are predicated on an income distribution that society may regard as unjust. While this claim cannot be refuted on logical grounds, steps can be taken to secure minimum standards of access to care for groups designated as economically disadvantaged. A number of methods have been suggested for accomplishing this; a few are noted at this point:

(1) If it is desired that all of module m receive intervention strategy d_i, set $X_m^{d_i} = 1$ in the constraint set.

(2) If it is desired that f percent of m receive d_i, set $X_m^{d_i} = f/100$.

(3) If it is desired that m receive some form of active intervention against disease d, but more flexibility is sought, establish the constraint

$$f/100 < \sum_{\substack{i=1 \\ (i \neq 0)}}^{S_d} x_m^{d_i} \leq 1.$$

It may be seen that to establish these additional requirements in the context of the full pay tax scheme is to imply that the total cost of all intervention strategies in the optimum solution cannot then be covered by taxes equal to the sum of the target population's willingness-to-pay expressions. Since under the demand-revealing plan the target population's programs are generally not self-supporting, it holds a fortiori that a policy of minimum benefit guarantees would require deficit financing.

Input Wage Rates

Throughout, it has been assumed that resource p was purchased at a constant price of c_p per time unit of acquisition. These wage (rental) rates were assumed to be determined competitively elsewhere in the economy and exogenously given to the target population. But given the mathematical programming framework in which this analysis has proceeded, it is possible to derive an implicit wage rate for each input which, in the optimum, would reflect the value-added (in willingness-to-pay terms) of the marginal unit of this input within the target population.

It should be noted that if resources are assumed to be infinitely divisible, both the full-pay and the demand-revealing schemes yield optimal solution sets in which all elements of

$$(R_p(t))_{e''}^{y''}$$

are fully utilized. If the resource allocation were in the form of a general (rather than integer) linear program, then it is well known (Baumol, 1969) that each $R_p(t)$ will be associated with a positive "shadow price" which can be interpreted as a summary measure of the population's willingness to pay for the next (marginal) unit of this input. Let c_p' be the shadow price of input p. Linear-programming theory then guarantees that

$$\sum_{p=1}^{Q} c_p' R_p(t)_{e''}^{y''} = \bar{B}(t,y'')^2.$$

That is, if each input were in fact charged its shadow price in the optimum, then total program expenditures would just equal aggregate willingness to pay. If each input were paid at the rate c_p', all inputs together would be remunerated an amount equal to the population's aggregate valuation of the services the inputs render. This suggests that c_p' is the

appropriate wage for input $R_p(t)$ when employed in intervention
strategies for this target population.

However, there are two issues that cloud this apparently neat result. The first arises because both tax
expenditure schemes discussed here were set in an integer-
programming framework. As Gomery and Baumol (1969) have
shown, positive (integer-valed) shadow prices do emerge from
such an integer-programming maximization model, but their
interpretation can be problematic: (1) For any given optimization model, these shadow prices need not be unique.
Rather, they will probably depend on which set of artificial
constraints (called Gomery cuts) are selected to convert the
original integer program into a new linear program with an
integer solution. In addition, positive shadow prices may
be imputed to one or more of these artificial constraints.
(2) A less mathematical complication relates to the manner in
which the optimum resource vector,

$$(R_p(t))_{e''}^{y''},$$

is selected by either tax expenditure scheme. In reviewing
this input selection process--and the procedure for choosing
the optimal solution vector,

$$\{\hat{x}_m^{d_i}\}^{y''}$$

--it is apparent that the exogenous market input prices, c_p,
play a crucial role. If they were altered sufficiently,
a new solution vector and associated least-cost resource set
would emerge. This implies that the shadow prices, to which
one hoped to attach some normative significance, are, ceteris
paribus, a function of their exogeneous real world counter-
parts, which are determined in competitive markets elsewhere
in the economy. The problem may initially arise from the
partial equilibrium manner in which the target population's
programs have been regarded here. A more general analysis
would require that each c_p be determined explicitly on the
basis of aggregate demand and supply conditions in all interacting markets.

SUMMARY

As Mishan and others have argued, the willingness-to-
pay approach to public program evaluation is the only
methodology that permits unambiguous assessment of resource
allocation decisions by the Pareto criterion. In health
program evaluation, a variety of other schemes have also
been implemented; these include, most recently, an interesting approach to predicting the impact of alternative budget
allocations on a somewhat arbitrarily defined social utility
function (Bush, 1973; Lipscomb, 1977; Torrance, 1973). By

mathematical programming techniques, an allocation of resources among competing programs and competing population subgroups can be determined so as to maximize the expected social
utility. However, a major strength of the allocation model--
its explicit incorporation of individual preferences into a
social decision-making construct--can also be regarded as a
major methodological weakness; for, in effect, classical
assumptions about the measurability and interpersonal comparability of utility must be invoked.

The purpose of this paper has been to suggest how the
willingness-to-pay approach might be integrated into this
resource allocation framework. Two tax expenditure schemes
were introduced. The first guarantees Pareto-efficient allocations under certain assumptions, the strongest of which
is that individuals truthfully report their willingness to
pay for program outcomes. The second scheme, derived in part
from Clarke's demand-revealing approach to public goods
assessment, does motivate each individual to express his true
preference, but, from society's perspective, it need not lead
to a Pareto-efficient set of health programs for the target
population. The resource allocation algorithm is structured
to permit philanthropic contributions by non-members of each
subgroup to the subgroup's welfare. Simple methods are also
introduced for the allocation of "minimal" benefit packages
to subgroups designated as economically disadvantaged.

In conclusion, it might be well to consider why, in
the first place, one would want to conduct cost-benefit
analysis from the multi-input, multi-output perspective af-
forded by mathematical programming. In this paper, the
choice of a structure for the allocation model was motivated
in part by earlier allocation models, which were based on
mathematical programming but which employed interval-scale
utility weights (or votes) as the social evaluation parameters
in the objective function. While cost-benefit analysis can
clearly be performed on a program-by-program basis, using
either the classical approach (Mishan, 1971) or the demand-
revealing process of Clarke (1971), there are at least two
advantages to the simultaneous-programs format inherent in
the programming models. First, because the intervention
strategies are determined jointly, the amount of each scarce
resource needed for the health system as a whole emerges
naturally from the computations. Second, along with the
programming solution comes a vector of shadow prices for the
resources used; these establish rates of remuneration that
are internally consistent with the contributing population's
aggregate (and implicit) assessment of the contribution of
each input to the improvement of target population health
status.

APPENDIX

Derivation of the Expected Period Prevalence
of a Health State for a Semi-Markovian Process

In his discussion of semi-Markovian concepts, Howard
(1971) makes a distinction between _real_ transitions (from
state i to another state j) and _virtual_ transitions (from i
to itself). However, there will be no advantage in maintaining this distinction here and the exposition is simplified
considerably by regarding all transitions as real. Thus,
define

$$P_{ii} = \begin{cases} 0, \text{ if } i \text{ is transient.} \\ 1, \text{ if } i \text{ is trapping (absorbing).} \end{cases}$$

To develop an expression for the prevalence of a health
state over some finite period t, define

$$x_{ij}(n) = \begin{cases} 1, \text{ if the individual is in state } j \text{ at} \\ \text{ time } n, \text{ given that he entered } i \text{ at} \\ \text{ time zero.} \\ 0, \text{ otherwise.} \end{cases}$$

Then, following Howard, the individual's total time in j over
t, given an entry to i at time zero, is $pp_{ij}(t) = \sum_{n=0}^{t} x_{ij}(n)$,
where the pp notation indicates period prevalence for the
individual. The expected value of this random variable is

$\overline{pp}_{ij}(t) = \sum_{n=0}^{t} \overline{x}_{ij}(n)$. But since $x_{ij}(n)$ is either zero or
unity, $\overline{x}_{ij}(n) = \phi_{ij}(n)$, the so-called "interval transition
probability" of _being in_ state j at time n, given an entry
into i at time zero. Thus, $pp_{ij}(t) = \sum_{n=0}^{t} \phi_{ij}(n)$. This

definition of period prevalence corresponds to what Kao

(1972) termed "time in recovery state" in his semi-Markovian model for predicting the recovery progress of coronary patients. From Kao, it is clear that the variance of $pp_{ij}(t)$ is $pp_{ij}(t) = \overline{pp}_{ij}(t)\ (2\ \overline{pp}_{jj}(t) - 1 - \overline{pp}_{ij}(t))$.

Now each $\phi_{ij}(n)$ is a function of all the transition probabilities and holding-time distributions, so that knowledge (or estimates) of these permits one to calculate (or estimate) $\overline{pp}_{ij}(t)$. For purposes here, the most useful expression for this interval transition probability is

$$\phi_{ij}(n) = \sum_{m=0}^{n} e_{ij}(m)\ ^{>}w_j(n-m)$$

where $e_{ij}(m)$ is the probability that an individual will enter state j at time m, given that he entered state i at time zero; and

$$^{>}w_j(n-m) = \sum_{r=n-m+1}^{\infty} \sum_{k=1}^{N} P_{jk}\ h_{jk}(r) = Pr(\tau_j > n-m),$$

the probability that the "waiting" time in j before the next transition is greater than (n-m) time units. The semi-Markovian "entrance" probabilities above (Howard, 1971) can be determined from the recursive equation,

$$e_{ij}(m) = \delta_{ij}\ \delta(m) + \sum_{s=1}^{N} \sum_{q=0}^{m} P_{is}\ h_{is}(q)\ e_{sj}(m-q),$$

where $\delta_{ij} = \begin{cases} 1, & \text{if } i=j \\ 0, & \text{otherwise} \end{cases}$ and $\delta(m) = \begin{cases} 1, & \text{if } m=0 \\ 0, & \text{otherwise.} \end{cases}$

Then, by substitution, the expression for expected prevalence becomes

$$\overline{pp}_{ij}(t) = \sum_{n=0}^{t} \sum_{m=0}^{n} e_{ij}(m)\ ^{>}w_j(n-m).$$

If i, the state of entry at period zero, is known with certainty, the above expression represents simply the expected
prevalence of j over period t. Otherwise, the expected prevalence of j must reflect the fact that each i attains with
only some probability at time zero. Kao handled this problem
by employing data in which the probability of being in each
coronary recovery state at the moment of hospital admission
was assumed known. In essence, the patient's recovery
progress was regarded as being governed by a semi-Markovian
process that went into effect, so to speak, only after the
patient's entry into the hospital.

In a more general view of disease prevalence, however,
an individual's disease state occupancy pattern would be assumed to be governed continuously by a semi-Markovian process.
However, this poses a fundamental difficulty in calculating
expected prevalence starting from some arbitrarily (randomly)
chosen point in time. As Howard notes, the probability that
the individual will be in i at this randomly chosen moment
is ϕ_i, the limiting interval transition probability for state
i. However, if the individual is found to be i, it is not
likely, of course, that he has just entered i; rather, one
must allow for the overwhelming likelihood that the individual
was observed in the midst of a holding time. (It should be
noted, though, that since a discrete time process is assumed,
the time remaining in the randomly entered state will be
integer.) Consequently, the probability that the next
transition will be to j and the length of holding time

remaining before that next transition will not be governed by
the p_{ij} and $h_{ij}(m)$ defined earlier. Rather, they will be
described by elements of the form (to use Howard's notation)
$_rp_{ij}$ and $_rh_{ij}(m)$, which acknowledge the random manner in
which the period of length t is initiated. Fortunately, as
Howard shows, these latter quantities can be derived from the
basic set of transition probabilities and holding time
distributions:

$$_rp_{ij} = p_{ij} \, \overline{\tau}_{ij} \, / \, \overline{\tau}_i = \text{the probability that an}$$

individual observed in
state i at a random mo-
ment will make his next
transition to j,

$$_rh_{ij}(m) = \sum_{s=m}^{\infty} h_{ij}(s) \, / \, \overline{\tau}_{ij} = \, ^{>}h_{ij}(m-1) \, / \, \overline{\tau}_{ij}$$

= the probability that an individual observed
in state i at a random moment will remain
there m more time units, given that his
next transition is to j.

Consequently, the expected prevalence of state j over a period
of length t whose starting point is randomly selected can be
expressed as

$$\overline{pp}_j(t) = \sum_{i=1}^{N} \phi_i \sum_{k=1}^{N} \sum_{m=0}^{t} \, _rp_{ik} \, _rh_{ik}(m)$$

$$\left[\delta_{ij} \, m + \sum_{n=0}^{t-m} \sum_{s=0}^{n} e_{kj}(s) \, ^{>}w_j(n-s) \right] ,$$

where $\delta_{ij} = \begin{cases} 1, & \text{if } i=j \\ 0, & \text{otherwise.} \end{cases}$

This formulation acknowledges that (1) without further
information, the state occupied at the randomly selected
starting moment will be i with probability ϕ_i; (2) the

probability that the next transition will be made m time units
later to k is $_r p_{ik} \cdot _r h_{ik}(m)$; (3) if i=j, the time before the
first observable transition is included in the prevalence of
j over t (thus the role of $\delta_{ij} \cdot m$); and (4) after the first
transition, the portion of the interval remaining for analysis
is t-m.

REFERENCES

Acton, Jan Paul
    1973   Evaluating Public Programs to Save Lives: The
            Case of Heart Attacks, R-950-RC. Santa Monica:
            The RAND Corporation.

Anderson, N. H.
    1970   "Functional measurement and psychophysical
            judgment." Psychological Review 77:153-170.

Baumol, William J.
    1969   Economic Theory and Operations Analysis. Engle-
            wood Cliffs, N.J.: Prentice-Hall.

Bush, J. W. and M. M. Chen
    1970   "Markovian analysis of disease history and the
            problem of equilibrium." Paper presented before
            the Statistics Section of the Annual Meeting
            of the American Public Health Association,
            Houston, Texas (October 28).

Bush, J. W., M. M. Chen, and D. L. Patrick
    1973   "Health status index in cost effectiveness:
            Analysis of PKU program." In Berg, Robert E.
            (ed.), Health Status Indexes. Chicago: Hospital
            Research and Educational Trust.

Bush, J. W., S. Fanchel, and M. M. Chen
    1972   "Analysis of a tuberculin testing program using
            a health status index." Socio-Economic Planning
            Sciences 6:49-69.

Chen, M. M. and J. W. Bush
    1977   "Maximizing health system output with political
            and administrative constraints using mathematical
            programming." Inquiry 13:215-227.

Chen, M. M., J. W. Bush, and Donald L. Patrick
    1975   "Social indicators for health planning and policy
            analysis." Policy Sciences 6 (March):71-89.

Chen, M. M., J. W. Bush, and J. Zaremba
    1975   "A critical analysis of effectiveness measures
            for operations research in health services."
            Operations Research in Health--A Critical
            Analysis. Baltimore: Johns Hopkins University
            Press.

Clarke, Edward H.
    1979   "Social valuation of life- and health-saving ac-
            tivities by the demand-revealing process." In
            Mushkin, Selma J. and David W. Dunlop (eds.),
            Health: What is it Worth? (this volume).

Clarke, Edward H.
    1971   "Multipart pricing of public goods." Public
            Choice (Fall).

Ehrlich, Isaac and Gary S. Becker
    1972   "Market insurance, self-insurance, and self-
            protection." Journal of Political Economy
            80:623-648.

Fischer, Gregory W.
    1977   "Willingness to pay for probabilistic improve-
            ments in functional health status: A
            psychological perspective." Working paper,
            Institute of Policy Sciences and Public Affairs,
            Duke University (August) (forthcoming).

Harsanyi, J. C.
    1956   "Approaches to the bargaining problem before and
            after the theory of games: A critical discussion
            of Zeuthen's, Hick's, and Nash's theories."
            Econometrica 24:144-157.

Howard, Ronald A.
    1971   Dynamic Probabilistic Systems. Vol. II: Semi-
            Markov and Decision Processes. New York:
            John Wiley and Sons.

Kao, Edward P. C.
    1972   "A semi-Markov model to predict recovery progress
            of coronary patients." Health Services Research
            (Fall):191-208.

Kaplan, Robert M., J. W. Bush, and Charles C. Berry
    1976   "Health status: Types of validity for an index
            of well-being." Health Services Research
            (Winter).

Lipscomb, Joseph
            "Health resource allocation and quality of care
            measurement in a social policy framework." In
            Policy Sciences (forthcoming).

Lipscomb, Joseph, Lawrence E. Berg, Virginia L. London, and
Paul A. Nutting
    1977   Health Status Maximization and Manpower Alloca-
            tion. Working paper #9761, Institute of Policy
            Sciences and Public Affairs, Duke University
            (April).

Lipscomb, Joseph and Richard M. Scheffler
    1975   "The impact of the expanded duty assistant on
            cost and productivity in dental care delivery."
            Health Services Research 10 (Spring):14-35.

Luce, R. Duncan and Howard Raiffa
    1971   Games and Decisions. New York: John Wiley
            and Sons.

Luce, R. Duncan and J. W. Tukey
    1964   "Simultaneous conjoint measurement: A new type
            of fundamental measurement." Journal of
            Mathematical Psychology 1:1-27.

Mishan, E. J.
    1971   "Evaluation of life and limb: A theoretical
            approach." Journal of Political Economy 79
            (July/August):253-271.

Musgrave, Richard A.
    1959   The Theory of Public Finance. New York:
            McGraw-Hill.

Pauly, Mark V.
    1972   Medical Care at Public Expense. New York:
            Praeger.

Tideman, T. Nicholas and Gordon Tullock
    1976   "A new and superior process for making public
            choices." Journal of Political Economy
            84:1145-1159.

Torrance, George W., David L. Sackett, and Warren H. Thomas
    1973   "Utility maximization model for program
            evaluation: A demonstration application." In
            Berg, Robert E. (ed.), Health Status Indexes.
            Chicago: Hospital Research and Educational
            Trust.

Torrance, George W., Warren H. Thomas, and David L. Sackett
    1972   "A utility maximization model for evaluation of
            health care programs." Health Services Research
            (Summer):118-133.

U.S. Department of Health, Education, and Welfare
    1974   P.S.R.O. Program Manual. Prepared by Office of
            Professional Standards Review (March).

6 Issues in the Conceptualization and Measurement of Value Placed on Health

John E. Ware, Jr.
JoAnne Young

Although the concept of health as a value has often been ignored by value theorists, it has received some attention in the theoretical and empirical literature relating to health care research. Health value measures have been accorded less attention, however, than those of other concepts, such as health status and patient satisfaction. There is a dearth of information about the reliability and validity of survey instruments for measuring the value placed on health and about population differences in valuing health.

Numerous theorists have offered arguments about the role that the value placed on health plays in health status models and models of health and illness behavior, among them Bull (1941), Goldstein (1959), Kenny (1963), Mechanic (1968), Andersen and Newman (1973), Rosser (1971), Freeman and others (1972), and proponents of the Health Belief Model (such as Becker and others, 1977). Conceptualizations of health as a value in relation to other values have attributed greatest importance to health (for example, Bull, 1941; Freeman and others, 1972). One investigator (Rokeach, 1973) has concluded that health as a value is too important to measure. Mechanic (1968) has argued, to the contrary, that despite health's high placement in the hierarchy of values, health is likely to be valued less when other essential values are seriously threatened (such as national security).

Theorists also have addressed the consequences of differences in the value placed on health. Rosser (1971), Andersen and Newman (1973), and Becker and others (1977) have argued, for example, that individuals' health values influence their actions. The last group has called attention to the problems of measuring the value that individuals place on health in testing such a hypothesis. According to Rokeach's (1973) conceptualization of the role of values, a personal system of health values derives from the forces that act on the individual, such as life stress events and perceptions of one's health status. This personal system of values serves

141

as a standard for decisions about health and illness behavior
(Ware and Young, 1976).

From this theory of the role of health values, it follows that, if health is highly valued, personal standards for
health care services would be high also. Thus, health as a
value would be positively associated with the importance
placed on desirable characteristics of health care services.
This theory also assumes that values have a strong motivational component and, therefore, serve as a guide to individual actions (such as when to use health care services). Thus,
differences in valuing health may account, at least in part,
for the historical differences between men and women in the
use of health care services--women may value health more than
men. Furthermore, it follows that those who are sick would
value health more than those who are in good health. Consistent with this hypothesis, there should be a positive relationship between age and the value placed on health, as
older persons are more likely to be ill.

Empirical tests have yielded some support for health
value theory (Anderson, 1968; Fabrega and Roberts, 1972;
Wallston and others, 1974; Ware and Young, 1976). Nevertheless, the usefulness of health value as a concept in applied
(as opposed to basic) research and the validity of health
value measures have not been demonstrated sufficiently.

Among the many methods that have been used to obtain estimates of personal values are rating and ranking tasks for
use in general population surveys. Rating tasks do not require complex instructions, and they allow respondents to
rate each construct on a value continuum without regard to
others. However, they allow the respondent to assign the
same importance to all values, potentially resulting in little
or no score variation. Ranking tasks, on the other hand, require more complex instructions, but they force respondents to
make finer value discriminations, thereby yielding greater apparent score variability.

The research reported in this paper employed both rating
and ranking tasks. Specifically, the following questions are
addressed: How important is health as a value? Is there
enough variability in the value placed on health to warrant
the inclusion of health in value surveys? Do populations
differ in their valuing of health? What is the dimensionality
of health values? Is it possible to distinguish values
placed on physical, mental, and social health components?
What are some of the methodological issues involved in
measuring the value placed on health?

Data were gathered through the use of standardized,
self-administered survey instruments. Over 2,000 persons were
surveyed in five field tests between 1973 and 1975. The survey instruments for all field tests included an 18-item

value-ranking battery; respondents were asked to rank the
items in order of importance. One item pertained to health
(that is, the value of physical and mental well-being). In
two field tests, respondents also answered a 22-item rating
battery. Respondents were asked to rate the importance they
placed on each of the 22 items (which described individual
characteristics relevant to health) by rating each on a five-
point scale. Four of the field tests involved samples drawn
from general populations in Franklin, Perry, Sangamon, and
Williamson counties in Illinois; East St. Louis, Illinois; and
Los Angeles County, California. The fifth field test involved
students at Southern Illinois University. Table 1 summarizes
the respondents' characteristics for the five field tests.
The methods of the research are described in detail in Ware
and Young (1976) and Ware and others (1974).

SCALING OF ITEMS

        Any study based on questionnaire data can be only as
good as the questionnaire items that are employed. Findings
regarding population differences, for example, reflect both
the soundness of theory underlying hypothesized relationships
and the adequacy of measures. Therefore, to achieve the best
possible measures, extensive evaluation of the value rating
and ranking items was performed using psychometric criteria.

        Rating items.--Fourteen of the 22 value-rating items
were grouped according to three health value constructs:
Physical Health (eight items), Mental Health (three items),
and Social Health (three items). The three constructs and
the specific groupings of the rating items were hypothesized
on the basis of the theoretical and empirical literature on
health status assessment. Eight of the 22 items were not
grouped since there was no prior theoretical or empirical
basis for hypothesizing the health value constructs measured
by them. (However, three of those items were later shown to
define a construct that we labeled the Value of Health Behavior). A complete list of the value-rating items and the
a priori hypothesized groupings is shown in figure 1.

        To determine the extent to which rating items in each
hypothesized grouping measured the same health value dimension and to explore the possibility that the items defined
one or more unhypothesized value dimensions, the 22 rating
items were subjected to factor analysis using data from two
field surveys (East St. Louis and Sangamon County). The
Alpha Method (Kaiser and Caffrey, 1965) was used to extract
principal factors. To further test items in the three hypothesized groupings and in the fourth grouping identified
during factor analysis, criteria of discriminant validity
were applied. All 17 items in the four health value groupings satisfied the criteria of factor analysis and discriminant validity of the multitrait scaling analysis. Factor

Table 1. Summary of Respondent Characteristics,
          Five Field Tests.

Characteristics	Field tests a/				
	TRC	ESL	SAC	LAC	UNS
Sample size	433	323	432	640	345
Sex					
Male (%)	24	19	22	63	64
Female (%)	76	81	78	37	36
Race					
White (%)	88	10	97	65	93
Non-white (%)	12	90	3	35	7
Age					
Minimum	16	17	17	18	17
Maximum	83	88	84	92	39
Median	52	43	45	43	21
Family income ($)					
Minimum	0	0	<2,000	0	b/
Maximum	20,000+	20,000+	20,000+	30,000+	b/
Median	7,400	5,400	11,900	9,500	12,000
Education (years)					
Minimum	2	3	3	0	13
Maximum	20	20+	20+	20+	18
Median	11	11	12	12	b/

a/ TRC = Tri-County (Franklin, Perry, Williamson counties)
    ESL = East St. Louis
    SAC = Sangamon County
    LAC = Los Angeles County
    UNS = University students.
b/ Not available.

solutions and detailed results of the discriminant validity
tests are presented in Ware and Young (1976).

     Ranking items.--The 18 value-ranking items are shown
in figure 2. Factor analyses of correlations between the
18 value-ranking items identified three dimensions of value
orientation. One was obviously health-related in that it
was associated with a high loading for the item pertaining to
relative value of health. The similarity of value-ranking

Figure 1.   Verbatim Items Contained in the Health-Value
            Rating Questionnaire.

Number a/	Item	Hypothesis b/
1	Being free of illness.	P
2	Understanding myself.	–
3	Having true friendship	S
4	Getting the right amount of sleep.	–
5	Adapting to changes in my life	–
6	Being able to fight off disease.	P
7	Getting affection from others.	–
8	Being safe from accidents and injuries.	P
9	Knowing how to take care of myself.	–
10	Getting along with the people I know.	S
11	Being well all of the time.	P
12	Having a healthy mind.	M
13	Eating well.	–
14	Being safe from disease.	P
15	Having good relationships with other people.	S
16	Being free from pain.	P
17	Accepting myself the way I am.	M
18	Having a comfortable life.	–
19	Having a regular medical checkup.	–
20	Having a healthy body.	P
21	Having peace of mind.	M
22	Knowing how to keep from getting sick.	P

a/ Indicates questionnaire placement.
b/ Hypothesized health value construct: P=Physical Health;
    M=Mental Health; S=Social Health; a blank indicates that
    a hypothesis was not stated in advance.

NOTE.—Items 4, 13, and 19 were used to score Prevention.

factors across field tests was studied by inspection and by
computing factor vector similarity coefficients, as suggested
by Kaiser and others (1971). Despite the tendency for factors
to be confirmed across field tests, they were difficult to
interpret. Value-ranking items were intended to be heteroge-
neous; thus, the major factors derived from correlations between the items defined very general value orientations. To
avoid confusion that might result from disagreement over interpretation, each value-ranking factor (VRF) was assigned a
roman numeral; for example, the first rotated factor was

Figure 2. Verbatim Items Contained in the Modified
           Rokeach Value Survey.*

A COMFORTABLE LIFE (a prosperous life)
AN EXCITING LIFE (a stimulating, active life)
A SENSE OF ACCOMPLISHMENT (lasting contribution)
A WORLD AT PEACE (free of war and conflict)
A WORLD OF BEAUTY (beauty of nature and the arts)
EQUALITY (brotherhood, equal opportunity for all)
FAMILY SECURITY (taking care of loved ones)
FREEDOM (independence, free choice)
HAPPINESS (contentedness)
HEALTH (physical and mental well-being)
INNER HARMONY (freedom from inner conflict)
MATURE LOVE (sexual and spiritual intimacy)
NATIONAL SECURITY (protection from attack)
PLEASURE (an enjoyable, leisurely life)
SALVATION (saved, eternal life)
SOCIAL RECOGNITION (respect, admiration)
TRUE FRIENDSHIP (close companionship)
WISDOM (mature understanding of life)

---

* This survey was modified and copied with the
   permission of Milton Rokeach.

labeled VRF-I. Further interpretation and labeling of these
factors was postponed pending studies of the validity of VRF
scores (see Ware and Young, 1976).

    Thirteen of the 18 value-ranking items tended to have
high loadings on the same VRFs across field tests; the five
items that did not were eliminated. Retained items were
enumerated so that 18 equaled the highest value score and one
equaled the lowest score. The items were grouped and the
simple algebraic sum of scores for items in each group was
computed, taking into account the sign that was consistently
associated with each item in the factor analyses across field
tests (see figure 3). For example, the highest possible
numeric score for VRF-II indicated that a high value had been
placed on health and salvation and that a low value had been
placed on exciting life and sense of accomplishment. The
lowest possible numeric score for VRF-II indicated the reverse value orientation, namely, low value for health and
salvation and high value for exciting life and sense of
accomplishment.

Figure 3. Items and Direction of Scoring for Value-Ranking
           Factor Scales.

Factor scales	Abbreviated item content	Scoring a/
VRF-I b/	Happiness	+
	Mature love	+
	Equality	−
	National security	−
	World at peace	−
VRF-II	Health	+
	Salvation	+
	Exciting life	−
	Sense of accomplishment	−
VRF-III	Inner harmony	+
	Wisdom	+
	Comfortable life	−
	Pleasure	−

a/   + indicates high value associated with high numeric
     score; − indicates high value associated with low
     numeric score.
b/   VRF = Value-ranking factor.

FINDINGS

Importance of Health

     Consistent with earlier hypotheses (Bull, 1941; Freeman
and others, 1972; Rokeach, 1973), results from all five field
tests strongly support the importance of health as a value.
However, high value was also consistently placed on happiness,
family security, and freedom in all surveys fielded during
the current research.* These values have been ranked high in
importance in other value surveys that did not include health
(Rokeach, 1973; Feather, 1975).

_____

*   Additional tabular data on analyses of the survey results
     are presented in the appended matter.

Table 2. Medians and Composite Rank Orders for Value Rankings, Five Field Tests.

	TC		ESL		SC		LAC		US	
Values	MED b/	CRO c/	MED	CRO	MED	CRO	MED	CRO	MED	CRO
Comfortable life	9.8	10	7.4	4	10.9	12	8.7	9	11.2	13
Exciting life	15.1	18	13.2	17	14.1	16	11.7	13	10.4	11
Sense of accomplishment	11.1	12	11.5	13	9.9	11	8.4	7	9.7	9
World at peace	5.4	4	8.6	8	8.3	8.5	8.5	8	9.2	8
World of beauty	14.6	17	14.4	18	14.4	18	13.2	15	12.5	15
Equality	10.6	11	8.3	7	11.6	13	11.5	12	10.6	12
Family security	4.3	3	5.4	3	3.9	2	4.1	2	10.1	10
Freedom	7.5	6	7.9	6	7.8	5	7.4	4	5.5	3
Happiness	6.2	5	5.1	2	5.7	3	5.5	3	5.5	2
Health	2.3	1	2.8	1	5.7	1	3.0	1	4.7	1
Inner harmony	9.3	9	11.1	12	8.1	7	8.2	6	5.6	4
Mature love	11.1	13	10.5	11	8.8	10	9.6	11	6.8	6
National security	11.1	14	12.8	15	13.1	14	13.5	16	16.2	18
Pleasure	14.0	15	12.8	14	13.6	15	12.4	14	12.4	14
Salvation	3.3	2	7.5	5	7.0	4	14.5	18	15.8	17
Social recognition	14.4	16	13.1	16	14.3	17	14.4	17	14.7	16
True friendship	9.1	8	9.6	10	8.3	8.5	9.0	10	7.1	7
Wisdom	8.7	7	8.7	9	8.0	6	8.1	5	6.4	5

Field tests a/

a/ TC = Tri-County (N=433); ESL = East St. Louis (N=323); SC = Sangamon County (N=432); LAC = Los Angeles County (N=525); US = University students (N=345).
b/ MED = Median.

Relative value of health.--The first analyses were performed to determine the importance of health in relation to
other value constructs and whether the variability in health
value scores was sufficient to warrant further study.
Table 2 presents the median (MED) rank and composite rank
order (CRO)* observed for health and for other values in the
18-item value-ranking instrument in each of the five field
tests. Median ranks for health ranged from 2.3 to 4.7; the
CRO for these medians was unity in all field tests. Thus, in
the aggregate, health was clearly valued most. However,
there was noteworthy variability in the rankings assigned to
health both within and between field tests. Health was
rarely ranked lowest in importance, but other values were
often ranked higher than health. As many as 40 percent and
as few as 20 percent of respondents (across field tests),
for example, did not include health in the first five ranks;
a value other than health was ranked highest the great majority of the time in all field tests. Included among the
values most frequently ranked higher than health were family
security, happiness, world at peace, and salvation (data not
reported here; see Ware and Young, 1976).

To facilitate comparisons of relative values across
field tests, means and standard deviations for the relative
value of health (RVH) item and the VRF-II that contained
the item were performed. For these analyses, RVH was
scored so that a high number indicated high value. Differences in RVH scores were significant; scores tended to
be lowest for university students, followed by urban blacks
in East St. Louis. The largest difference in RVH between
university students and respondents in a general population was approximately two-thirds of a standard deviation.
Differences between the general populations with regard to
RVH tended to be smaller; the largest difference (approximately one-third of a standard deviation) was observed between East St. Louis and Los Angeles County (higher for the
latter).

A somewhat different picture was apparent when relative
value orientations were viewed in terms of VRF-II, which contained the RVH item and three other items (as defined earlier
in figure 3). Los Angeles County respondents tended to score
lowest by as much as two-thirds of a standard deviation. This
discrepancy in results between the RVH item and VRF-II was
traced to the tendency of Los Angeles County respondents to
assign lower value to salvation.

Health value ratings.--Noteworthy differences in value
placed on health were also apparent in comparisons of mean

---

* The composite rank order, which was computed independently
  in each field test, is the rank order of medians across
  18 values.

scores for the four value-rating scales fielded in Sangamon
County and East St. Louis (see table 3). Specifically, East
St. Louis respondents tended to assign greater importance to
both physical health and health behavior than respondents in
Sangamon County. In the case of physical health, the magnitude of difference in mean scores was approximately one-third
of a standard deviation. In the case of health behavior, the
magnitude of mean difference was approximately two-thirds of
a standard deviation. Differences in the value placed on the
three components of health status and health behavior defined
by rating scales were also observed within each field test
when scale scores were expressed as percentages of the total
possible score (see percentage of possible score, table 3).
The pattern of results also clearly differed across field
tests. For white middle-class respondents in Sangamon County,
highest value was placed on mental health, followed by
physical health, social health (both approximately one-half
of a standard deviation lower), and health behavior (approximately a full standard deviation lower). For urban
blacks in East St. Louis, both physical health and mental
health were valued highly, followed by social health and
health behavior (both approximately two-thirds of a standard
deviation lower).

     With respect to differences in value scores between
field tests, conclusions were not the same for the RVH measure as they were for health-value ratings. Physical health
was clearly rated higher in value by East St. Louis respondents than by Sangamon County respondents. When forced to
view health in relation to other values, however, East St.
Louis and Sangamon County respondents did not differ.

     The variability of rating and ranking scores obtained
with health value surveys is clearly sufficient to warrant
measurement of value placed on health in surveys using these
methods. Whereas greatest importance was placed on health
more often than any of the other 17 values included in the
modified Rokeach (1973) Value Survey, there was considerable
variability in health value rankings. Health was assigned
highest value by no more than 31 percent of the respondents
across field tests (only 18 percent of the university
students ranked health highest). Health was assigned the
first two or three ranks about half of the time, and was
ranked fifth or lower in importance by as many as one-third
of the respondents across field tests. Subgroups of interest
within general populations (for example, men, the very young,
and the more educated) assigned even less relative importance
to health. Considerable variability was also observed in
ratings of the importance of specific health status components (for example, physical, mental, and social health).
Thus, while improvements in health value surveys are necessary to achieve precise tests of hypotheses regarding health
values, current study findings clearly indicate that

Table 3. <u>Means and Standard Deviations (in Parentheses) for
Value Rating Scores, Two Field Tests</u>.

| Value dimension | Scoring method | | | | |
| | Raw score | | Percentage of possible score | | |
	ESL <u>a</u>/	SAC <u>a</u>/	ESL	SAC	F <u>b</u>/
Physical health	29.0 (6.5)	26.8 (6.0)	72.5 (16.2)	67.0 (15.4)	23.0*
Mental health	11.4 (2.6)	11.2 (2.2)	76.0 (17.3)	74.7 (14.8)	1.2
Social health	9.8 (2.8)	10.0 (2.2)	65.3 (18.2)	66.7 (14.7)	1.1
Health behavior	10.1 (2.5)	8.5 (2.3)	67.3 (16.2)	56.7 (15.0)	81.2*

<u>a</u>/ ESL = East St. Louis (N=320); SAC = Sangamon County
     (N=424).
<u>b</u>/ F-ratio for one-way analysis of variance.
* $p < .001$.

variability in health value scores is sufficient to warrant
inclusion of health value constructs in value surveys.

Population Differences

     When demographic and socioeconomic variables were
studied in relation to health values, some consistent results
and large differences were observed. All health constructs
were valued more by women, people who were older, and those
with lower income. Some group differences in health values
are large and consistent across populations and across rating
and ranking methods. In the case of education, however, discrepancies in results were observed across field tests. These
population differences should be studied further before generalizing conclusions about the relationships in question.

     These correlations suggest that health value measures
may be useful in understanding better why socio-demographic
variables have been linked to differences in the use of
health care services. Another implication of these findings
concerns the development of a population health index. When
health status assessments are scaled by means of health
value preferences, it may be necessary to account for

differences by age, sex, education, and income in the value
placed on health. Current study findings do not support the
practice of generalizing average-value preference weights to
all persons for health status constructs.

Conceptual and Methodological Issues

    Dimensionality of health values.--The psychometric
studies of health value-rating items suggest that health
values can be conceptualized along the lines of physical,
mental, and social components of health status and that it
is possible to construct scales to distinguish between the
values placed on those components. Although there was a
tendency for people who place high value on their health
to value physical, mental, and social health status components, it is clear that different population groups do
not value a given health status component the same, and
that individuals often place different value on the components of health status.

    Reliability.--The failure of health value surveys (par-
ticularly those employing ranking tasks) fielded during the
current research to achieve consistently high reliability is
a noteworthy constraint on their use in general populations.
In the current research, test-retest reliability coefficients
for value rankings were in the moderate to high range for
university students and were comparable to those reported by
others for similar questionnaires (Rokeach, 1973; Feather,
1975). However, the same value-ranking tasks yielded much
lower test-retest reliability coefficients in general populations (particularly those involving respondents with less
than a high school education). Scores for scales to measure
general health perceptions and patient satisfaction tended to
be much more reliable in these populations (Ware and Karmos,
1976; Ware and others, 1976); thus, this measurement dilemma
is somewhat unique to health value constructs and current
study methods. Perhaps less complicated ranking tasks would
result in improved reliability for health value scores. For
example, relative health values could be estimated by asking
respondents to rank health and a smaller number of other
values than 17 (as required in the current research). Another solution to the reliability problem may be to construct
health value scales from multiple measures of the value of
each health component (for example, the value-rating scales
that were constructed during the current research).

    These reliability findings have implications for the
interpretation of statistical parameters for health values.
First, confidence intervals about estimates of central
tendency for health values (particularly those computed from
the 18-item ranking task) are likely to be large. In addition
to this loss of precision, substantial downward bias in correlation coefficients used to estimate associations between

health values and other variables should be anticipated (due
to poor reliability), particularly in disadvantaged populations. These effects and biases can be taken into account
during statistical analyses if reliability estimates are
obtained.

Second, given the substantial difference in reliability
estimates for health value scores between university students
and respondents in general population surveys (particularly
those based on ranking tasks), the practice of generalizing
reliability estimates obtained for students to general populations (Rokeach, 1973; Feather, 1975) is questionable.
In the absence of satisfactory reliability estimates, lack of
perfect reliability should always be considered as an alternative explanation for insignificant differences and weak
associations in studies of health values.

Validity.--The significant relationships observed between the relative value of the health-ranking item and the
physical health-rating scale constitute convergent evidence
of validity. However, the relationships were weak in the two
field tests where both the rating and ranking tasks were used.
These results exemplify one consequence of poor reliability,
namely, inadequate precision for purposes of hypothesis
testing.

Given that the rank assigned to health was significantly
related only to ratings of physical health and that insignificant trends for health value rankings and ratings of mental
health and social health were observed in both directions,
rankings of the relative value of health may reflect primarily physical health. This interpretation of health is
consistent with other findings, for example, results indicating that people tend to focus more on their physical
(rather than mental) health when asked to rate "health in
general" (Ware, 1976; Johnston and Ware, 1976). The relative
value of mental health appears to have been better tapped by
value-ranking factors that were not associated, or were only
weakly associated, with the health value-ranking item.

It may be, also, that the importance of health as defined by value ratings and the relative importance of health
as defined by value rankings or resource allocation tasks*
should be treated differently in a conceptualization of health
values. Health value-rating measures may reflect absolute
value and not the current priorities or the importance of
health when tradeoffs are involved. Thus, the results of

---

* Resource allocation tasks require respondents to indicate
  how they would spend a fixed amount of money (that is,
  how much for health care, recreational facilities, crime
  prevention, vocational training, etc.). Value is in-
  ferred from the proportions.

ranking tasks (like the 18-item battery in the current research) and resource allocation tasks should agree more with
each other than either would agree with the results of value-
rating tasks. The findings of an experiment with university
students support this hypothesis (Ware and Young, 1976). It
remains to be determined whether ratings or rankings are more
sensitive to the health-related forces that act on individuals
and which of the two health value constructs--absolute value
or relative importance--is more influential in health care
decision making.

     Empirical tests of the scale placement of value-rating
items substantially confirmed operational definitions of
physical, mental, and social health values. Given the clarity
and consistency of results across field tests, the scaling
studies support the construct validity of the value-rating
scales. Significant relationships between health value-rating
scores, age, and sex were also consistent with predictions
from theory (that is, health increased in value with age and
was valued more by women). Hence, the construct validity of
these survey measures is also supported by findings regarding
population differences in health values.

     The validity of health value measures, however, has by
no means been thoroughly addressed in the analyses that were
described. Forty hypotheses derived from value theory were
tested during the current research to provide an empirical
basis for further development of value theory and to test the
validity of measures of value rating and ranking; findings
are reported elsewhere (Ware and Young, 1976). Briefly, results were consistent with value theory and constituted at
least weak support for the construct validity of current study
measures.

SOME SUGGESTIONS FOR FUTURE RESEARCH

     In the absence of established criteria for the value of
health, comparisons between measures based on different
methods will contribute to a better understanding of both the
validity of health value scores and the appropriate interpretation of specific measures. For these studies, health
value constructs should be defined at the same degree of
specificity across methods. This will allow the isolation of
the effects of the methods on scores and the testing of convergent and discriminant validity. Unfortunately, in the
current research the rating scales focused on more specific
health constructs than the ranking items did.

     To the extent practical, health value surveys should be
fielded in general populations. Since overall data quality,
and particularly the reliability of ratings and rankings,
appear to be lower for general populations than for university
students, methodological research should emphasize the former.

Other characteristics of the respondent samples should be kept in mind when interpreting the results of methodological studies. For instance, university students appear to have substantially different value orientations from those observed for persons outside the university.

While health care researchers interested in the role of values naturally would think first of health values, a more nearly comprehensive conceptualization of value orientation will probably result in the best predictions (Ware and Young, 1976). Thus, future health value surveys should include measures of value constructs that do not pertain explicitly to health, as well as those that do.

Finally, although the review of the literature conducted during the current research was not exhaustive (see Ware and Young, 1976), it suggests that a well-specified theoretical model of the antecedents and consequences of differences in health value orientation is lacking. An improved theoretical conceptualization of health values would greatly facilitate future research.

Acknowledgments.

Data gathering and analyses were performed pursuant to Contract No. HSM 110-72-299, National Center for Health Services Research, U.S.DHEW. Additional analyses and the preparation of this paper were supported by the Health Insurance Study, a grant from U.S.DHEW.

APPENDIX TABLES

Table A-1. Summary of Test-Retest and Internal-Consistency
            Reliability Coefficients for Health Value
            Measures

Table A-2. Frequency Distributions of Ranks Assigned to
            Health, Five Field Tests

Table A-3. Means and Standard Deviations (in Parentheses)
            for Health Value Rankings, Five Field Tests

Table A-4. Mean Health Value Rankings and Rating Scores
            by Age, Four Field Tests

Table A-5. Mean Health Value Ranking and Rating Scores
            by Education, Four Field Tests

Table A-6. Mean Health Value Ranking and Rating Scores
            and Standard Deviations by Sex, Four Field Tests

Table A-7. Mean Health Value Ranking and Rating Scores by
            Income, Four Field Tests

Table A-1. Summary of Test-Retest and Internal-Consistency
            Reliability Coefficients for Health Value
            Measures.

Measure/	Test-retest a/			Internal consistency a/			
value dimension	#	H	M	L	#	H	M	L
Value rankings								
Single item	4	.53	.46	.30	b/	–	–	–
VRF-II	3	.72	.50	.44	4	.55	.45	.30
Other VRF scales	6	.68	.50	.34	8	.56	.54	.39
Value ratings								
Physical health	0	c/	–	–	2	.90	d/	.86
Mental health	0	–	–	–	2	.76	–	.73
Social health	0	–	–	–	2	.78	–	.76
Prevention	0	–	–	–	2	.68	–	.67

a/ # = number of coefficients across field tests; H =
    highest coefficient; M = median; L = lowest.
b/ Not applicable to single-item measures.
c/ Not studied.
d/ Not applicable; estimated in only two field tests.

Table A-2.   Frequency Distributions of Ranks Assigned to Health, Five Field Tests.

Ranks	Tri-County f	cum. %	Students f	cum. %	East St. Louis f	cum. %	Sangamon County f	cum. %	Los Angeles f	cum. %
					Field tests					
1	130	30.7	63	18.3	82	25.6	127	29.7	136	27.3
2	106	55.8	41	30.1	66	46.2	73	46.7	84	44.1
3	51	67.8	33	39.7	39	58.4	55	59.6	59	55.9
4	38	76.8	31	48.7	31	68.1	50	71.3	51	66.1
5	17	80.9	29	57.1	21	74.7	28	77.8	39	73.9
6	20	85.6	29	65.5	11	78.1	26	83.9	31	80.2
7	15	89.1	19	71.0	8	80.6	12	86.7	21	84.4
8	10	91.5	20	76.8	8	83.1	11	89.3	15	87.4
9	10	93.9	19	82.3	14	87.5	8	91.1	16	90.6
10	4	94.8	11	85.5	12	91.2	9	93.2	15	93.6
11	3	95.5	14	89.6	6	93.1	9	95.3	8	95.2
12	4	96.5	14	93.6	6	95.0	6	96.7	9	97.0
13	4	97.4	6	95.4	2	95.6	6	98.1	5	98.0
14	5	98.6	7	97.4	5	97.2	2	98.6	1	98.2
15	2	99.1	3	98.3	5	98.7	4	99.5	2	98.6
16	3	99.8	4	99.4	1	99.1	1	99.8	3	99.2
17	1	100.0	0	99.4	3	100.0	1	100.0	2	99.6
18	0	100.0	2	100.0	0	100.0	0	100.0	2	100.0
Total	423	100.0	345	100.0	320	100.0	428	100.0	499	100.0

Table A-3. Means and Standard Deviations (in Parentheses)
            for Health Value Rankings, Five Field Tests.

| Health value measures | Field tests a/ | | | | | F b/ |
	ESL	SAC	TRC	LAC	UNS	
RVH	14.7	15.2	15.5	15.9	13.5	27.7*
	(3.8)	(3.3)	(3.2)	(3.5)	(3.8)	
VRF-II	48.3	48.6	53.6	41.5	c/	72.2*
	(13.1)	(11.5)	(9.8)	(12.1)		

a/ ESL = East St. Louis; SAC = Sangamon County; TRC =
    Tri-County, LAC = Los Angeles County; and UNS =
    University Students.
b/ F-ratio for one-way analysis of variance.
c/ Not studied.
*   p < 0.01 (one-tailed test).

Table A-4. Mean Health Value Rankings and Rating Scores by Age, Four Field Tests.

Field test/ health value measure	Age groups a/							F b/	r c/
	17-24	25-34	35-44	45-54	55-64	65-74	75-84		
Tri-County									
Rank of health d/	15.0	14.8	15.7	16.2	15.3	16.1	15.2	1.7	.07
VRF-II e/	47.7	52.0	53.9	55.3	54.7	53.4	54.8	2.9*	.13*
Los Angeles County									
Rank of health	13.4	14.1	14.9	15.7	15.2	15.1	16.0	3.4*	.16*
VRF-II	35.7	39.4	41.5	42.0	40.5	46.1	48.1	5.0*	.21*
East St. Louis									
Rank of health	14.8	14.0	15.2	14.5	15.2	14.8	-- f/	<1	.05
VRF-II	43.1	45.2	50.4	47.9	49.7	53.4	--	4.3*	.23*
Physical health	29.9	29.3	28.4	28.4	29.9	28.1	--	<1	-.06
Mental health	11.9	11.5	11.0	11.4	11.3	11.2	--	<1	-.08
Social health	9.4	9.5	9.3	10.1	10.1	10.4	--	1.4	.12*
Health behavior	10.3	9.8	9.8	10.0	10.3	10.4	--	<1	.04
Sangamon County									
Rank of health	14.0	14.8	15.4	15.2	15.7	15.9	14.8	1.6	.09**
VRF-II	43.2	45.8	50.0	48.8	51.1	51.9	51.9	4.1*	.19*
Physical health	27.7	25.7	26.5	26.1	28.2	28.0	27.9	1.9	.10**
Mental health	11.4	11.1	11.3	11.6	11.2	10.9	10.7	<1	-.04
Social health	10.3	9.8	10.0	9.9	10.2	10.2	10.2	<1	.03
Health behavior	8.4	8.2	8.2	8.4	9.0	9.0	9.6	2.1	.14*

a/ N for age groups ranged from 19 to 113; the median of 27 groups was 57. Standard deviations ranged from
    2.6 to 4.4 for rank of health, from 8.4 to 13.3 for VRF-II, from 5.2 to 7.0 for physical health, and
    from 1.8 to 3.2 for mental health, social health, and health behavior.

b/ F-ratio for one-way analysis of variance.

c/ Product-moment correlation between age and health value.

d/ Single-item health value ranking; scored so that high number defined high value.

e/ Second value-ranking factor (see text).

f/ Not computed due to small sample size.

* $p < 0.01$.

** $p < 0.05$.

Table A-5. Mean Health Value Ranking and Rating Scores by Education, Four Field Tests.

Field test/ health value measure	Education in years a/					F b/	r c/
	0-8	9-11	12	13-16	17+		
Tri-County							
Rank of health d/	15.7	15.7	15.5	15.1	-- f/	<1	-.03
VRF-II e/	54.4	54.4	53.8	51.1	--	1.5	-.14*
Los Angeles County							
Rank of health	15.7	14.5	14.8	14.9	14.7	1.1	-.05
VRF-II	50.5	44.2	41.8	39.5	36.3	13.8*	-.32*
East St. Louis							
Rank of health	14.4	15.1	14.8	14.2	--	<1	.04
VRF-II	49.4	48.8	48.1	45.8	--	<1	-.10**
Physical health	28.4	28.5	29.3	30.3	--	1.1	.11**
Mental health	10.9	10.9	11.6	12.4	--	4.7*	.18*
Social health	9.8	9.5	9.8	10.0	--	<1	.01
Health behavior	10.2	10.2	10.0	9.9	--	<1	.00
Sangamon County							
Rank of health	15.7	15.2	15.5	15.0	13.6	2.6**	-.12*
VRF-II	51.1	48.8	51.4	47.3	37.1	13.9*	-.28*
Physical health	28.2	28.3	26.8	26.7	23.5	4.0*	-.19*
Mental health	10.8	11.6	10.9	11.6	11.3	2.3	.06
Social health	9.9	10.2	9.8	10.4	9.8	1.6	.00
Health behavior	8.7	9.4	8.5	8.5	7.2	4.7*	-.19*

a/ N for education groups ranged from 31 to 181; the median for 18 groups
    was 72. Standard deviations ranged from 2.8 to 4.1 for rank of health,
    from 9.1 to 13.6 for VRF-II, from 5.2 to 4.1 for rank of health, from
    9.1 to 13.6 for VRF-II, from 5.2 to 7.0 for physical health, and from
    1.8 to 3.0 for mental health, social health, and health behavior rating
    scales.
b/ F-ratio for one-way analysis of variance.
c/ Product-moment correlation between education and health value.
d/ Single-item health value ranking; scored so that high number defined
    high value.
e/ Second value-ranking factor (see text).
f/ Not computed due to small sample size.
* $p < .01$ (one-tailed test).
** $p < .05$ (one-tailed test).

Table A-6. Mean Health Value Ranking and Rating Scores and
            Standard Deviations by Sex, Four Field Tests.

Field test/ health value measure	Males a/		Females a/		
	Mean	SD	Mean	SD	F
Tri-County					
Health value rank b/	15.4	3.7	15.6	3.1	<1
VRF-II c/	50.9	11.0	54.4	9.2	9.8*
Los Angeles County					
Health value rank	14.3	3.8	15.8	2.7	19.2*
VRF-II	40.1	12.4	44.2	11.4	12.8*
East St. Louis					
Health value rank	14.2	4.1	14.9	3.7	1.8
VRF-II	42.9	14.8	49.5	12.4	12.7*
Physical health	29.4	6.1	28.9	6.6	<1
Mental health	11.5	2.6	11.3	2.6	<1
Social health	10.2	2.7	9.7	2.8	1.5
Health behavior	10.0	2.6	10.1	2.5	<1
Sangamon County					
Health value rank	14.5	3.7	15.3	3.2	4.1
VRF-II	43.7	12.8	49.9	10.8	21.5*
Physical health	26.1	5.9	26.9	6.1	1.4
Mental health	10.8	2.2	11.4	2.3	5.1*
Social health	9.7	2.0	10.1	2.2	2.6**
Health behavior	8.1	2.1	8.6	2.4	3.4**

a/ Sample sizes for males and females, respectively, were
    102 and 320 in Tri-County, 315 and 168 in Los Angeles,
    60 and 259 in East St. Louis, and 89 and 339 in
    Sangamon County.
b/ Single-item health value ranking scored so that a high
    number indicated high value.
c/ Second value-ranking factor, which included health
    (see text).
* $p < 0.01$.
** $p < 0.05$.

Table A-7. Mean Health Value Ranking and Rating Scores by Income, Four Field Tests.

Field test/ health value measure	Annual income a/					F b/	r c/
	$0-4,999	$5,000-8,999	$9,000-14,999	$15,000-19,999	$20,000+		
Tri-County							
Rank of health d/	15.6	15.5	15.8	14.9	14.6	<1	-.04
VRF-II e/	54.2	52.5	54.5	52.4	49.6	1.7	-.06
Los Angeles County							
Rank of health	14.9	14.4	14.6	15.3	15.2	<1	.05
VRF-II	44.8	42.2	39.7	39.6	39.6	4.1*	-.16*
East St. Louis							
Rank of health	14.9	14.5	15.0	--f/	--	<1	-.01
VRF-II	48.3	47.2	50.9	--	--	1.1	-.02
Physical health	29.1	28.8	29.7	--	--	<1	-.04
Mental health	11.3	11.4	11.8	--	--	<1	.05
Social health	9.8	9.4	10.0	--	--	<1	.00
Health behavior	10.3	10.1	10.1	--	--	<1	-.08
Sangamon County							
Rank of health	14.7	16.1	15.1	15.2	15.0	1.3	-.02
VRF-II	49.9	49.1	49.6	49.1	44.3	3.3**	-.11*
Physical health	27.8	28.3	27.2	26.2	25.7	2.3	-.13*
Mental health	11.0	11.5	11.3	11.4	11.3	<1	.03
Social health	10.2	10.0	10.2	9.9	10.1	<1	-.02
Health behavior	9.3	9.2	8.3	8.6	8.0	3.6*	-.16*

a/ N for income groups ranged from 20 to 166; the median of 18 groups was 77. Standard deviations ranged from 2.3 to 4.4 for rank of health, from 7.9 to 13.8 for VRF-II, from 5.7 to 6.7 for physical health, and from 1.9 to 2.8 for mental health, social health, and health behavior.

b/ F-ratio for one-way analysis of variance.

c/ Product-moment correlation between income and health value.

d/ Single-item health value ranking; scored so that high number defined high value.

e/ Second value ranking factor (see text).

f/ Not computed due to small sample size.

* p < 0.01.

** p < 0.05.

REFERENCES

Andersen, R.
    1968   A Behavioral Model of Families' Use of Health
            Services. Research Series No. 25. Chicago:
            University of Chicago.

Andersen, R. and J. R. Newman
    1973   "Societal and individual determinants of medical
            care utilization in the United States." Health
            and Society 51:95-124.

Armor, D. J.
    1974   "Theta reliability and factor scaling." In
            Costner, H. L. (ed.), Sociological Methodology,
            1973-1974. San Francisco: Jossey-Bass
            Publishers.

Becker, M. H., D. P. Haefner, S. V. Kasl, J. P. Kirscht,
L. A. Maiman, and I. M. Rosenstock
    1977   "Selected psychological models and correlates of
            individual health-related behaviors." Medical
            Care 15:27-46.

Bull, N.
    1941   "The biological basis of value." The Scientific
            Monthly 53:170-174.

Fabrega, H., Jr. and R. E. Roberts
    1972   "Social-psychological correlates of physician
            use by economically disadvantaged negro urban
            residents." Medical Care 10:215-223.

Feather, N. T.
    1975   Values in Education and Society. New York:
            The Free Press.

Freeman, H. E., S. Levine, and L. G. Reeder
    1972   Handbook of Medical Sociology. Englewood Cliffs,
            N.J.: Prentice-Hall.

Goldstein, K.
    1959   "Health as a value." In Maslow, A. (ed.), New
            Knowledge in Human Values. Chicago: Henry
            Regnery Co.

Johnston, S. A. and J. E. Ware, Jr.
    1976   "Income group differences in relationships among
            survey measures of physical and mental health."
            Health Services Research 11:416-429.

Kaiser, H. F. and J. Caffrey
    1965   "Alpha factor analysis." Psychometrika 30:1-14.

Kaiser, H. F., S. Hunka, and J. C. Bianchini
    1971   "Relating factors between studies based upon
            different individuals." Multivariate Behavioral
            Research 6:409-422.

Kenny, M.
    1963   "Social values and health in Spain: Some pre-
            liminary considerations. Human Organizations
            21:280-285.

Mechanic, D.
    1968   Medical Sociology: A Selective View. New York:
            The Free Press.

Rokeach, M.
    1975   Personal communication (April 23).

    1973   The Nature of Human Values. New York:
            The Free Press.

Rosser, J. M.
    1971   "Values and health." The Journal of School
            Health 41:386-390.

Wallston, K. A., S. A. Maides, and B. A. Wallston
    1974   "Health care information seeking as a function
            of health locus of control and health value."
            Nashville: Vanderbilt University (mimeographed).

Ware, J. E., Jr.
    1976   "Scales for measuring general health percep-
            tions." Health Services Research 11:396-415.

Ware, J. E., Jr. and A. H. Karmos
    1976   Development and Validation of Scales to Measure
            Perceived Health and Patient Role Propensity:
            Volume II of a Final Report. Carbondale, Ill.:
            University School of Medicine.

Ware, J. E., Jr., M. K. Snyder, and W. R. Wright
    1976a   Development and Validation of Scales to Measure
            Patient Satisfaction with Health Care Services:
            Volume I of a Final Report. Part A: Review of
            Literature, Overview of Methods, and Results
            Regarding Construction of Scales. Carbondale,
            Ill.: Southern Illinois University School of
            Medicine.

    1976b   The Development and Validation of Scales to
            Measure Key Health Concepts. Methodological
            Appendix: Volume IV of a Final Report.
            Carbondale, Ill.: Southern Illinois University
            School of Medicine.

Ware, J. E., Jr. and J. Young
    1976   Conceptualization and Measurement of Health as
            a Value: Volume III of a Final Report.
            Carbondale, Ill.: Southern Illinois University
            School of Medicine.

Ware, J. E., Jr., J. Young, M. K. Snyder, and W. R. Wright
    1974   The Measurement of Health as a Value. NTIS
            publication no. PB-230-616/AS. Springfield,
            Va.: National Technical Information Service.

7 Willingness to Pay for Probabilistic Improvements in Functional Health Status: A Psychological Perspective

Gregory W. Fischer

Previous efforts to develop health status indexes have explicitly avoided attaching dollar values to health states or to health state transitions. Instead, Bush, Chen, Fanshel, Torrance, and others have used psychometric procedures to directly scale subjective preferences for various functionally defined health states. These scale values can then be incorporated in mathematical programming procedures to maximize "total (expected) health status," subject to a set of input constraints (for example, Bush and others, 1973). But while existing health status indexes may provide a suitable basis for performing cost-effectiveness analyses (that is, determining the optimal allocation given fixed resource constraints), these indexes cannot be used to answer the larger questions: Should society be devoting more or fewer resources to a given health care activity? Is society already devoting too many resources to health care activities, or are we, in fact, too miserly with regard to health care? As policy makers display increasing concern over the rapidly mounting costs of health care services, these larger questions assume ever greater importance.

Because the stakes are so large, many technical analysts are inclined to leave these larger allocation questions to the political process, focusing their own efforts on the task of maximizing health status within politically generated constraints. Other analysts adopt this same stance simply because they doubt that formal analytical exercises will ever have a substantial impact on the political processes which ultimately determine the amount of public resources devoted to health and safety activities. This pessimism is not universal. Some policy analysts, most of them trained in economics, believe that formal cost-benefit analysis can and should be used as a basis both (1) for deciding whether an activity is worth undertaking at all and (2) for allocating public resources to activities with different objectives (for example, health versus education). Ordinary health status indexes and other measures of

167

effectiveness used in cost-effectiveness analyses are inadequate for both tasks. Because they do not attach a dollar
value to benefits, they cannot be used to answer a basic
question: Do the social benefits of this program exceed its
social opportunity costs? In addition, because health status
indexes are incommensurable with, for example, the measures
of effectiveness used in education, these indexes cannot be
used to resolve tradeoffs between different program areas.
By contrast, if one is willing to accept the assumptions
underlying cost-benefit analysis, these shortcomings are
eliminated. They are eliminated because cost-benefit analysis
reduces all costs and benefits to dollars. With this simpli-
fication, not only can one readily eliminate from consideration all programs whose opportunity costs exceed their benefits, but one can also directly compare programs with different objectives, allocating marginal resources to programs
which produce the greatest marginal net benefit.

        This paper investigates the feasibility of applying
the willingness-to-pay principle to cost-benefit analysis for
the evaluation of health and safety programs. While the
paper derives from an economic approach to cost-benefit
analysis, it is written from a "behavioral decision theory"
perspective. Behavioral decision theory is a subdiscipline
of psychology which attempts to integrate the insights of
the rational sciences--economics, decision theory, and
statistics--with the empirically-based insights of modern
cognitive psychology. In the present context, the behavioral
decision theory perspective leads me to be relatively
pessimistic about the possibility of obtaining meaningful
measures of willingness to pay for health and safety programs.
This skepticism derives from two observations. First, a
formal analysis of decisions involving tradeoffs between
health status and other forms of material consumption reveals
that the structure of these decisions is very complex.
Second, a large body of psychological research suggests that
people show little facility for dealing with decisions of
such complexity.

        The remaining sections of this paper all contribute,
in one way or another, to these conclusions. The second
section sets the stage by briefly outlining the theoretical
justification for the willingness-to-pay approach to social
decision making. The third section then provides a discussion of how a "rational individual" might decide on how much
he would be willing to pay for probabilistic improvements
in health status. This discussion suggests that if an
individual is to make informed willingness-to-pay decisions
in the health and safety arena, he must be able to
evaluate complex multi-period lotteries (gambles) over
multiple outcome variables. The fourth section briefly surveys the findings of psychological studies of intuitive decision making and judgment. This discussion documents the
rather substantial limitations of intuitive inferential and

decision-making processes. The final section uses the insights and empirical generalizations developed in the previous
sections to critically evaluate a variety of approaches to
the assessment of willingness to pay for the consequences of
health and safety programs.

COST-BENEFIT ANALYSIS AND THE
WILLINGNESS-TO-PAY PRINCIPLE

Given the objective of attaching a dollar value to a
health or safety program,* two separate subtasks may be
identified. First, a dollar value must be attached to the
public and private resources consumed by the program. While
this is by no means a trivial task, I have nothing to contribute to this question; I happily leave it in the hands of
the economists. Second, a dollar value must be assigned to
program-induced changes in health status. Here, two approaches may be identified. The first is a crude offshoot of
the human capital theory developed by Becker (1964) and
others. The second is based on the willingness-to-pay principle of cost-benefit analysis.

The Human Capital Approach

When applied policy analysts have attempted to attach
a dollar value to the losses associated with mortality or
morbidity, they have almost always used discounted foregone
wages as an indicator of the societal opportunity cost. To
the extent that wages accurately reflect an individual's contribution to society, this approach has a certain intuitive
appeal. Nevertheless, this procedure has been subjected to
harsh theoretical and pragmatic criticism (see, for example,
Acton, 1973; Jones-Lee, 1976; Mishan, 1971; and Schelling,
1968). From a theoretical standpoint, the human capital approach's main weakness (as a societal decision criteron) is
that it has no normative justification in modern welfare
economics. In the absence of such justification, the following specific criticisms are extremely damaging:

> (1) The approach necessarily attaches less value
> to the health and lives of the poor than the
> affluent. In fact, it attaches no value to
> the lives of those who earn no wages. (To
> avoid putting housewives in this category,
> human capital accountants value the efforts
> of housewives by crediting them with the
> wages of a domestic worker.)

---

* To simplify this discussion, I treat different levels of
investment in a given program as if they were different
programs.

(2)   The approach attaches no value to health
      and survival per se, though most members
      of society presumably do.

(3)   The approach attaches no value to the pain
      and suffering associated with disease and
      injury.

(4)   The approach attaches no value to the
      emotional pain experienced by those who
      love a seriously ill or deceased individual.

(5)   The values generated by the approach have
      no obvious relationship to the preferences
      of the individuals comprising our society.

The Willingness-to-pay Approach*

     The willingness-to-pay approach to valuing the social
costs of mortality and morbidity is, in contrast to the
earnings-based method, firmly based in modern welfare
economics. This is not to say that the willingness-to-pay
principle is uncontroversial, but simply that it has a clearly
understood philosophical rationale. Consider a status quo
state of the world, X^O, and an alternative state, X'. Under
what conditions should a society that wishes to base its collective decisions on the preferences of its individual members choose to move from X^O to X'? The Pareto principle provides a widely accepted, but rarely applicable, answer to
this question. If at least some members of society prefer X'
to X^O, and no one prefers X^O to X', then society should choose
X'. Intuitively, if some people are better off with the
change, and no one is worse off, then society as a whole
clearly profits from the change.

     As stated, the Pareto principle contributes nothing to
the resolution of social choice dilemmas in which some members
of society prefer X^O and others X'. Fortunately, the domain
of the Pareto principle can be greatly expanded by introducing side payments whereby those who prefer X' to X^O are given
the opportunity to compensate those who prefer X^O to X'.
Assuming that these side payments can be made without cost,
and that all side payments are made in a common unit (say
dollars), it is easy to derive the conditions under which the
Pareto principle will lead society to choose X' or X^O. Suppose that the i-th individual in society prefers X' to X^O,
and let b_i denote that individual's maximum buying price, or
the most he would be willing to pay to move from Xo to X'.

_____

*   This section relies heavily on Mishan's (1973) discussion
    of the willingness-to-pay basis of cost-benefit analysis.

Suppose that the j-th individual prefers X^O to X', and let s_j denote that individual's <u>minimum selling price</u>, or the smallest compensation he would be willing to accept for moving from X^O to X'.* Then assuming m individuals prefer X^O to X', and n individuals prefer X' to X^O, society will choose X' to X^O if and only if

$$(1) \quad \sum_{i=1}^{n} b_i > \sum_{j=1}^{m} s_j.$$

This result follows directly from the Pareto principle because, when (1) holds, those who prefer X' can compensate those who prefer X^O, and still have something left over. Thus, after compensation, nobody will be worse off and some people will be better off, so society should, according to the Pareto principle, choose X' over X^O, <u>provided that the compensation is actually carried out</u>. Unfortunately, except in very small groups, the implementation of the side payment procedure will be extremely costly if not totally unfeasible. Moreover, if side payments are actually to be carried out, individuals may have n incentive to misrepresent their actual preferences.** Thus, even with the introduction of side payments, the Pareto principle is of no value for the real world decision maker.

One resolution to this dilemma was suggested by the economists Nicholas Kaldor and Sir John Hicks. They argued that if $\Sigma b > \Sigma s$, then society should choose X' over X^O, <u>even if no compensation is actually made</u>. While this Kaldor-Hicks criterion is sometimes justified on the grounds that it creates the potential for a Pareto principle improvement, this argument is hardly compelling given that without compensation the change is not such an improvement (some members of society will be worse off because of the change). A more common justification of the Kaldor-Hicks criterion is that it leads to decisions which are economically "efficient" in much

---

* Technically, the maximum buying prices and minimum selling prices should leave all individuals indifferent between X^O and X'. That is, for those who prefer X^O to X', $(X'+s) \sim (X^O)$; for those who prefer X', $(X'-b) \sim (X^O)$, where "$\sim$" denotes indifference.

** If the number of individuals in society is large, those who prefer X' to X^O should understate b. In so doing, they are unlikely to change society's ultimate decision, and if X' is chosen, they will pay less than they would be willing to pay, thus getting a "bargain." Through a similar logic, those who prefer X^O to X' may be motivated to overstate s.

the same sense that decisions generated by competitive markets are efficient. But like competitive markets, the Kaldor-
Hicks criterion ignores issues of distributive justice. Thus,
the criterion can lead to public decisions which favor the
rich at the expense of the poor. All that is required is
that the benefits to the rich outweigh the costs to the poor.

       The Kaldor-Hicks criterion has other shortcomings as
well. For example, it confers dictatorial powers upon any
individual who prefers the status quo and for whom no compensation is sufficient to induce a voluntary move from the
status quo. Also, it can be shown that the rule can lead
society to choose state X' over state X^o, but then, given the
altered distribution of resources in X', move back to X^o.
Nevertheless, the Kaldor-Hicks criterion and the economic
efficiency argument provide the theoretical justification
for cost-benefit analyses based on the willingness-to-pay
principle. Many people are unpersuaded by these arguments
and thus reject the cost-benefit criterion as a social decision rule. But even if one rejects the cost-benefit approach, willingness-to-pay information may be of considerable
interest. By separately estimating the costs and benefits
experienced by various subgroups of the population, the
analyst may be able to use willingness-to-pay data to achieve
distributional goals. For example, such data could be used
to evaluate the attractiveness of alternative in-kind transfers aimed at a given target population: Would they rather
have better schools or better health? Here I simply take the
position that willingness to pay for marginal changes in
health status probabilities ought to be of some interest to
any policy maker who expends resources with the goal of
achieving improvements in overall societal health status.

WILLINGNESS TO PAY FOR HEALTH STATUS:
A DECISION THEORY PERSPECTIVE

       Conceptually, an individual's life may be represented
by the outcome vector $[(H_1, C_1), (H_2, C_2, ..., (H_n, C_n))]$,
where H_t denotes the individual's health status in period t,
C_t his consumption level in period t, and n the number of
remaining periods in the individual's life.* From the individual's perspective, this outcome vector is subject to
substantial uncertainty. The individual is uncertain as to
how many periods he will survive. Assuming that he survives
to period t, he is also uncertain regarding that period.
He is unsure as to his health status and as to his consumption level. These sources of uncertainty are not independent of one another. The individual's probability of

---

*   To simplify this discussion, I do not consider bequest
    motives for the legacy the individual leaves to his
    heirs.

surviving period t is clearly conditional on his health
status in period t-1, and possibly in earlier periods.
Similarly, because earning power may depend on health status,
the individual's consumption level in period t is conditional
on his health status in that period and, possibly, earlier
periods. Thus, from the individual's point of view, the effect of alternative health and safety policies is to alter the
joint probability distribution over health status and consumption for each of the possible future periods of his life.

Consider a completely selfish individual who values
health and safety programs only to the extent that they benefit or harm him, and assume that the individual is rational in
the sense that he bases decisions on the "expected utility
principle" (von Neumann and Morgenstern, 1944; Savage, 1954).
The expected utility principle is a formal decision rule which
can be derived from an intuitively appealing set of normative
guidelines for decision making in the presence of risk or uncertainty (see Raiffa, 1968).* In particular, if $(A^1, A^2,$
$..., A^m)$ is a mutually exclusive and exhaustive set of
possible consequences of those alternatives, and $p_j{}^i$ denotes
the conditional probability that consequences X_j
will occur if act A^i is selected, then the <u>expected utility</u>
of act A^i, denoted by $E[U(A^i)]$, is

$$E[U(A^i)] = \sum_{j=1}^{n} p_j{}^i \, U(X_j).$$

If the individual's preferences satisfy the normative axioms
alluded to above, then it can be shown that:

(1) $U(\cdot)$ is defined on an interval scale;

(2)   the individual will choose that alternative
      which maximizes expected utility.

Consider now the simplest willingness-to-pay dilemma
which might confront our rational but purely egocentric
decision maker. First, assume that the policy alternatives
affect the individual's outcome probabilities only for the
next period. Second, suppose that health status is a binary
variable, for example, life versus death. Assume that under
the status quo, the individual experiences consumption level
c^o and faces a p^o chance of dying. Thus, his status quo
option may be represented by the lottery

---

* Here I ignore the potential distinction between "risk" and
  "uncertainty," assuming that all uncertainty can be expressed in the form of (possibly subjective) probability
  distributions.

$$A^o \equiv \left\langle \begin{array}{l} \underline{\quad 1-p^o \quad} \quad (C^o, \text{ Live}) \\ \\ \underline{\qquad\qquad} \quad (C^o, \text{ Die}) \\ \quad p^o \end{array} \right.$$

with expected utility

$$E[U(A^o)] = (1-p^o)U(C^o, \text{ Live}) + p^o U(C^o, \text{ Die}).$$

Suppose that an alternative policy A' reduces the individual's chances of dying by some amount $\delta (\delta \leq p^o)$, but that the individual will be forced to sacrifice x dollars of consumption to obtain this reduction in his chances of dying. Schematically

$$A' \equiv \left\langle \begin{array}{l} \underline{\quad 1-(p^o-\delta) \quad} \quad (C^o-x, \text{ Live}) \\ \\ \underline{\qquad\qquad\qquad} \quad (C^o-x, \text{ Die}) \\ \quad (p^o-\delta) \end{array} \right.$$

Then his maximum willingness to pay for a δ reduction in mortality is given by x* such that

$$(1-p^o)U(C^o, \text{ Live}) + p^o U(C^o, \text{ Die}) = [1-(p^o-\delta)]$$

$$U(C^o-x^*, \text{ Live}) + (p^o-\delta)U(C^o-x, \text{ Die}).$$

For if $x < x^*$, A' is preferred to A^o, and if $x > x^*$, A^o is preferred to A'.

Four points are worth noting here. (1) Willingness to pay for a reduction in mortality obviously depends on the initial level of consumption, C^o. Other things being equal, it seems reasonable to expect that the greater C^o, the greater the willingness to pay for a δ reduction.* (2) Not so obviously, willingness to pay for a δ reduction should also depend on the initial risk level, p^o. For example, I would be willing to pay more to reduce my chances of dying from .002 to .001 than to reduce them from .500 to .499, even though the incremental change in risk level is the

---

* This result can also be derived from a variety of sets of plausible assumptions about preferences. See, for example, Jones-Lee (1976) and Weinstein and others (1975).

same.* The fact that willingness to pay for incremental
changes in risk is dependent on both initial risk level and
initial consumption level considerably complicates the problem of empirically assessing willingness to pay. For it
means that we must study the effects of variation in C^o, p^o,
and δ. (3) Even in this single period formulation, multi-
period considerations are implicitly involved. In particular,
single period tradeoffs between consumption and risk of mortality should depend on expectations about future mortality
levels. For example, I would be less willing to sacrifice
current period consumption for marginal reductions in current
mortality risk if I knew that I had a terminal illness doom-
ing me to sure death in the near future. Thus, single period
willingness-to-pay formulations implicitly assume that the
decision maker considers probable future outcomes in evaluating current outcomes. Finally, it should be noted that the
analysis developed above is equally applicable to the case
of increases in risk of death. Here the alternative policy
may be represented by

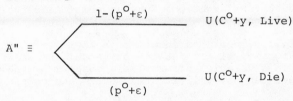

where ε is the added risk of death and y is the compensation
price offered to induce the decision maker to accept the additional risk. It is, in principle, straightforward to re-
lax the restrictive assumptions made above. For example, if
we wish to use a fuller health status measure--say one involving 50 possible outcomes instead of two--then each single
period lottery will involve 50 branches and 50 outcomes instead of just two.

When the consequences of alternatives ripple through
future periods, the single period formulation is no longer
adequate. For example, from an individual's standpoint, the
enforcement of stricter environmental quality standards is
likely to have a depressive effect on both his short-
run and long-run consumption levels (relative to what they
would be in the absence of such standards). But the health

---

* Jones-Lee (1976) and Weinstein and others (1975) prove
  that willingness to pay for a given decrement in risk
  should depend on the initial risk level. Interest-
  ingly, however, their proofs violate my intuition.
  In particular, they prove that willingness to pay for
  a given decrement in risk should (given plausible
  assumptions about preferences) be monotonically increasing with initial risk level.

status benefits to the individual are likely to be confined
primarily to the long run. Thus, an appropriate
willingness-to-pay analysis of programs with delayed consequences necessarily requires that the individual consider the
joint probability distribution over time of consumption level
and health status. In practice, the decision trees associated with multi-period decision problems with uncertain consequences tend to be extremely complex--so complex that often
such decision problems can only be represented, stored, and
solved by computer. To the applied mathematician, such complexity is inconvenient but challenging. To the intuitive
decision maker, it is simply overwhelming.*

     Willingness-to-pay problems become even more complex
when we introduce the possibility of altruism. For if an
individual cares about the health and safety of others, then
his total willingness to pay for a program will also be a
function of the probabilistic impact of the program on the
present and future health status of those for whom the buyer
cares. Such considerations further complicate the structure
of the decision tree.

     It is by now apparent that in the context of health and
safety programs, willingness to pay should be based on a
reasoned consideration of extremely complex probabilistic re-
lations between several variables over many points in time.

PSYCHOLOGICAL STUDIES OF JUDGMENT AND CHOICE:
IMPLICATIONS FOR THE ASSESSMENT OF WILLINGNESS TO PAY

Some Basic Limitations of Human Information Processing

     Beginning with the pioneering work of Miller
(1956), cognitive psychologists have attempted to establish
the fundamental constraints governing human reasoning
processes. Miller's most well-known contribution to this
literature was his discovery of the "magic number 7, plus or
minus 2." First, he found that ordinary human beings can
store at most five to nine "chunks of conceptual information"
in short-term memory.** Thus, for example, unfamiliar long

---

*   Throughout this paper, I use the adjective intuitive to
     characterize inferences and decisions that are made with-
     out resort to formal mathematical analysis.

**   With efficient coding schemes, a "chunk" may contain many
     "bites" of information. However, the more complex coding
     scheme, the smaller the number of chunks which can be
     stored. Also, the more complex the logical operations ap-
     plied to chunks, the smaller the number of chunks which
     can be stored.

distance telephone numbers of 10 digits strain the limits of
our short-term memory. Second, Miller found that when humans
are asked to classify stimuli varying along a pure perceptual
continuum, they are able to reliably use only five to nine
categories.* Although memorizing simple lists and classifying pure stimuli may seem far removed from complex decision
processes, important relationships do exist. All rational
models of choice assume that people implicitly trade off one
outcome attribute against another, weight outcomes by their
likelihoods, and so forth. Implicitly, then, these models
assume that human beings are able to manipulate many pieces
of information at the same time. Miller's findings suggest
that people cannot. Further, when people form subjective
expectations (probabilities) about future events, they must,
in essence, categorize events along a pure continuum--
likelihood. Similarly, complex choices implicitly force the
decision maker to categorize many outcomes in terms of their
relative desirability or subjective utility. Miller's findings suggest that intuitive expectations and preferences are
much less finely grained than the formal probability and
utility models of economists, statisticians, and decision
theorists.

Numerous investigators have attempted to statistically
model intuitive forecasting, inference, and decision-making
processes, in both laboratory and field settings. These
studies (many of which are reviewed by Slovic and
Lichtenstein, 1971) are universally consistent with Miller's
findings. In most cases, three or fewer variables explain
80 percent or more of the predictable (non-random) variance
in individual behavior. And to my knowledge, no study has
found evidence that individuals systematically respond to
more than eight to ten "chunks" of information.

The Pitfalls of Intuitive Inference and Prediction

Almost all interesting choice dilemmas force decision
makers to choose between alternatives whose consequences are
uncertain. This is clearly the case for most decisions affecting health and safety. Under such circumstances, the intuitive decision maker must--if he is to behave at all
rationally--attempt to consider the uncertainties involved.
Numerous laboratory and field studies have examined the
quality of intuitive inferences and predictions in uncertain
environments. Here I briefly summarize some of the major
findings of these studies, organizing this summary around a
series of properties which should characterize the behavior
of a "good intuitive statistician."

---

* People can make much finer discriminations when they are
  simply asked to make paired comparison judgments between
  stimuli.

(1) The inferences and predictions of a good intuitive statistician should be "coherent" in the sense of
satisfying the basic laws of probability theory. For example, conditional and joint probability assessments should
be appropriately related. The probabilities assigned to sets
of mutually exclusive events should satisfy the summation
rule. When prior probabilities are revised in light of new
data, the revision process should be consistent with Bayes's
theorem. Some investigators have found an impressive degree
of correspondence between the organization of subjective beliefs and the laws of probability theory (see, for example,
Wyer, 1975). But many others have found systematic discrepancies. Recent review papers by Slovic and Lichtenstein
(1971) and Tversky and Kahneman (1974) document the following
major shortcomings of intuitive statistical judgments. First,
when people revise their beliefs in light of new information,
their inferences show little relation to the prescriptions of
Bayes's theorem. Sometimes they alter their beliefs too
much; at other times too little. At times, intuitive inferences systematically violate even the ordinal implications
of Bayes's theorem. People also seem unable to adjust their
inferences when presented with unreliable (or noisy) data.
Often they ignore the unreliability problem altogether, treating the information as error free. People also fail to adjust for redundancy. The consistency of redundant data
sources leads people to extract too much information from redundant data. By contrast, people fail to give enough weight
to surprising or unexpected events. Given that an unexpected
event is often very informative, the human tendency to ignore
events which are inconsistent with currently favored hypotheses is far from adaptive. In short, human inference
processes are frequently incoherent in the sense of deviating
rather drastically from the prescriptions of probability
theory.

(2) The predictions of a good intuitive statistician
should be "well-calibrated" in the sense that, on the average,
of all the events assigned a p probability of occurrence,
(100 p) percent of those events should occur. For example,
aggregating over all those days on which your weather fore-
caster says there is a .25 chance of rain, you might reasonably hope that there would be rain on roughly 25 percent of
those days. In fact, recent studies indicate that U.S.
Weather Service forecasters are remarkably well-calibrated
when making short-term precipitation forecasts. But a review paper by Lichtenstein and others (1976)
indicates that the excellent calibration of weather forecasters is a glaring exception. In general, intuitive
probability forecasts are characterized by extreme "overconfidence." Specifically, people assign excessively high
probabilities to events which they view as relatively likely;
they assign excessively low probabilities to events which
they view as unlikely. For example, numerous studies have
found that 25 percent or more of events fall beyond the

bounds of intuitively-assessed 99 percent confidence intervals. Consequently, people should very often be sur-
prised by the events which occur about them. Why do they not
learn from experience to temper the confidence of their predictions? First, learning is possible only when unambiguous
feedback is available. Often it is not. Second, if feedback
is delayed, people may "forget" their earlier predictions.
In fact, Fischoff and Beyth (1975) conducted a longitudinal
study which shows that when people are given delayed (several weeks) outcome feedback, they conveniently distort their
recollections and recall making forecasts which are consistent
with the actual outcome. This bias effectively eliminates the
possibility of learning from experience. The excellent calibration of weather forecasters may well be attributable not
only to the fact that they receive immediate feedback, but
also to the fact that the public nature of their forecasts
forces them to acknowledge the surprises which do occur.
These, certainly, are the ideal conditions for eliminating
the overconfidence bias.

    (3) The good intuitive statistician must be able to
make fine discriminations between the relative likelihoods of
rare events. This capacity is crucial if the intuitive
statistician is to be able to respond rationally when confronted with low probability catastrophic events. Decisions
affecting health or safety are often of this nature.
Realizing that very large samples of data are needed to accurately estimate small probabilities, anyone with a rudi-
mentary knowledge of sampling theory might quickly surmise
that people cannot make such discriminations. In fact,
Slovic and others (1976) have found that people are quite
poor at assessing very small probabilities. The researchers presented subjects with pairs of causes of
death--for example, lung cancer and stomach cancer--and
asked them (1) to judge which was the more likely cause of
death and (2) to estimate the relative odds. Only when
the true (actuarial) odds of the more or less likely cause
of death exceeded 2:1 were the subjects able to make even
reliable ordinal discriminations. The investigators also
found that subjects systematically overestimated the likelihood of highly publicized or feared causes of death--for
example, fires, homicide, and cancer.

Decisions in the Presence of Uncertainty

    Most well-controlled studies of decision making (given
uncertainty) have considered only very simple forms of behavior, for example, choices between pairs of two-outcome
gambles. In general, these studies have shown that the expected utility model typically provides an excellent approximation to the gambling behavior of individual subjects
(Davidson and others, 1957; Tversky, 1967). But even
for very simple risky decisions, systematic violations

of the expected utility model have been observed. In two
separate studies, one conducted in a Las Vegas casino,
Lichtenstein and Slovic (1973, 1971) obtained systematic
discrepancies between gambles and statements of willingness
to pay for gambles. In particular, a subject might bid $10
for gamble A and $7 for gamble B, yet when offered the option
to play either A or B at no cost, choose B over A.* This
result was explained by the fact that subjects pay more attention to the odds of winning when they choose between types
of gambles, but focus more on the amounts to be won or lost
when bidding for gambles. This is a particularly disturbing
finding because it brings into question the validity of the
preference concept which underlies all rational models of
choice.

When we move from simple gambles to choices between
complex alternatives, the descriptive power of rational choice
models is further diminished. When subjects are asked to perform search tasks, sequential sampling tasks, or to make production and inventory decisions under well-controlled experimental conditions, their behavior often does not even re-
motely approximate that of the optimal mathematical programming model (for a review, see Rappoport and Wallsten,
1970). This is true even when subjects are motivated by substantial financial costs and payoffs and when experienced
businessmen have performed the inventory and production
tasks. Apparently people are unable to cope with the full
complexity of these tasks, using simple heuristic decision
rules which often completely ignore crucial aspects of the
decision problem (see Payne, 1976).

Further evidence for this proposition is provided by
Kunreuther's (1976) study of insurance purchases by 3,000
households in areas prone to earthquake and flood. The expected utility model can be readily applied to prescribe or
predict the amount of insurance purchased. In Kunreuther's
formulation, the optimal purchase level was a function of
four variables: the cost per dollar of insurance protection,
the probability of disaster, the dollar loss if disaster
occurs, and the percent tax write-off on uninsured losses.
Kunreuther conducted his household survey in order to
evaluate this model (and others). The results of the survey
cast severe doubt on the descriptive validity of the expected utility model: (1) Despite the fact that the survey
was conducted only in (relatively) high risk areas where appropriate disaster insurance was available, only two-thirds
of the residents were even aware of the existence of such
insurance. Even larger proportions of the population were
unaware of the cost of this insurance. (2) Despite the

---

* In fact, many people refused to admit that they had made a
  mistake when confronted with this obvious inconsistency in
  their behavior.

relatively homogeneous risk levels confronting individual
households, respondents varied enormously (by over a factor
of 10,000) in their assessments of the probability of
disaster.

As the above facts make clear, the expected utility
model provides no insight whatsoever into the behavior of a
substantial proportion (over one-third) of Kunreuther's
respondents simply because they lacked the information necessary to make an informed choice.* Further, Kunreuther's
analyses suggest that a substantial proportion of those respondents who did possess the necessary information made
choices which were irrational inasmuch as they violated the
expected utility model. In short, Kunreuther's findings are
extremely damaging to the expected utility model of behavior
in the face of low-probability, high-risk events.**

Conclusion

In brief, psychological studies of inference, pre-
diction, and choice lead to the conclusion that human beings
are at best adaptively rational, relying on relatively simple
heuristic rules and adjusting their behavior through a process
of trial and error. Unfortunately, this fact means that
people are poorly equipped to respond to situations involving
either complex probabilistic processes or small probabilities
of catastrophic events. Nor are they well-equipped to make
decisions whose consequences extend far into the future. For
such decisions, if they are to be made rationally, require
that the decision maker explicitly consider complex lotteries
over several variables at many points in time. That task
easily exceeds the limits of human intuitive reasoning
powers.

OPERATIONAL PROCEDURES FOR ASSESSING WILLINGNESS TO PAY

In discussing possible strategies for actually assessing willingness to pay for health and safety programs, or for
the health-related consequences of stricter environmental
standards, it is useful to classify procedures along two
dimensions. First, we may distinguish between procedures
which attempt to directly assess willingness to pay for

----

* One might try to defend the rational model by arguing
that many individuals rationally chose not to pay the
costs of acquiring this information. Without support-
ing evidence, however, this argument is not compelling.

** Kunreuther is now in the process of testing a variety
of heuristic models of such behavior.

programs or stricter standards per se, and those which attempt
to assess willingness to pay for program outcomes. When assessment is with respect to outcomes, the policy analyst
simply computes the individual's willingness to pay for
various programs, based on the analyst's assumptions about
what the program consequences will be. Second, we may distinguish between two types of assessment procedures: (1)
those which infer willingness to pay based on real decisions
in the market place and (2) those which infer willingness to
pay based on hypothetical decisions or answers to hypothetical
willingness-to-pay questions.

    In discussing alternative assessment methods, it is
also useful to distinguish between three criteria which may
be used to evaluate methods. First, a good assessment procedure should be reliable in the sense of being relatively
free of random error. If the reliability we need is only at
an aggregate level, then the central limit theorem implies
that we need not be excessively concerned about random variation at the individual level.* Second, the measurement procedure should be unbiased in the usual statistical sense.
And third, the procedure should be valid in the sense of reflecting the "true preferences" of individuals.

    While the distinction between true as opposed to ap-
parent preferences is tenuous at best, I believe that the
following conditions are necessary (though not sufficient)
for valid preference assessment. First, either the individual
whose preferences are being assessed must accurately perceive
the probabilistic relationships between acts and outcomes,
or the preference assessor must be aware of the individual's
information state. For if the individual's information state
differs from that of the observer who measures his
preferences, serious inferential errors may occur. For example, suppose that an individual refuses to employ a car's
shoulder harness system simply because he believes that this
system increases the chances of death or serious injury. An
external observer, unaware of the individual's information
state, might easily make the incorrect inference that the individual viewed the trivial costs of buckling up as more than
offsetting the benefits associated with a reduced probability
of death or serious injury. Second, valid preference assessment is possible only if the behavior of the individual whose
preferences are being assessed is "coherent" in the sense of
satisfying the usual axioms of rational choice. For example,
we cannot measure the preferences of an individual who claims
to prefer A to B, B to C, and C to A, for, quite literally,

---

* This will normally be the case in cost-benefit analyses,
   since we will be summing over many individuals.

that person does not know what he wants.* Similarly, we cannot measure the preferences of a person who claims to prefer
X to Y, but is willing to pay more for Y than for X. Only
when behavior is coherent can we make inferences about
preferences.**

Using these ideas and drawing upon the arguments developed in previous sections of this paper, we are now in a
position to evaluate a variety of strategies for operationally
measuring willingness to pay for improvements in health and
safety.

Market-revealed Willingness to Pay

Given the choice, most economists would prefer to use
actual market decisions as a basis for making inferences about
willingness to pay. The bias toward market-based inferences
seems to reflect the intuitively plausible belief that if a
decision is "real" (that is, has "real" consequences), then
the individual will take it seriously, and his behavior will
therefore reveal true preferences. By contrast, when an interviewer presents the individual with a hypothetical decision, nothing is at stake, so the possibility arises that
the individual will either not take the decision seriously or
will simply tell the interviewer what he thinks the interviewer wants to hear.***

Unfortunately, serious practical problems arise when
one actually attempts to infer willingness to pay from market
behavior. Among these are the following:

(1) The statistical procedures employed gen-
     erally lead to valid inferences only in
     perfectly competitive markets. If market
     imperfections are substantial, statistical
     inferences may be seriously in error.

(2) In many cases, the "good" in question has
     never been sold on a market.

---

*   Technically, this person's choices violate the transi-
     tivity axiom, one of the basic premises of all rational
     theories.

**   For a more formal elaboration of this argument, see
     Coombs and others (1970, pp. 7-30).

*** This latter possibility also arises for self-reports
     of actual behavior.

(3)   It is extremely difficult to accurately
      assess the information states of the in-
      dividuals participating in markets.
      Typically, the statistician must assume
      that these individuals have the same in-
      formation he does. If this assumption
      is false, inferences about preferences
      per se may be seriously in error.

Despite these and other problems, economists have attempted to obtain market-based estimates of willingness to
pay for reductions in mortality probability. In essence,
such efforts (1) reduce health status to a binary outcome
variable and (2) attempt to estimate the marginal rate of
substitution between income (or wealth) and yearly survival
probability. To illustrate this approach, we shall briefly
discuss Thaler and Rosen's (1975) widely cited study of the
wage premiums paid to persons employed in hazardous occupations. Thaler and Rosen begin by explaining the dynamics of
a perfect competitive market in which workers demand a wage
premium in exchange for performing hazardous work, and employers offer wage premiums to the extent that premiums are
more profitable than investing in safety improvements. Ignoring the rather substantial market imperfections introduced
by government safety requirements and union-negotiated safety
clauses, Thaler and Rosen estimate these wage premiums by re-
gressing weekly wage rates on a series of dependent variables,
including the following: (1) the added annual probability of
death associated with the job in question;* (2) a set of
worker characteristics, including age, education, and family
status; (3) a set of job characteristics, including unioni-
zation, industrial sector, and the nature of the job; and
(4) dummy variables for region of the country and urban versus
rural. With the exception of the occupational risk variable,
all data were obtained from a large University of Michigan
cross-sectional survey of lower income male-headed households in 1967. The occupational risk data were obtained from
a separate 1967 study of job-specific mortality rates. Using
these data, and employing a variety of model specifications,
Thaler and Rosen conclude that in 1967 workers demanded an
average annual wage premium somewhere between $140 and $260 in
return for accepting an incremental increase of .001 in their
annual probability of dying. These numbers have been widely
cited as providing a reasonable basis for bracketing the
social value of incremental changes in mortality rates.

From a psychological standpoint, that conclusion seems
most debatable; for the validity of Thaler and Rosen's procedure rests on the assumption that individual workers accurately perceive the objective (actuarial) risks which

---

* Only riskier-than-average jobs were studied.

confront them.* In fact, the added risk of death associated
with the occupations studied ranged from .00002 per year (for
linemen and servicemen) to .00267 per year (for guards and
watchmen). These are very small incremental changes by any
standard, and the experimental results cited earlier suggest
that people simply cannot reliably discriminate between such
small probabilities. And to the extent that subjective perceptions of risk deviate from objective reality, an "errors
in variables" problem arises which results in biased inference. More fundamentally, the psychological findings cited
earlier suggest that decisions to accept hazardous jobs may
reflect little understanding of the risk involved, for people
are simply not capable of accurately perceiving very small
differences between probabilities. Consequently, I am of the
opinion that market-based inferences about willingness to pay
for marginal reductions in mortality or morbidity rates will
seldom (if ever) be valid as defined at the beginning of this
section.

Survey-based Inferences about Willingness to Pay

        All willingness-to-pay studies relying on responses to
hypothetical questions are subject to the following criticisms: First, because nothing is at stake, respondents may
fail to take the questions seriously, or they may simply give
what they believe are socially desirable responses, which will
elicit the interviewer's approval. This is a real problem,
but as Mishan (1971) has argued, imperfect survey data may
well be better than no data at all. Second, critics have
argued that hypothetical judgments are particularly difficult
when dealing with small probabilities of catastrophic events
such as death. As Schelling (1968) has noted, however, even
real decisions involving small probabilities of death (say
buckling a seat belt) have a strangely hypothetical aura to
them; these decisions are often made hastily with little
calculation. Thus, it is not obvious that real behavior
necessarily provides a better indicator of true preference.
Also, survey procedures permit the investigator to control
the information upon which respondents base their decisions,
thus eliminating a potentially major source of inferential
error.

        Willingness to pay for programs.--It is at least
imaginable that a public official might commission a survey
research organization to poll the residents of a region and
ask the following: "What is the most you would be willing
to pay per year to have an additional fully-equipped 250-bed
hospital in this county?" I suspect that people would agree

---

*   These objective risks are used as the independent variable
    "risk."

to answer such a question, and that it would be possible to
devise reliable procedures for eliciting their responses.
Quite possibly an individual's response might even provide a
valid measure* of willingness to pay for the new hospital
program, given the individual has a correct perception of
the planned changes. But it is extremely unlikely that
responses to such a question would provide a valid measure
of willingness to pay for the likely consequences of the
new hospital program. For it is virtually unimaginable that
an ordinary lay person could comprehend the impact of a complex health or safety program on his life, or on the lives
of those for whom he cares. This impact would typically
involve very small changes in the health state transition
probabilities confronting the individual and those for whom
he cares; because people would misperceive these small
changes, their stated willingness to pay for the program
itself would not provide an accurate reflection of what they
would be willing to pay if they correctly perceived the program's likely impact.

     Willingness to pay for health status transitions.--
Given two well-defined health states, H' and H", such that
H' is preferred to H", one might attempt to approach the
willingness-to-pay problem by asking citizens to state the
largest sum they would be willing to pay in order to spend
one (or more) periods in the preferred state H', rather than
in state H". This approach is straightforward and would be
perfectly appropriate if decisions concerning allocations
in the health and safety sector were made with "perfect
information." If it were possible, that is, to specify with
certainty the sequence of health states that each member of
the target population would experience under each alternative
policy proposal. But from an individual's point of view, the
consequences of health and safety programs are almost in-
variably uncertain. And, unfortunately, there is no simple
relationship between willingness to pay for sure health
status transitions and willingness to pay for changes in
probabilistic health status transitions. For example, assume
that a period is one week in duration, that H' denotes a
state of "perfect" (complete functioning, symptom-free)
health, and that H" denotes a state of home confinement to
bed or chair, suffering the aches, fever, sore throat, and
head congestion of a respiratory virus. Assume that I am
given the option of paying for a state of H' rather than
state H". Given the activities I have planned for the coming
week, I think I would be willing to pay roughly $200

---

* The term valid measure, used here and subsequently in
  this section, is meant to be defined as it is at the
  beginning of this section. A measurement is valid
  only (1) if the observer is aware of the individual's
  information state and (2) if the individual's behavior is coherent.

to spend that week in state H' rather than in state H". More
realistically, however, I might be facing a .10 chance of
spending next week in state H". Imagining that I have the
option of reducing that probability from .10 to 0, I can ask
the following: "What is the most I would be willing to pay
to eliminate any possibility of my having a respiratory
virus next week?" One might attempt to infer my willingness
to pay from the fact that I would give up $200 to avoid a
sure week in bed. For example, it might be argued that I
should be willing to pay .10 x $200 ($20) to avoid a 10 percent chance of spending next week in bed with the flu. But
no accepted principle of rational choice states that $20 must
be my maximum willingness to pay. In fact, assuming that I
am a "risk averse" expected-utility maximizer,* $20 will not
be my maximum willingness to pay. I should be willing to
pay more. In fact, I am, probably up to $25. Consequently,
my stated willingness to pay for sure changes in health status
provides no exact information about my willingness to pay for
probabilistic changes in health status. The problem is particularly acute when death is one of the relevant health
states. I would be willing to sacrifice all of my current
assets plus everything I could borrow to avoid the certainty
of dying tomorrow. But I would be willing to pay almost as
much to avoid a 50-50 chance of dying tomorrow. Clearly,
information about willingness to pay for sure health state
transitions is not helpful when the actual outcomes are uncertain and death is one of those outcomes.

Willingness to pay for changes in health status
transition probabilities.--The arguments developed above
strongly suggest that what is needed is information concerning people's willingness to pay for marginal changes in
health status transition probabilities. Numerous analysts
have recognized this fact (for example, Schelling, 1968;
Acton, 1973; Conley, 1976; Lipscomb, 1976). From a practical
standpoint, however, there remains the unresolved question:
Can we devise a valid procedure for obtaining such information? In the simplest possible case, the willingness to pay
for health status transition probabilities can be confined to
a single period, and the health status variable can be
dichotomous, for example, life or death. The question we
might wish to ask is the following: What is the most that
an individual would be willing to pay to achieve a .001 reduction in his probability of dying next year?

This is, of course, the type of question which Thaler
and Rosen attempted to answer by analyzing the wage premiums
paid to persons employed in hazardous occupations. Acton

---

* Among other things, a risk-averse-expected-utility maximizer will always prefer the expected monetary value of
  a gamble to the gamble itself. See Raiffa (1968).

(1973) addressed the same question using a direct survey procedure. In particular, he attempted to determine how much
people would be willing to pay for emergency coronary care
services which reduced the probability that a heart attack
victim would die as a direct consequence of the heart attack.
The questionnaire that Acton used provided most of the information that a rational (expected-utility-maximizing) individual would need in order to give an informed willingness-
to-pay judgment. In particular, the respondent was given an
assumed level of risk of heart attack per year (.01 and .05)
and an assumed risk of death if he experienced a heart attack
(.40).   The respondent was also given the effectiveness level
of the new emergency care system. With two initial risk
levels and two effectiveness levels, the respondents evaluated
four scenarios. Assuming a low initial risk of heart attack
(.01), they gave willingness-to-pay statements for emergency
care systems which had either a .001 or .002 chance of saving
their life; and assuming a high initial risk level (.05),
they evaluated systems having either a .005 or .01 chance of
saving their life.

Acton administered his questionnaire to three separate
groups of respondents. The first was a small (n=36) strati-
fied random sample of residents of three communities in the
metropolitan Boston area. The second and third were groups
of trade union leaders (n=21) and advanced management personnel (n=36) attending short courses at the Harvard Business
School. For the community sample, questionnaires were orally
administered by trained interviewers. For the trade union
and advanced management samples, questionnaires were
self-administered.

Acton's questionnaire was carefully developed and pre-
tested. The questions he asked made good theoretical sense.
Not surprisingly, his study has often been viewed as demon-
strating the feasibility of obtaining direct statements of
willingness to pay for marginal reductions in mortality rates.
It is this conclusion which I wish to question.

Testing Acton's respondents by the two necessary conditions for valid preference measurement, there do not seem
to be any major difficulties. First, the respondent must
correctly perceive the probabilistic relationships between
acts and outcomes. Assuming that Acton's respondents understood all of the probabilities he provided, the first necessary condition for valid preference measurement appears to
have been fulfilled. Of course, it is by no means obvious
that his respondents did understand the information he
provided.

The second validity criterion--namely, that the behavior of respondents be coherent or rational--is easier to
test. For example, under almost any reasonable assumption,
a rational person should be willing to pay something (perhaps

not very much) to avert a small chance of dying. Also,
willingness to pay for reductions in mortality rate should be
a non-decreasing function of the magnitude of that reduction.
That is, other things being equal, a person should not pay
more for a small reduction in mortality than for a large one.

While these seem to be very minimal criteria for es-
tablishing the coherence of behavior, it is apparent that a
substantial proportion of Acton's respondents failed to
satisfy them. He describes 10 response patterns, only two of
which satisfy both of the criteria. While Acton (1973, p. 91)
laments the fact that the desired patterns were not more common, he gives no breakdown on the number of respondents dis-
playing each pattern. We can make some rough guesses, however, from data he provides in his paper.* First, four of
the 36 community sample respondents gave one or more zero
responses, as did seven of the 21 trade union leaders. Also,
only 14 of the 36 advanced management course sample members
gave responses which were a non-decreasing function of the
probability that their life would be saved. Finally, of the
46 community and trade union sample members who made no zero
responses, only 20 satisfied the non-decreasing function
criterion. In short, well over half of Acton's respondents
gave incoherent responses. This fact suggests that many respondents were unable to "understand" the task set for them.
If so, I would argue that their responses are uninformative
as to their preferences, and, thus, that the Acton measurement procedure fails to provide a valid measure of willingness
to pay.

This conclusion is quite disturbing for two reasons.
First, Acton went to considerable lengths to develop and pre-
test his questionnaire. His respondents' inconsistent behavior cannot be attributed to a slipshod effort. (Of course,
it is possible that other ways of asking the same questions
would lead to better results.) Also, Acton's poor results
arose in the simplest possible willingness-to-pay problem of
interest--namely, the single period, two health states problem (see the preceding section). If a substantial proportion
of potential respondents give inconsistent responses even in
this relatively simple case, it seems extremely unlikely that
respondents would be able to respond consistently to hypothetical multi-period lottery decisions. Thus, my interpretation of Acton's data suggests that preference assessment
procedures, based on explicit statements of willingness to
pay, are unlikely to meet the two necessary conditions for
valid preference measurement.

---

* These data are obtained by noting the number of respondents Acton excludes from various analyses and noting
  the reasons for their exclusion.

The decision analysis approach to willingness to pay.
--All of the approaches discussed so far implicitly assume
that people know what they want and that the policy analyst's
only problem is to devise procedures for measuring these
preferences. But given the complexity of most willingness-
to-pay questions in the health and safety area, it is not
obvious that people are capable of intuitively responding to
such questions. For example, it is possible that the incoherent behavior of Acton's respondents was due not to some
fault of his survey procedure, but rather to the fact that
even his relatively simple willingness-to-pay questions exceeded the limits of many of his respondents' intuitive
reasoning powers.

Decision analysis is a subdiscipline of applied mathematics which provides a set of procedures for explicitly
analyzing complex decision problems and choosing according to
the expected utility principle (see, for example, Raiffa,
1968). While an economist may feel uncomfortable with the
assertion that people do not know their own preferences, the
applied decision analyst routinely assumes that people are
incapable of intuitively comprehending complex choice
problems. Decision analysts advise decision makers as to
what their preferences for acts should be, given: (1) that
the decision maker wishes to choose according to the expected
utility principle, (2) a probability model, linking acts to
outcomes, which the decision maker accepts as providing a
valid representation of his beliefs, and (3) a utility model,
defined over the set of possible consequences, which the
decision maker accepts as providing a valid representation
of his preferences. Given these preconditions, selection of
an appropriate course of action reduces to a computational
exercise.

Because willingness-to-pay problems relating to health
and safety may often exceed the limits of people's intuitive
reasoning power, it seems natural to consider what a decision
analyst might do in advising an individual on some complex
willingness-to-pay problems. Here I simply assume that the
individual wishes to base his decisions on the expected
utility principle and is willing to let the "experts" supply
the model specifying the probabilistic linkages between acts
and outcomes. Thus, the primary task confronting the
decision analyst is that of specifying a utility function
$U(\cdot)$, defined over all possible streams of future consumption
and health. For, given such a function, the determination
of willingness to pay reduces to a (possibly complex) optimization exercise.

The first stage in specifying $U(\cdot)$ is to determine
a functional form. One particularly appealing form is the
additive utility model,

$$U [(H_1, C_1),\ldots, (H_n, C_n)] = \sum_{t=1}^{n} a_t [U_h(H_t) + U_h(C_t)]$$

where $U_h(\cdot)$ and $U_c(\cdot)$ are comparably scaled utility functions defined over health status and consumption, respectively, and where a_t are scaling constants reflecting the relative weight to be given to each time period. Decision theorists have developed relatively simple procedures for directly assessing the parameters of additive utility models; recent experimental evidence demonstrates that when preferences are additive (or nearly so), these procedures generate a very accurate representation of people's preferences (Fischer, 1977). Unfortunately, a priori considerations suggest that additive models will seldom provide an accurate representation of preferences over time, at least not when uncertainty is involved. This assertion can best be supported using a simple example. Again, let H' denote a state of perfect (complete functioning and symptom-free) health, and H" denote a day of home confinement to bed or chair, suffering from the aches, fever, and congestion of a respiratory virus. Letting a period be a day in duration, we now consider two lotteries defined over the next five-day work week:

$$L_1 \equiv \begin{cases} .20 & (H_1", H_2', H_3', H_4', H_5') \\ .20 & (H_1', H_2", H_3', H_4', H_5') \\ .20 & (H_1', H_2', H_3", H_4', H_5') \\ .20 & (H_1', H_2', H_3', H_4", H_5') \\ .20 & (H_1', H_2', H_3', H_4', H_5") \end{cases}$$

$$L_2 \equiv \begin{cases} .20 & (H_1", H_2", H_3", H_4", H_5") \\ .80 & (H_1', H_2', H_3', H_4', H_5') \end{cases}$$

Viewed from one perspective, these two health status lotteries are very different. With L_1, you are sure of spending one (but only one) of the next five days sick in bed, and the only question is which one. With L_2, by contrast, there is one chance in five that you will spend the whole week sick in bed and four chances in five that you will escape without ever contracting the flu. From another perspective, however, these two lotteries are very similar. In particular, for each day of your coming work week, each lottery gives one chance in

five of home confinement with the flu, and four chances in
five of perfect health. It can easily be shown that if a
decision maker's preferences are inter-temporally additive,
then he will always be indifferent between any two lotteries
which have an identical probability distribution over outcomes in each period.* Since L_1 and L_2 have identical outcome distributions for each day of the week, one's preferences
for the health states in question are inter-temporally additive only if one is indifferent between L_1 and L_2. A casual
survey of seven of my colleagues suggests that most people
are not. Six of the seven preferred option L_1; the other,
option L_2. No one professed indifference despite the fact
that I explicitly included that as an option. Two commented
that missing five days of work was more than five times as
bad as missing one. Another said that he could "use a day
off," but that he could not afford a one-in-five chance of
losing a whole week. Each of these arguments favoring option
L_1 results in a form of inter-temporal risk aversion which
is inconsistent with any inter-temporally additive utility
model. I suspect that such inter-temporal risk aversion is
common among those subgroups of the population for whom any
protracted illness would be extremely disruptive.

Meyer (1970) and Richard (1972) have developed non-
additive multi-period utility models which are capable of
reflecting tastes that are either temporally risk-averse or
temporally risk-seeking. Moreover, they have devised procedures for specifying the parameters of these non-additive
multi-period utility models. Unfortunately, these procedures
require the decision maker to respond to a series of hypothetical choice dilemmas which appear to me to be much more
difficult to think about than direct willingness-to-pay
questions.** Thus, the validity of the responses that people
give to these questions is in doubt. Also, it seems to me
most unlikely that an "ordinary person on the street" could
even begin to comprehend the meaning of these questions. A
good background in decision theory and applied mathematics
seems to be an essential prerequisite for understanding the
hypothetical choices used in specifying the parameters of
non-additive inter-temporal utility models.

By contrast, model specification is quite simple if
one is willing to invoke the inter-temporal additivity

---

* Fishburn (1965) proved a general result for all multi-
  dimensional utility models. Here I simply apply his
  result to the special case of multi-period utility models.

** For a good introduction to the literature on multi-period
   utility models, and for a description of the scaling procedures, see Keeney and Raiffa (1976).

assumption. Fischer and Vaupel (1976) fitted relatively
simple temporally additive utility models to directly stated
preferences for outcomes, described by length of life and
average consumption level. Here the respondents demonstrated
a very high level of consistency and the additive models generally provided an excellent approximation to the respondents'
behavior. The major shortcoming of this study lies in the
fact that the outcomes in question were sure things rather
than lotteries. Because temporal additivity in the absence
of risk does not imply temporal additivity in the presence
of risk, this study must be viewed as inconclusive.*

SUMMARY AND CONCLUSIONS

        I began this paper by arguing that it would be very
useful to have good data on consumers' willingness to pay
for probabilistic improvements in health status. Next, I
provided an intuitive description of how a rational consumer
would analyze a willingness-to-pay question. This discussion
suggested that in order to make an informed statement of
willingness to pay, a consumer must be able to intuitively
evaluate multi-period lotteries over multiple outcome variables. I next reviewed the psychological literature relevant to the following question: Can people make informed
decisions when confronted by complex multi-period lotteries?
The answer, I argued, is no; people cannot. Such decision
tasks simply overwhelm the limited human capacity for
reasoned choice.

        In the final section of this paper, I surveyed a
variety of approaches for obtaining empirical estimates of
willingness to pay for probabilistic improvements in health
status. In my judgment, each of the approaches surveyed has
serious shortcomings; these shortcomings have much less to
do with the inadequacies of the measurement procedures than
they do with the inherent difficulty of the questions being

----

*   Actually, respondents began by rank-ordering the set of 20
    sure outcomes. They then assigned relative utility values
    to these 20 outcomes using a "standard gamble" utility as-
    sessment procedure. Because the respondents were all stu-
    dents in a decision analysis course, they were supposed to
    be familiar with this assessment procedure. Had they em-
    ployed the procedure correctly, their responses should have
    reflected their "attitude toward risk," and thus could pro-
    vide a valid measure of preference for risky outcomes.
    As one of the authors of the study, however, I have
    serious doubts as to whether the self-administered utility
    assessment procedure truly captured the respondents' at-
    titude toward risk. Instead, I believe that they may have
    used the utility scale as a simple 0 to 100 riskless
    rating scale.

asked, for example, the following question: How much are
consumers willing to pay for a given incremental improvement
in health state transition probabilities? When we ask this
question, we implicitly assume that each consumer has a consistent set of preferences for various combinations of health
status and other forms of consumption and that the consumer
can reveal these preferences through some form of behavior.
While it is a tautology to assert that an individual will
display preferences when confronted with complex probabilistic
tradeoffs between health status and consumption (after all, an
individual must choose), it is by no means certain that the
individual's behavior will reveal a consistent set of preferences. Yet only when behavior is consistent can we make
meaningful inferences about willingness to pay. In this
paper, I have argued that people often behave inconsistently
when confronted with health or safety-related willingness-
to-pay decisions; people do so because the issues involved
are so complex that they cannot respond to them in an informed or systematic fashion. When this is the case, the
numbers we are looking for simply do not exist. When behavior
is inconsistent, preferences do not exist, at least not in
the usual rational sense. If one accepts this logic, then it
follows that the question above (How much are consumers willing to pay for a given incremental improvement in health
state transition probabilities?) will often have no answer.
It will have no answer whenever the issues are so complex that
consumers behave inconsistently. To anyone committed to the
principle that social choice should be based on the preferences of the individuals comprising society, this is a most
disturbing conclusion. What can be done to eliminate this
unfortunate state of affairs?

My bias is that of the decision analyst. When confronted by individuals choosing inconsistently (irrationally)
between complex alternatives, the decision analyst is not
dismayed, but instead sees it as an opportunity to apply the
tools of his discipline. The decision analyst begins by confronting the decision maker with some very simple choices
which the decision maker can easily understand; the decision
analyst uses these choices to assess the decision maker's
preferences for the basic outcomes at stake. Then by modeling the decision alternatives available, the decision analyst
selects the optimal course of action, assuming that the decision maker wishes to choose rationally (consistently) in
the sense of satisfying the expected utility principle. The
decision maker who follows the advice of his decision analyst,
in essence, discovers, rather than reveals, his preferences
for complex alternatives.

Applying this logic to questions of willingness to pay
for probabilistic improvements in health status, we need a
very simple prototypal decision dilemma, which will tell us
a great deal about an individual's preferences. The single
period tradeoff between consumption and risk of death seems

to represent a logical starting point. I suspect that Acton's
method of direct questioning about willingness to pay will not
work well. Finding the exact break-even point, the absolute
most one would be willing to pay, is not easy. Personally, I
find simple paired comparisons judgments much easier to think
about. For example, if presented with the alternatives

$$A^O \equiv \begin{cases} .999 & \text{(Live, \$20,000)} \\ .001 & \text{(Die)} \end{cases}$$

$$A' \equiv \begin{cases} .99 & \text{(Live, \$30,000)} \\ .01 & \text{(Die)}, \end{cases}$$

I would have no difficulty whatsoever in choosing A^O, but I
would have a very difficult time specifying the minimum value
of X such that I would be indifferent between A^O and the
lottery

$$A'' \equiv \begin{cases} .99 & \text{(Live, X)} \\ .01 & \text{(Die).} \end{cases}$$

Although individual paired comparisons judgments convey much
less information than a single indifference judgment, if one
is willing to make some plausible assumptions about the functional form of a utility model, a small number of (consistent)
paired comparisons judgments will provide a great deal of information about the parameters of the model. While I have
yet to do this experiment, I am sure that some procedure can
be devised which will lead to consistent respondent behavior.
The single period consumption level versus mortality rate
question is simply not that complex. It is difficult to believe that people cannot behave consistently when confronted
with such a simple choice, provided that the probabilities
involved differ by magnitudes which people can intuitively
comprehend.

     If the problem of obtaining meaningful measures of
single period reductions in mortality proves tractable, the
problem of dealing with more complex multi-period, multi-
health-state tradeoffs will again arise. As I have

repeatedly argued in this paper, there is a great deal of
evidence to suggest that people do not behave rationally when
confronted with decisions of such complexity. The resolution
of this dilemma is not apparent to me. As an heuristic
solution, I suspect that a "quality-adjusted life years" approach might be adequate. That is, the quality-adjustment
function could be used to transform choices between complex
vectors involving many health states into equally valued,
but relatively simple, vectors involving only "normal health"
and death.

In the short run, however, I believe that attempts to
measure willingness to pay for probabilistic health status
improvements should focus on the simple consumption versus
mortality question. For not only is that the simplest of the
willingness-to-pay questions which the health policy analyst
would like to see answered, it may well also be the most
important.

REFERENCES

Acton, Jan Paul
    1973   Evaluating Public Programs to Save Lives: The
            Case of Heart Attacks. R-950-RC. Santa Monica:
            The RAND Corporation.

Becker, G. S.
    1964   Human Capital. New York: National Bureau
            of Economic Research.

Bush, J. W., M. M. Chen, and D. L. Patrick
    1973   "Health status index in cost effectiveness:
            Analysis of PKU program." In Berg, R. E. (ed.),
            Health Status Indexes. Hospital Research and
            Educational Trust.

Conley, B. C.
    1976   The Value of Human Life in the Demand for Safety.
            Research Report, Center for Public Economics.
            San Diego: California State University.

Coombs, C. H., R. M. Dawes, and A. Tversky
    1970   Mathematical Psychology: An Elementary
            Introduction. Englewood Cliffs, N.J.:
            Prentice-Hall, Inc.

Davidson, D., P. Suppes, and S. Siegel
    1957   Decision Making: An Experimental Approach.
            Stanford University Press.

Fischer, Gregory W.
    1977   "Convergent validation of decomposed multi-
            attribute utility procedures for risky and
            riskless decisions." Organizational Behavior
            and Human Performance 18:295-315.

Fischer, Gregory W. and J. Vaupel
    1976   "A lifespan utility model: Assessing preferences
            for consumption and longevity." In Vogt, W. G.
            and M. H. Mickle (eds.), Modeling and Simulation
            7(2):1139-1144.

Fischoff, B. and R. Beyth
    1975   "I knew it would happen: Remembered probabili-
            ties of once-future things." Organizational
            Behavior and Human Performance 13:1-16.

Fishburn, P. C.
    1965   "Independence in utility theory with whole
            product sets." Operation Research 13:28-45.

Jones-Lee, M. W.
    1976   The Value of Life: An Economic Analysis.
            University of Chicago Press.

Keeney, R. L. and H. Raiffa
    1976   Decisions with Multiple Objectives. New York:
            John Wiley and Sons, Inc.

Lichtenstein, S., B. Fischoff, and L. D. Phillips
            "Calibration of probabilities: The state of the
            art." In Jungerman, H. and G. de Zeeum (eds.),
            Decision Making and Change in Human Affairs.
            Amsterdam: D. Reidl (in press).

Lichtenstein, S. and P. Slovic
    1973   "Response-induced reversals of preference in
            gambling: An extended replication in Las Vegas."
            Journal of Experimental Psychology 101:16-20.

    1971   "Reversals of preference between bids and choices
            in gambling decisions." Journal of Experimental
            Psychology 89:46-55.

Lipscomb, J. L.
    1976   The Willingness-to-pay Criterion and Public
            Program Evaluation in Health. Durham, N.C.:
            Institute of Policy Sciences and Public
            Affairs, Duke University (October).

Meyer, R. F.
    1970   "On the relationship among the utility of assets,
            the utility of consumption, and investment
            strategy in an uncertain, but time invariant
            world." In Lawrence, J. (ed.), OR 69: Proceed-
            ings of the Fifth International Conference on
            Operational Research, Tavistock Publications.

Miller, G. A.
    1956   "The magical number seven plus or minus two:
            Some limits on our capacity to process in-
            formation." Psychological Review 63:81-97.

Mishan, E. J.
    1973   "Welfare criteria: Resolution of a paradox."
            Economic Journal (September).

    1971   "Evaluation of life and limb: A theoretical
            approach." Journal of Political Economy 79
            (July/August).

Payne, J.
    1976   "Task complexity and contingent processing in
            decision making: An information search and
            protocol analysis." Organizational Behavior
            and Human Performance 16:366-387.

Raiffa, H.
    1968   Decision Analysis. Reading, Mass.: Addison
            Addison Wesley Publishing Co.

Richard, S. F.
    1972   Optimal Life Insurance Decisions for a Rational
            Economic Man. Unpublished doctoral disserta-
            tion, Graduate School of Business Administration,
            Harvard University.

Savage, L. J.
    1954   The Foundations of Statistics. New York:
            John Wiley.

Schelling, T. C.
    1968   "The life you save may be your own." In Chase,
            S. (ed.), Problems in Public Expenditure
            Analysis. Washington, D.C. The Brookings
            Institution.

Slovic, P., B. Fischoff, and S. L. Lichtenstein
    1977   "Behavioral decision theory." Annual Review of
            Psychology.

    1976   "Cognitive processes and societal risk taking."
            In Carroll, J. S. and J. W. Payne (eds.),
            Cognition and Social Behavior. Lawrence
            Erlbaum Associates.

Slovic, P. and S. L. Lichtenstein
    1971   "Comparison of Bayesian and regression approaches
            to the study of information processing in
            judgment." Organizational Behavior and Human
            Performance 6:649-744.

Thaler, R. and S. Rosen
    1975   "The value of saving a life: Evidence from the
            labor market." In Terleckyj, N. (ed.), House-
            hold Production and Consumption. New York:
            National Bureau of Economic Research.

Tversky, A.
    1967   "Additivity, utility, and subjective probabil-
            ity." Journal of Mathematical Psychology
            4:175-202.

Tversky, A. and D. Kahneman
    1974   "Judgment under uncertainty: Heuristics and
            biases." Science 185:1124-1131.

von Neumann, J. and O. Morgenstern
    1944   Theory of Games and Economic Behavior.
    1953   Princeton, N.J.: Princeton University Press.

Weinstein, M. C., D. S. Shepard, and J. S. Pliskin
    1975   Decision-Theoretic Approaches to Valuing a Year
            of Life. Center for the Analysis of Health
            Practices, Harvard School of Public Health
            (January).

Wyer, R. S., Jr.
    1975   "The role of probabilistic and syllogistic
            reasoning in cognitive organization and
            social inference." In Kaplan, M. F. and
            S. Schwartz (eds.), Human Judgment and
            Decision Processes. New York: Academic
            Press, Inc.

Returns to
Biomedical Investments

8 Measuring Returns to Technical Innovation in Health Care: The Utility Theory Approach

S. Y. Wu

This paper explores a new method, the utility theory approach, for the computation of the social rate of returns derived from investments in biomedical research. However, this paper represents only a preliminary report of ongoing research. Since the research is still in its infantile stage, no empirical results are available; therefore, only the conceptual portion of the research is outlined here. In order to keep the technical development tractable and to show how concrete implications can be drawn from the results, the presentation is in the context of pharmaceutical innovations. The proposed technique is, however, sufficiently general that it can be applied to other biomedical research as well as other consumer-product innovations.

In the pharmaceutical industry, there has been a long-standing controversy over the relationship between profit-making and innovation (involving improvement in the quality of an existing drug or introduction of a new drug). In this industry, according to some observers, the rate of returns to innovation has, traditionally, been extremely high. Whether or not this is true, it is possible to argue that high rates of return in this industry are justified for the following reasons: (1) The introduction of drug-therapeutic techniques for the treatment of a disease typically reduces the overall costs of treatment. Alternative medical treatments often involve complex and expensive equipment and inputs of highly trained personnel. In an age of soaring medical costs, it is rational to encourage the development of relatively cheaper drug therapy; in order to do this, it is necessary to offer strong incentives for drug innovation. (2) A high profit rate for pharmaceutical manufacturers is warranted by the extraordinary research and development (R&D) expenditures associated with drug innovations. It has been pointed out that, unlike many other major industries, in the drug industry, the vast majority of funds for R&D comes from private rather than public sources. This, combined with the high-risk nature of pharmaceutical research, implies that without the incentive

of a high rate of return, capital will shun the pharmaceutical
industry, thus causing under-development in drug quality and
reduction in the types of new drugs produced. Because improvement of public health is currently a primary public concern, contraction in the flow of capital into the pharmaceutical industry would be contrary to the public interest.

Others, however, contend that the high profit of the
drug manufacturers is a result of the existing market structure. They say that a small number of firms, shunning competition with each other, use innovation as a means to develop brand loyalty (impeding the entry of other firms) and
to reap high monopolistic profits.

Is the rate of return to R&D in the drug industry
higher than that for other investments in the economy? Has
innovation been a primary method used to create brand loyalty
and prevent diffusion? In general, have drug innovations
contributed to social welfare or have they led to divergence
between private and social returns? In order to answer these
and other questions, we must collect more information on the
social and private rates of returns from pharmaceutical innovations and analyze the distribution between consumer-
benefits and producer-benefits. This information is vital in
clarifying public debates and is essential for defining public
issues. Only when these issues are clearly formulated will
the question of market intervention be answered in terms of
a rational public policy.

Unfortunately, there does not exist a body of knowledge
sufficient to guide a rational formulation of public policies
toward pharmaceutical innovations. Worse yet, there does not
even exist a suitable method by which to calculate social
benefits and the social rate of returns from innovations in
the drug industry. In order to generate the much needed information to obtain accurate measures relating to product
innovation, an appropriate technique must be devised. The
first part of this paper briefly summarized the commonly used
techniques for calculating social benefits and the social
rate of returns, and discusses the limitations of these techniques. The second portion of the paper outlines a new technique for obtaining a more satisfactory rate of returns from
pharmaceutical innovations. The last part summarizes the
findings and points out the tasks that remain.

EXISTING TECHNIQUES AND THEIR LIMITATIONS

In measuring benefits derived from innovative activities, economists traditionally employ cost-benefit analysis
and compute the internal rate of returns to R&D expenditures.
The internal rate of return, r, is found by solving the following equation:

$$(1) \quad \sum_{t=0}^{T} \frac{R_t - B_t}{(1 + r)^t} = 0$$

where R_t denotes the R&D expenditures incurred in period t, and B_t denotes the streams of net social benefits derived during period t, $t = 0,\ldots,T$. Although the convention adopted for assigning R&D expenditures is not without controversy, that problem is not discussed here. This paper simply adopts the conventional wisdom that only the direct costs associated with the development of the drug in question is included in the R&D expenditures; other costs, such as those associated with the development of unsuccessful drugs, pure research, and that part of the administrative cost not directly related to the R&D activities of the drug in question, are excluded. Thus, the discussion is limited to the question of how B_t is obtained.

There are two approaches used by economists to obtain a representation of social benefits derived from innovative activities. In the context of pharmaceutical innovations, the first is the human capital approach; the second is the consumer's surplus approach.

Human Capital Approach

Two seminal studies on prescription drugs, Weisbrod (1971) on polio vaccine and Peltzman (1973) on tranquilizers, measure the benefits derived from treatment or prevention of a disease as the opportunity costs saved. These opportunity costs include a direct and indirect component: the direct cost includes the actual costs that would have been incurred in order to find, treat, and rehabilitate the victims from the disease; the indirect costs include the income foregone because a loss in productivity is attributable to the disease. Although in principle favorable effects in whatever form derived from the drug should be included in computing the social benefits, in practice, the measure of benefits is generally limited to the pecuniary costs mentioned above. For example, Weisbrod limits his measured benefits to "...only the sum of (i) the market value of production lost because of premature mortality due to polio, (ii) the market value of production lost as a result of morbidity--illness and disability--caused by polio, and (iii) the cost of resources devoted to treatment and rehabilitation of polio victims" (Weisbrod, 1971). The advantage of the human capital approach lies in the fact that the data required by it is more readily available; however, it does have some inherent limitations.

The shortcomings of the human capital approach stem from its emphasis on the opportunity cost saved. The resultant computation has a tendency to yield a measure of

social benefits biased toward income and to neglect the non-
pecuniary benefits of innovations. When the non-pecuniary
benefits are related to reduction in pain and suffering, the
resultant social benefit measure is concerned only with the
employed; it ignores the welfare accrued to the unemployed and
the elderly.

Mishan (1971), for a different reason, criticized the
human capital approach employed to calculate the benefits
derived from changes in incidents of mortality and morbidity.
He objected to the fact that this approach uses the total
production loss of the individual, less consumption expenditure, to calculate the present value of net production loss
due to death or illness. Mishan argued that this computation
method is incorrect because it is inconsistent with the Pareto
criterion underlying the existing allocation theory and cost-
benefit analysis. The criterion that should be used is the
well-known compensation principle: A project should be undertaken if the sum of the gains and losses from the project is
positive. Thus, after adjusting the income effect, the correct measure of the benefits derived from a new drug is the
maximum amount that the beneficiaries are willing to pay for
the drug.

But what is the value that a beneficiary would be willing to pay? One would presume that an individual with a fatal
disease would be willing to pay an amount equal to his total
wealth (or an infinite amount, if that were possible). The
willingness-to-pay question is especially troublesome when
payment is made by a third party. Mishan suggested that the
amount an individual would pay to save his life after the
occurrence of a disease is not an appropriate measure for
benefits. The appropriate measure should be assessed before
the illness; it should be the amount that an individual is
willing to pay for a drug that reduces the risk of contracting, becoming very ill from, or dying from a particular disease. Mishan admitted that obtaining accurate information
from individuals on this willingness-to-pay question may be
very difficult.

Consumer's Surplus Approach

A more refined approach, frequently used by economists
to compute social benefits, employs the concept of consumer's
surplus. This concept is, of course, a controversial one
(Willig, 1976, 1973). But given the current theoretical
know-how, it is hard to engage in applied welfare economic
studies without adopting some concept of this type. Yet to
date, the consumer's surplus approach has not been applied
widely in computing social benefits associated with pharmaceutical innovations. The only exception has been a work by
the author (Wu, unpublished). This paper follows Mansfield
(1977) and calculates the social benefits as the consumer's

surplus derived from substituting a brand name drug with its
generic equivalent. Mansfield, in studying the social rate
of return of 17 manufacturing industries, calculates the
social benefits as the consumer's surplus derived from lower-
ing the price of the products following an innovation, plus
the value of the resources saved. The latter is equivalent
to the profits of the innovator plus the profits of the
imitators, less the profit that would have been made if innovation had not taken place.

The Mansfield technique is mainly designed to measure
benefits derived from cost-saving process innovations and is
inappropriate when applied to a broader class of product innovations. The underlying assumption for using this technique is that innovation does not change the consumer's demand
curve for the product. Thus, the Mansfield method, though
suitable for those industries selected by him and for the
case of generic substitution for brand name drugs, is not
adequate for pharmaceutical innovation in general. The nature
of pharmaceutical innovation is much more complicated. Innovations in drugs take place when production and marketing of
a drug replace an old drug in the treatment of a given disease, extend the capability of treating additional diseases,
or make it possible to treat a disease hitherto untreatable
by another drug.

In the case of the old drug X being replaced by the
new drug Y, the economically relevant possibilities are that
Y may be

  (a) equally effective but cheaper;

  (b) more effective but equal in cost;

  (c) more effective but more costly;

  (d) more effective and less costly; and

  (e) less effective and less costly.

Except in case (a), the industry demand curve for the product
shifts following an innovation. A more general method to
calculate social benefits via consumer's surplus is therefore
needed. Difficulty arises from several sources:

  (i)   the demand curves for the new and old drug
        differ;

  (ii) the more effective drug may reduce pain and
        suffering;

  (iii) innovation also reduces income foregone
        through reduction in illness and death; and

(iv)   it may even increase the consumer's enjoy-
       ment of other goods and services.

    From the above discussion, we see that the existing
techniques are severely limited in providing us with comprehensive information regarding the extent of social rate of
returns derived from a broad class of product innovations.
Considerable work must be done to improve the methods of
computing social benefits and to actually obtain these
measurements. A recent development in consumer demand theory
(Lancaster, 1971) offers us the hope of developing a more
adequate measure.

SOCIAL BENEFITS BASED UPON THE UTILITY THEORY APPROACH

    It is well-known that traditional demand analysis,
based upon the utility of goods, cannot cope with either a
change in the quality of goods or a change in the number of
goods consumed. When a drug innovation represents either an
improvement in quality or an introduction of a new product,
then the measurement of the consumer's surplus cannot be
calculated on the basis of a demand function that is assumed
to be derived from the traditional utility function. In order
to provide the theoretical foundations for the calculation of
consumer's surplus under these circumstances, we propose that
a Lancasterian utility function be used. Lancaster's departure from the traditional utility theory is that satisfaction is derived from the characteristics possessed by the
goods rather than from the goods themselves. The Lancaster
model can be summarized as:

(2)   To maximize $U(\underset{\sim}{Z})$

        Subject to $\underset{\sim}{Z} = \underset{\sim}{B}\underset{\sim}{X}$ (the household production
                                    function)

                     $M = \underset{\sim}{P}'\underset{\sim}{X}$ (the income constraint)

where Z is a column vector denoting characteristics, X is a
column vector denoting the goods, P' is a row vector denoting
the prices of the goods, B is a matrix denoting the consumption technology, and M a scalar denoting the consumer
income.

    The advantages of the Lancaster approach are obvious.
First, it represents a generalization of the traditional approach. The traditional model is merely a special case of
the Lancasterian Model with $B = I$ where I is the identity
matrix. Second, the traditional model confounds tastes and
technology; a change in demand attributable to a change in
technology is designated as a change in tastes. The
Lancaster approach, however, distinguishes between these two
sources. Finally, either an increase in the efficiency of a

drug or an introduction of a new drug can be viewed as a
change in the consumption technology. When the number of
characteristics in the utility function remains unchanged,
the effect of changes in consumption technology on consumer's
surplus, in terms of characteristics, is well-defined.

Demand for Characteristics Under Certainty

    <u>Some assumptions</u>.--Let the consumption technology be
of the form:

$$\underset{\sim}{B} = \begin{bmatrix} \underset{\sim}{B}_1 & \underset{\sim}{0} \\ \\ \underset{\sim}{0} & \underset{\sim}{B}_2 \end{bmatrix}$$

Let $\underset{\sim}{B}_1$ be a 2 x 2 submatrix. The above technology matrix $\underset{\sim}{B}$
indicates that the goods X_1 and X_2 do not produce characteris-
tics other than Z_1 and Z_2; and Z_1 and Z_2 are not produced by
any goods other than X_1 and X_2. This assumption makes it possible to apply theorems relating to separable utility functions and to simplify the presentations (Strotz, 1957).
Specifically, it permits one to ignore the substitution effect between goods belonging to the groups $\{x_1, x_2\}$ and
$\{x_3, \ldots, x_n\}$, or between characteristics belonging to the two
groups $\{z_1, z_2\}$ and $\{z_3, \ldots, z_m\}$. Consequently, only the
following problem is examined:

    (3)   To maximize $V(\underset{\sim}{Z}_1)$

           Subject to $\underset{\sim}{P}'_1 \underset{\sim}{X}_1 = M_1$

                        $\underset{\sim}{B}_1 \underset{\sim}{X}_1 = \underset{\sim}{Z}_1$

where $\underset{\sim}{Z}_1 = \begin{pmatrix} z_1 \\ z_2 \end{pmatrix}$, $\underset{\sim}{X}_1 = \begin{pmatrix} x_1 \\ x_2 \end{pmatrix}$, $\underset{\sim}{P}_1 = \begin{pmatrix} P_1 \\ P_2 \end{pmatrix}$ and $\underset{\sim}{B}_1 = \begin{bmatrix} b_{11} & b_{12} \\ b_{21} & b_{22} \end{bmatrix}$.

In the interest of notational clarity, we further ignore all
vector subscripts.

    Let $\underset{\sim}{X} = \underset{\sim}{B}^{-1} \underset{\sim}{Z}$. By combining the constraints in (3) by
eliminating $\underset{\sim}{X}$, the consumer's maximization problem now
becomes:

    (4)   To maximize $V(\underset{\sim}{Z})$

           Subject to $\underset{\sim}{P}' \underset{\sim}{B}^{-1} \underset{\sim}{Z} = M$.

It can easily be shown that the problem represented by (4) is equivalent to the following problem:

(5)   To maximize $V(\underset{\sim}{Z})$

Subject to $\underset{\sim}{\pi}'\underset{\sim}{Z} = M$

where $\underset{\sim}{\pi}'$ is a row vector of characteristic prices.

To show equivalence of (4) and (5), it is necessary only to show that $\underset{\sim}{P}'\underset{\sim}{B}^{-1} = \underset{\sim}{\pi}'$. Suppose X_1 alone is consumed. From the constraints in (3) it is shown that, the total amount of characteristics derived from X_1 is

$$(z_1', z_2') = \left(\frac{M}{P_1}b_{11}, \frac{M}{P_1}b_{21} \right).$$

Substitute these values into the constraint of (5), and we obtain:

(6)(i) $\pi_1 b_{11} + \pi_2 b_{21} = P_1.$

Likewise, if X_2 alone is consumed, the amount of characteristics derived is

$$(z_1'', z_2'') = \left(\frac{M}{P_2}b_{12}, \frac{M}{P_2}b_{22} \right).$$

Substitute these values into the constraint in (5), and we get:

(6)(ii) $\pi_1 b_{12} + \pi_2 b_{22} = P_2.$

(6)(i) and (6)(ii) together state $\underset{\sim}{B}'\underset{\sim}{\pi} = \underset{\sim}{P}$ or $\underset{\sim}{\pi}' = \underset{\sim}{P}'\underset{\sim}{B}^{-1}$. Thus, given P_1, P_2 and the matrix $\underset{\sim}{B}$, the values of π_1 and π_2 are uniquely determined.

Let λ denote the Lagrange multiplier associated with (5); the first order maximization condition for (5) is:

(7) $V_1 - \lambda\pi_1 = 0$

$V_2 - \lambda\pi_2 = 0$

$\pi_1 z_1 + \pi_2 z_2 = M.$

Given the values π_1, π_2 and M, the equilibrium quantities of z_1 and z_2 are determined.

As shown in figure 1 (below), $\overline{OX_1}$ and $\overline{OX_2}$ represent the production process associated with X_1 and X_2.

Figure 1.

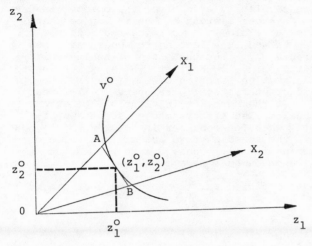

If the consumer spent all his income on X_1, as has been shown,
(z_1', z_2') amount of characteristics would be obtained. In
figure 1, let $A = (z_1', z_2')$. Similarly, let $B = (z_1'', z_2'')$ represent the situation in which the consumer spent all his income on X_2. $\overline{AB}$ thus represents the consumer's budget constraint in the (z_1, z_2)-plane. The consumer's utility is
maximized at (z_1^o, z_2^o) where $\overline{AB}$ is tangent to the indifference
curve v_o.

Algebraically, z_1^o and z_2^o can be expressed as a function
of π' and M:

(8) $z_j = g^j (\pi', M; B)$ $j = 1,2$

g^1 and g^2 are the demand functions for the characteristics Z_1
and Z_2, respectively. This demand function exhibits all the
properties of the traditional demand function: It is
homogeneous of degree zero in π' and M. and has the usual
properties associated with the income and substitution
effects.

Demand for Characteristics Under Uncertainty*

Uncertainty, for two reasons, is intimately related to
the demand for medicine. (1) Illness strikes without warning;
its appearance is, therefore, uncertain. (2) Once a person

_____

* See Arrow (1973) and Balch and Fishburn (1974).

becomes ill, the utilization of a drug and a physician's
services need not be completely effective; the outcome is uncertain. Thus, the consumer's state of health can be characterized as a random variable, and medicine and a doctor's
services can best be viewed as affecting the consumer's health
prospect in a favorable way. Let the state of health be represented by an index h, hϵ [0, 1] and let $F(h; x_1, x_2, \theta)$ denote
the probability distribution function of h; x_1 and x_2, together with θ (a set of statistical parameters), all appear
as parameters of F. Furthermore, it is plausible to assume
that the state of health also affects the consumer's preference. For example, when the consumer is healthy, he is not
interested at all in the speed of cure and may not value comfort as much as when he is ill. Thus, h also enters into the
consumer's utility function as a parameter.

The consumer's expected utility function thus can be
summarized as:

$$(9) \quad \int_0^1 u(z_1, z_2; h) \; dF(h; x_1, x_2, \underset{\sim}{\theta})$$

and his choice problem now becomes: to maximize (9) subject
to $\underset{\sim}{B}\underset{\sim}{X} = \underset{\sim}{Z}$ and $\underset{\sim}{P}'\underset{\sim}{X} = M$. Again, by using the relation $\underset{\sim}{X} = \underset{\sim}{B}^{-1}\underset{\sim}{Z}$
and by defining $\underset{\sim}{\pi}' = \underset{\sim}{P}\underset{\sim}{B}^{-1}$, the above choice problem
becomes:

$$(10) \quad \text{To maximize} \quad \int_0^1 u(\underset{\sim}{Z}', h) \; dF(h; \underset{\sim}{Z}'\underset{\sim}{B}'^{-1}, \underset{\sim}{\theta})$$

Subject to $\underset{\sim}{\pi}'Z = M$.

Let μ denote the Lagrange multiplier associated with (10).
The first order maximization condition for the above problem
is:

$$\int_0^1 u_1 dF + \int_0^1 u(b_{22} dF_{x_1} - b_{21} dF_{x_2}) - \mu\pi_1 = 0.$$

$$(11) \quad \int_0^1 u_2 dF + \int_0^1 u(b_{11} dF_{x_2} - b_{12} dF_{x_1}) - \mu\pi_2 = 0$$

$$\pi_1 z_1 + \pi_2 z_2 = 0.$$

The expected demand functions for Z_1 and Z_2 now can be expressed as:

$$(12) \quad z_j = f^j(\underset{\sim}{\pi}', M; \underset{\sim}{B}, \theta) \qquad j = 1, 2.$$

Again this demand function exhibits all the properties of the traditional demand function. It is homogeneous of degree zero in π' and M and has the usual properties associated with the income and substitution effects. Comparing (12) and (8), one can see that, except for the addition of the parameters θ, the presence of uncertainty has not affected the consumer's demand for the characteristics Z_1 and Z_2 in an essential way.

Empirical Estimation Procedure

Assume the time series of x_1, x_2, P_1, and P_2. By using the relationship $\underset{\sim}{B}\underset{\sim}{X} = \underset{\sim}{Z}$ and $\underset{\sim}{\pi}' = \underset{\sim}{P}'\underset{\sim}{B}^{-1}$, the time series of z_1, z_2, π_1, and π_2 can be constructed.* In theory, therefore, each transaction over time yields an observation on characteristic prices, quantities of characteristics, and exogenous shift variables. The shift variables are, for example, income and the consumption technology on the demand side and the factor prices on the supply side. This set of derived data can be used to estimate separate demand and supply equations for each characteristic in the usual manner. The underlying demand and supply functions are:

$$(13) \quad \pi_1 = D^1(z_{1t}, z_{2t}, \underset{\sim}{k}_t)$$

$$\pi_2 = D^2(z_{1t}, z_{2t}, \underset{\sim}{k}_t)$$

$$\pi_1 = S^1(z_{1t}, z_{2t}, \underset{\sim}{l}_t)$$

$$\pi_2 = S^2(z_{1t}, z_{2t}, \underset{\sim}{l}_t)$$

where D^1 and D^2 are the demand functions and S^1 and S^2 are the supply functions for the characteristics Z_1 and Z_2, respectively, and k_t and l_t are vectors of demand and supply parameters. In obtaining estimates for the functions in (13), the usual estimation procedures are used for simultaneous equation systems and the usual identification conditions are adopted.

Observe that the consumption technology is not only central to the Lancasterian demand theory, but also crucial in enabling us to derive the unobservable time series z_1, z_2, π_1 and π_2 from the observable time series x_1, x_2, P_1 and P_2.

---

* An explanation of how to estimate $\underset{\sim}{B}$ is given later.

A word concerning the matrix B is in order. Since B
defines the consumption technology, it is assumed to be objective in the sense that it is the same for all consumers.
Because X_1 and X_2 are medically related products and Z_1 and Z_2
are medically related characteristics, B can be estimated by
using the assistance of physicians and pharmacists and by
analyzing the patients' hospital records.

In order to demonstrate the procedure used to empirically estimate matrix B, denote

z_1 = a comfort index

z_2 = reduction in degree of illness

and

x_1 = quantity of a drug used

x_2 = amount of physician services employed.

Furthermore, let z_{ij}, i, j = 1,2 denote the amount of Z_i contributed by the input X_j, $z_{ij} \geq 0$. Then

$$(14) \quad z_1 = z_{11} + z_{12} = \left(\frac{z_{11}}{x_1}\right)x_1 + \left(\frac{z_{12}}{x_2}\right)x_2$$

$$z_2 = z_{21} + z_{22} = \left(\frac{z_{21}}{x_1}\right)x_1 + \left(\frac{z_{22}}{x_2}\right)x_2 .$$

Assume $\frac{z_{ij}}{x_j} = b_{ij}$, i, j = 1,2, where b_{ij} is a constant. The
equation can be written as $Z = \hat{B}X$, where $\hat{B}$ is an estimate of
the consumption technology matrix.

By examining the patients' records in the hospital,
with the assistance of physicians and pharmacists, we can
assign values for z_{ij} and calculate the matrix $\hat{B}$. Likewise,
after a drug innovation has taken place following the same
procedure, we can assess empirically how the matrix B has
changed.

Computing Consumer's Surplus

The following is a procedure by which the consumer's
surplus is computed: An innovation either improves a drug's
efficiency or reduces its price. Suppose it improves drug
X_2's efficiency in producing the characteristic Z_1.
Specifically, let the consumption technology change from B_1
to B_1', where all b_{ij} remain the same except that $b_{12}' >$
b_{12}. According to the definition of π, it may be concluded
that

$$\frac{\partial \pi_s}{\partial b_{12}} < 0 \text{ for } s = 1,2.$$

Since the demand curve for Z_1 and Z_2 are negatively sloped, an improvement in X_1's efficiency with respect to the production of the characteristic Z_1 increases not only the quantity of Z_1 demanded, but the quantity of Z_2 demanded. The shaded area between π_1^0 and π_1^1 and between π_2^0 and π_2^1 in figure 2 thus represents the consumer's surplus derived from an improvement in drug X_1 regarding the characteristics Z_1 and Z_2. The total increase in consumer's surplus is the sum of consumer's surplus accrued to both characteristics. Suppose Z_1 represents reduction in pain and suffering; the consumer's surplus thus obtained also includes his evaluations of the gains on this attribute.

Suppose, on the other hand, a process innovation decreases the cost of producing X_1 and it, in turn, decreases the price of X_1. Again, according to the relationship $\pi' = P'B^{-1}$,

$$\frac{\partial \pi_1}{\partial P_1} > 0 \text{ and } \frac{\partial \pi_2}{\partial P_1} < 0.$$

The shaded areas under the demand curves in figure 2, between π_1^0 and π_1^1 and π_2^1 and $\pi_2^{1'}$, thus represent the increment and the decrement in the consumer's surplus, derived from the characteristics Z_1 and Z_2, respectively. The total consumer's surplus resulting from a reduction in P_1 is the net sum of the consumer's surplus accrued to these characteristics.

Figure 2.

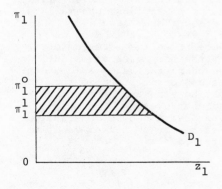 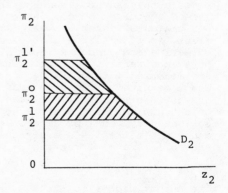

        If the innovation also increases the innovator's per
unit profit, then the social benefits derived from innovation
become the sum of the consumer's and the producer's surpluses.
Of course, if this innovation also replaces products, profits
from displaced products must be deducted.   Once social benefits derived from the innovation are computed, the internal
rate of return can be calculated as usual.

SUMMARY AND CONCLUSION

        The Lancasterian utility theory enables us to compute
consumer's surplus derived from pharmaceutical innovations in
the form of a quality improvement or a new product.   The only
restriction is that the number and the nature of the characteristics remain the same.   If some of the characteristics
are non-pecuniary attributes, for example, reduction in pain
and suffering, then the consumer's surplus so derived will
include a monetary imputation for these attributes.   The resultant social benefits will no longer be biased toward income, and the difficulties observed in item (ii) in the first
part of the paper are, therefore, overcome.   Moreover, in the
case of uncertainty (when the health state is assumed to affect the consumer's enjoyment of characteristics), the expected consumer's surplus, derived from the consumer's expected demand functions for characteristics, will also include
an imputation for the drug's contribution to the consumer's
enjoyment of other goods and services.   This result, at least
in part, avoids the difficulties associated with item (iv)
in the first major part.   It is hoped that better measurement
of social benefits derived from innovative activities will
ultimately lead to the formulation of wiser public policies
toward product innovations.

        Having pointed out the many advantages associated with
the Lancasterian utility theory, one must not lose sight of
the many difficulties that remain.   For example, how can one
be sure that an unbiased household production function will
indeed emerge by merely interviewing physicians, pharmacists,
and patients?   When a physician prescribes a drug for a patient, is it not true that he believes that this drug is more
effective and produces fewer side effects and more comforts?
More importantly, how are some of the characteristics defined
and measured?   Suppose one of the characteristics is comfort.
Can a meaningful comfort index be designed?   Even if the
answer is affirmative, how can one be sure that the data obtained are unbiased?   It is hoped that eventually a more
satisfactory model of experimental design can be constructed
and a set of reliable empirical estimates of social benefits
and social rate of returns be obtained.

Acknowledgments.

The author wishes to thank E. K. Choi for helpful discussion
and to thank NSF PRA/76-18777 for financial support.

REFERENCES

Arrow, K. J.
    1973   Optimal Insurance and Generalized Deductibles.
            Santa Monica: The RAND Corporation (February).

Balch, M. and P. C. Fishburn
    1974   "Subjective expected utility for conditional
            primitives." In Balch, M., D. McFadden, and
            S. Wu (eds.), Essays on Economic Behavior
            Under Uncertainty. Amsterdam: North-Holland
            Publishing Co.

Harberger, A. C.
    1971   "Three basic postulates for applied welfare
            economics: An interpretative essay." Journal
            of Economic Literature 9:785-797.

Lancaster, K.
    1971   Consumer Demand: A New Approach. New York:
            Columbia University Press.

Mansfield, E., E. Rapoport, R. Wagner, and J. Bearsely
    1977   "Social and private rate of returns from in-
            dustrial innovations." Quarterly Journal of
            Economics 91:221-240.

Mishan, E. J.
    1971   Cost-Benefit Analysis: An Introduction.
            New York: Praeger Press.

    1971   "Evaluation of life and limb: A theoretical
            approach." Journal of Political Economy
            79:687-705.

Peltzman, S.
    1973   "The benefits and costs of new drug regulation."
            In Landau, R. L. (ed.), Regulating New Drugs,
            The University of Chicago Center for Policy
            Study 113-213.

Strotz, R. H.
    1957   "The empirical implication of a utility tree."
            Econometrica 25:264-280.

Weisbrod, B. A.
    1971   "Cost and benefit of medical research: A cost
            study of poliomyelitis." Journal of Political
            Economy 79:827-844.

Willig, R. D.
    1976   "Consumer surplus without apology." American
            Economic Review 66 (September):589-597.

Willig, R. D.
    1973   "Consumer's surplus: A rigorous cashbook."
            Technical Report 98, Economic Series, Institute
            for Mathematical Study in the Social Sciences,
            Stanford University.

Wu, S. Y.

            "On optimal product imitation: A case study of
            selected pharmaceuticals." (unpublished).

9 Economics and Epidemiology: Application to Cancer

William Schulze
Shaul Ben-David
Thomas D. Crocker
Allen Kneese

It is extremely difficult to identify substances in
the environment which cause chronic illness and to quantify
their effects. Often there are multiple substances involved.
In addition, there may be a long latency period before effects are seen, and the amount and time of exposure is often
unknown. There are two broad general approaches to identifying such substances and quantifying their impact--both highly
imperfect. In the first approach, laboratory animals are fed
large doses of the suspect substance, and if effects appear,
an effort is made to extrapolate them to the human population.
How to extrapolate these effects to the human population is,
however, not well established. In the second approach,
cross-sectional data are developed, usually for cities, on a
number of variables that might be associated with chronic
illness; regression analysis is then used to see whether any
statistically significant relationships appear. Combining
these two broad approaches, a third approach uses animal
studies to develop hypotheses about relationships between exposure to potentially harmful substances and chronic illness.
Statistical information on human populations is then used to
try to refute such hypotheses; if they are not refuted, the
coefficients of the variable in the regression equation are
estimated; that is, what is the magnitude of the coefficients'
effects? This is the approach discussed in the present paper.
Statistical analysis is used to consider some methodological
and data problems. These problems include the following
facts: populations are mobile and therefore many persons are
exposed to multiple environments; chronic diseases often
display long latency periods so that present environmental
conditions may not be good indicators of exposure; the
analysis entails various kinds of simultaneous equation bias.
While this paper is primarily about methodology, an application is made to cancer.

That cancer is largely an environmental disease has
now achieved universal acceptance. A major problem for
health economics then becomes the determination of the

benefits of cancer prevention. The connection between
various categories of cancer and the broad array of inputs to
the human biosystem from air, water, and food deserve strong
attention simply because of the dimensions of the problem.
Cancer accounted for 365,000 deaths in 1975, or about 20 percent of total deaths. While the overall incidence of cancer
has not risen significantly in the past 25 years, this is the
result of offsetting trends among the several categories of
cancer. Lung cancer has been increasing and stomach cancer
declining, although recently the decline in the latter has
turned around and some increase has been registered. However, because cancer is believed to have a latency period between 15 and 25 years, we have not yet seen the effects of
the recent introduction of thousands of chemicals into the
natural environment, and into work places, households, and
most food products. Many of these have never been tested for
carcinogenesis. Yet the list of known carcinogens is growing; this gives rise to the suspicion that there may be increases in cancer rates. Although there is a need to learn
better ways of treating cancer, the heavy orientation of
medical research toward "cures" seems misplaced when contrasted with efforts aimed at cancer prevention.

     The first part of the paper discusses methodological
problems and approaches associated with measuring the cost
of risk of death and the role of economics in epidemiology.
The second part is an application of these findings to a
preliminary assessment of the cost of risk from
environmentally-induced cancer.

ECONOMICS AND EPIDEMIOLOGY

     The methodological approach recently advocated by
economists for evaluating the costs of disease resulting from
environmental exposures is straightforward although difficult
to quantify (see, for example, Kneese and Schulze, 1977):
First, the population at risk must be known. Second, the increased risk of mortality associated with environmental exposures must be quantified either through epidemiology or
through extrapolation from animal experiments. Third, the
amount of money, or the value that individuals place on
avoiding increased risk, must be known. Multiplying these
three values together then gives an approximation of the
incremental cost to society of increased environmental exposures or the incremental benefits of reducing such exposures. This cost or benefit is not in any way related to
a "value of life" which is, most likely, unmeasurable; this
cost or benefit focuses, rather, on the concept of "cost of
risk" imposed on individuals where such risks are statistically small.

     Mishan (1971) was the first to distinguish between
the concept of cost of risk, which is, perhaps, ethically

acceptable, and earlier efforts to value human life based on
lost earnings. The latter measure of the "value" of human
life has now been universally rejected by economists both on
theoretical and ethical grounds. Thaler and Rosen (1975)
were the first to estimate the cost of risk as determined
by wage differentials between jobs varying in the level of
job-associated risk of death. Unfortunately, however, their
study dealt with a high risk class of individuals. The
Thaler and Rosen estimate suggests that in current dollars a
small reduction in risk over a large number of individuals
which saves one life is worth about $340,000. Another study
(Blumquist, 1977),* which examines seat-belt use, suggests
that the figure might be $260,000, but it may be biased down-
ward because individuals do not seem to properly perceive
risks which involve an element of personal control, such as
driving an automobile. Finally, Smith,* based on work done
in 1975 relating industrial wages to job-related risk, has
suggested that, for a more typical population and for job-
related risks, the figure may be about $1 million.**
Clearly, the cost of risk is not precisely known, and perhaps
will never be since attitudes (risk preference) can, presumably, change over time, between groups, and even
in different situations. However, we have, at least, a range
of values with which to make order of magnitude estimates of
the cost of environmental risks.

The theoretical basis of the cost of risk concept can
be shown briefly as follows: Assume that an individual has
a utility function, $U(Y)$, where utility is an increasing
function of income, Y. If risk of death in any period is π,
expected utility in that period is $(1-\pi) U(Y)$. If we hold
expected utility constant, we have $(1-\pi)U(Y) =$ constant, and
the total differential of this equation is:

$$(1) \quad -U(Y)d\pi + (1-\pi)U'(Y)dY = 0$$

where the prime denotes differentiation. Holding utility
constant then implies that the increase in income necessary
to offset an increase in risk is:

---

* Both the Blumquist (Department of Economics, Illinois
  State University) and Smith (Department of Labor Re-
  lations, Cornell University) results were obtained from
  the authors by personal communication with W. Schulze.

** All these studies consider voluntarily-incurred risk,
   which entails a benefit to the risk taker. This is
   usually not true of environmentally imposed risk. There
   are thus grounds for believing that involuntary risks
   carry a larger net disbenefit to the party incurring
   them than do ones that are voluntarily accepted.

(2) $dY/d\pi + U/(U'(1-\pi))$.

This is the compensating variation measure of the cost to an
individual attributable to an increased risk of death.
Analysis of the last expression can be simplified if we assume a constant elasticity of utility with respect to income,
η, such that $U(Y) = Y\eta$ and consequently $\eta = \dfrac{dU}{dY} \dfrac{Y}{U}$. Then (2)
can be rewritten as:

(3) $dY/d\pi = Y/(\eta(1-\pi))$.

The right-hand side of equation (3) suggests several interesting points about the cost of risk. First, if we assume that
the elasticity of utility is less than one, people are risk
averse. This, in turn, implies that since the risk of death
is positive ($\pi > 0$), then $dY/d\pi > Y$. In other words, if an
individual is risk averse, his life, in terms of the risk
premium necessary to get him to accept risk, is worth more to
him than his income. Second, from (3), as income increases,
the risk premium required to accept an increase in risk voluntarily, $dY/d\pi$, increases proportionally. Finally, if we
take η as constant, then, since risk of death, π, increases
with age for adults, $dY/d\pi$ must then increase with age,
ceteris paribus. Thus, one would expect older people to act
in a more risk-averse manner than younger individuals, both
because of increased income and because of increased risk of
death.

     This model contrasts, for a number of reasons, with
the value of lost earnings approach often used in economic
analysis. First, if lost income itself is the measure, the
value of life measured through lost earnings cannot, obviously, exceed income. Second, increased income will increase the lost earnings measure as well as the cost of risk
measure. However, the cost of risk measure may not increase
proportionately if a different utility function is used.
Third, the lost earnings measure must decrease with age, at
some point, as individuals get older because the expected
remaining earnings must decrease, while the cost of risk, as
we argued above, must increase. Finally, it is clear from
(3) that as π approaches unity, $dY/d\pi$ approaches infinity.
In other words, the compensation required to induce an individual to accept a certainty of death voluntarily is infinite. The lost income measure has no similar property.
Nevertheless, the implication is that small increases in
risk may be valued in terms of compensation required to induce individuals to accept such risks voluntarily. Individuals, of course, rationally accept small risks on a
daily basis, presumably on the basis of some monetary or
psychic return.

     Given the analysis above, the current ad hoc methodol-
ogy of multiplying cost of risk numbers times
epidemiologically determined environmental risks can then be

justified as follows: Assuming a utility function U(Y) where
Y is income, if risk of death is π, the marginal cost of risk
as derived earlier is $(dY/d\pi)\overline{U} = U/(U'(1-\pi))$. If risk is a
function of health services, h, and pollution, X, where utility functions are identical for N individuals, one would wish
to maximize expected utility,

$$(4) \quad N \cdot 1-\pi(h,X) \; U(Y),$$

subject to a constraint on total income $(\overline{Y})$,

$$(5) \quad \overline{Y} - Nph - NY - C(X^O-X) - 0$$

which is allocated to health expenditures (Nph where p is the
price of health services), individual incomes (NY), and cost
of controlling environmental pollution from the initial level
X^O, $C(X^O-X)$. Noting that $\pi_h < 0$, $\pi_X > 0$ and $C' > 0$, the
first order conditions (where λ is the multiplier on (5) and L
denotes the Lagrangian) are

$$\partial L/\partial h = N\pi_h U - \lambda Np = 0$$

$$\partial L/\partial Y = N(1-\pi)U' - N\lambda = 0$$

$$\partial L/\partial X = -N\pi_X U + \lambda C' = 0$$

and imply first

$$(6) \quad U/(U'(1-\pi)) = -p/\pi_h,$$

or that the marginal cost of risk equals the marginal cost of
health improvement through health services, and second that

$$(7) \quad N \cdot [U/(U'(1-\pi))] \; \pi_X = C'$$

or that the number of individuals, N, times the marginal cost
of risk $[U/(U'(1-\pi))]$, times the marginal effect of pollution
on risk, π_X, equals the marginal cost of control, C'.
Clearly, this model abstracts from many welfare theoretic
problems, but it does suggest that calculation of the LHS of
(7) is a legitimate procedure for social decision making regarding environmental risks. Just as important, however,
are the implications of (6). That result implies that individuals subject to high risk circumstances may well demand
more health care than those in lower risk circumstances;
humans are not stones--they are likely to adjust to their
risk standing. Unfortunately, most epidemiological studies
fail to account for such adjustments.

THE CANCER APPLICATION

        Where sufficient experimental evidence (or adequately
detailed epidemiological data) on human exposures and health

impacts are lacking, and that is almost always, the task of
risk assessment is difficult. Both epidemiologists and
health economists have used rather gross statistical methods
to correlate environmental factors with mortality. For example, Lave and Seskin (1972) have attempted to determine
both the impact of air pollution on human health and the
quantification of the economic losses attributable to those
effects. Their methodology employed a cross-sectional regression analysis of the statistical relationships between
specific measures of air pollution and the incidence of morbidity and mortality. Similar statistical methods have recently been employed, using cross-sectional data for 60 U.S.
cities, in an effort to identify environmental factors that
show correlations between food consumption patterns and cancer mortality (Kneese and Schulze, 1977).

        The cancer study to be presented in this paper, the
Kneese and Schulze data, contains some methodological innovations. An effort was made to account for mobility, with
its attendant effects on exposure, by including population
change as an independent variable. An estimate of smoking
was included in the regression; variables that could be related to cancer were lagged to take account of cancer's long
latency period. The introduction of these considerations
into the statistical analysis have entailed large impacts on
the significance of the variables included. For example,
some variables which were not significant when introduced at
their current values were highly significant when lagged 16
years (the longest lag the data permitted).

        Nevertheless, several statistical problems merit
emphasis. First, simultaneous equation bias is likely
to be present. This is so because, as was suggested at
the end of the first section, human behavior may adapt
to risk situations. For example, if people in polluted
cities demand more medical care and if this reduces mortality, the estimated impact of pollution alone on mortality
rates will be underestimated using cross-sectional data from
cities. In this case, estimation of the true impact of
pollution would require the specification of a multi-equation
model that explicitly included the role of medical services.
Another example of simultaneous equation bias arises because
of multiple causes of death (see next part). Cities with
high coronary death rates may likely have lower cancer death
rates because people die of heart attacks before they have a
chance to die of cancer. In this situation, factors that
are positively correlated with coronary disease may have a
spurious negative correlation with cancer rates. Second,
multicollinearity is a problem in epidemiologic studies
where explanatory variables are themselves highly correlated,
and this problem may be serious for particular data sets.
Our example application of the methodology to cancer has this
problem but, as indicated later in this paper, some measures
have been taken to try to deal with it.

Aside from these particular problems, the usual caveats concerning such studies still apply; these relate chiefly to problems of causality. For example, if heart attacks are actually related to cigarette consumption, but smoking is correlated with coffee consumption for behavioral reasons, a spurious positive correlation might be shown between heart attacks and coffee consumption, especially if cigarette consumption is excluded from an estimated statistical relationship. In other words, correlation does not prove causation, and statistical hypothesis testing can never confirm, but only reject, a maintained hypothesis. Turning to an example more pertinent to the present study, if most nitrite ingestion is through consumption of pork products (70 percent of pork is cured), one might suspect, given the hypothesis of in vivo nitrosamine formation, that cancer mortality and pork consumption would be correlated. If such a correlation can be shown (as it has in the Kneese-Schulze work), then the only valid conclusion is that we do not reject the hypothesis that pork consumption (and, perhaps, in turn, nitrite ingestion) is related to human cancer. If, alternatively, one accepts the maintained hypothesis on a priori grounds, and no bias exists in the estimation procedure, regression analysis, using ordinary least squares, can give the best linear estimate of the actual relationship in the sample population; for example, between cancer mortality and a dietary factor such as nitrite ingestion. However, regression analysis cannot prove causality; casuality must be assumed in this procedure. This is why it is so important to have hypotheses concerning causality before a regression equation is specified. In studies, such as the one to be presented, the best source of such hypotheses appears to be animal studies.

QUANTITATIVE ASPECTS OF THE STUDY

The variables used in the regression analysis fall into five categories: (1) cancer mortality, (2) socioeconomic factors, (3) air and water pollutants, including radiation measures, (4) nutrients and other dietary factors, and (5) cigarette smoking. In all, data for 60 cities on some three dozen potential factors in cancer were included. Table 1 describes a selected set of the data and indicates the sources. An analysis of aggregate cancer mortality for all body sites was done for this study, but several subcategories have also been analyzed; these include digestive, respiratory, breast, genital, urinary, leukemic, and other cancers. The socioeconomic factors that were tested include the change in population from 1960 to 1970, the percent nonwhite population, and the median age (table 1). Not included in table 1, but also tested, were median age raised to various powers, median income, employment in primary metals, and employment in chemicals and allied industries. Median age raised to powers added no explanatory power to

Table 1.   Selected Set of the Data and Sources.

Variable		Year	Units	Mean	S.D.	Sources
CANC	Cancer Mortality	1972	deaths/1,000	1.96	0.42	1/
DPOP	Change in Population	1960-70	percent	4.71	18.46	2/
NONW	Non-white Population	1969	fraction	0.23	0.15	3/
MAGE	Median Age	1969	year	28.82	2.74	4/
AMMN	Atmos. Ammonium	1966	ug/m3	1.15	1.42	5/
GAMA	Terres. Gamma Rad.	1958-63	urem/yr/cap	40.22	10.78	6/
NTRI	Nitrites in Food	1955	g/yr/cap	1.27	0.14	7/ 8/ 10/
NTRA	Nitrates in Food	1955	g/yr/cap	69.86	9.05	7/ 8/ 10/
SFAT	Saturated Fatty Acids*	1955	g/yr/cap	16,220.00	874.65	8/ 9/ 10/
PROT	Protein*	1955	g/yr/cap	26,557.00	1,314.00	8/ 9/ 10/
CHOL	Cholesterol*	1955	g/yr/cap	234.81	6.98	8/ 9/ 10/
CVIT	Vitamin C**	1955	g/yr/cap	16.96	1.46	8/ 9/ 10/
COFF	Coffee	1955	kg/yr/cap	5.82	0.70	8/ 10/
CIGS	Cigarettes	1956	packs/yr/cap	110.23	18.41	11/

* Includes only animal products.
** Includes only fruits and vegetables eaten fresh.

1/ National Center for Health Statistics. Vital Statistics of the United States: 1972, vol. II, Mortality, part B, tables 7-9.

2/ U.S. Bureau of the Census. U.S. Census of Population: 1970, vols. 1-50.

3/ See 2, tables 23, 27, 31.

4/ See 3, table 24.

5/ U.S. Department of Health, Education, and Welfare. Air Quality Data from the National Surveillance Network and Contributing State and Local Networks, table 16, 1966.

6/ U.S. Environmental Protection Agency. Natural Radiation Exposure in the United States, report no. ORP/SID 72-1, table A-1, 1972, 1974 reprint.

7/ White, Jonathan W., Jr. "Relative significance of dietary sources of nitrate and nitrite." Journal of Agricultural and Food Chemistry 23:5, table VI, 1975, p. 890.

8/ U.S. Department of Agriculture. Household Food Consumption Survey, 1955, report nos. 2-5.

9/ Watt, Bernice K. and Annabell L. Merrill. Composition of Foods: Raw, Processed and Prepared, U.S. Department of Agriculture, Agricultural Handbook no. 8, 1968.

10/ U.S. Bureau of the Census. U.S. Census of the Population: 1960, vol. I, tables 140, 148.

11/ Tobacco Tax Council. Cigarette Taxes in the U.S., table 15, 1956.

the equation and the other excluded variables were not significant. Among the air and water quality variables tested,
only atmospheric ammonium and terrestrial gamma radiation
(effective absorbed dose) showed statistical significance
and are presented in table 1. Nitrogen-related variables
included, but not found significant, were atmospheric nitrates, nitrogen dioxide, and nitrates in water. Also
tested, and not found significant, were particulates, atmospheric beta, ultraviolet and cosmic radiation, and water
hardness.

     Table 1 also presents the nutrients that were found
significant: nitrates and nitrites in food, saturated fatty
acids and protein in food from animal sources, cholesterol,
and vitamin C (abscorbic acid); calories and vitamin A were
found not significant. In addition, coffee, alcohol, and
cigarette consumption were tested; only coffee and cigarettes were found to be significant.

     All of the nutrient variables were lagged, usually,
for 16 years, because that was the longest lag the data set
permitted. The significance of introducing the lag, to reflect the latency period of cancer, is shown by the fact
that some of the most significant variables found have no
explanatory power when introduced at their current values.
The dietary variables had to be constructed since there are
no direct data available. For example, for each of the
states that included sample cities, cigarette consumption
was estimated on the basis of cigarette tax revenues and
tax rates for each state.

     The procedure used in the construction of the nu-
trient and dietary data is worth describing in some detail,
as it is somewhat involved. Food consumption data for the
60 cities were first constructed from food consumption and
family size of a 1955 sample of 2,832 urban households distributed among eight income brackets for four regions of the
United States (see sources, table 1). The result obtained
for each city is a weighted average of food consumption in
each income bracket for the region of the city, multiplied
by the fraction of the city's population in each of the income brackets. Nutrient data for each city were then generated by multiplying the quantities of 49 foods, constructed as described, by their respective concentrations of a
given nutrient. Several regional patterns are observable
in the final results of this procedure. For example, people
in southern cities, in 1955 at least, appear to have consumed more nitrites and nitrates, but less protein, less
alcohol, and fewer cigarettes than people of other regions.
In the northeast, people consumed fewer nitrites, but more
cigarettes, than people of other regions.

     The independent variables included in the cancer mor-
tality regression analysis are based on several hypotheses

that relate them directly or indirectly to cancer. A simple
positive association between consumption of meat and cancer
rates has long been noted. However, this association may
be due to a number of simultaneous factors, including protein, fats, and preservatives. Thus, for example, ingestion
of meats cured with nitrite may result in formation of a
potent class of carcinogens known as nitrosamines. In vivo
formation of nitrosamines may then, in the main, be determined by the levels of lunch meat and cured pork which are
consumed. Ascorbic acid constructed from freshly eaten
fruit and vegetable data is hypothesized to block formation
of nitrosamines in vivo. Thus, a significant negative relationship between ascorbic acid and cancer may lend additional credence to a nitrite variable. Hypotheses involving
possible connections between the other variables and cancer
include protein and fat as well as caffeine in the diet,
exposure to radiation, and smoking.

The following equation is a result of the inclusion
of all the variables listed in table 1 (t-coefficients are
given in parentheses):

(8)   CANC = -8.500 - 0.00438 DPOP + 0.620 NONW
             (-3.17)   (1.97)   (2.26)

        + 0.101 MAGE + 0.0661 AMMN + 0.00194 GAMA
          (7.33)   (2.50)   (0.54)

        + 4.688 NTRI + 0.000687 PROT - 0.204 CVIT
          (3.32)   (3.05)   (-2.21)

        + 0.00271 CIGS + 0.0207 NTRA
          (1.20)   (0.96)

        - 0.000642 SFAT - 0.0380 CHOL
          (-1.57)   (-1.58)

        + 0.710 COFF
          (2.13)

R^2 = 0.787 D.F. = 46.

The negative signs on SFAT and CHOL were not expected, although they are significant at the 95 percent level. It may
be speculated, however, that these variables contribute to
competing causes of death, such as cardiovascular disease,
and thus indirectly affect cancer mortality. This is a

possible example of simultaneous equation bias.* If these
two variables are removed, then COFF and NTRA become insignificant (t $\leq$ 1.00). The following equation has all four
removed:

$$(9) \quad CANC = -9.593 - 0.00470 \text{ DPOP} + 0.332 \text{ NONW}$$
$$ (-4.08) \quad (-2.32) (1.49)$$

$$+ 0.0979 \text{ MAGE} + 0.0651 \text{ AMMN}$$
$$(7.23) (2.63)$$

$$+ 0.00418 \text{ GAMA} + 2.69 \text{ NTRI}$$
$$(1.26) (4.07)$$

$$+ 0.000338 \text{ PROT} - 0.249 \text{ CVIT}$$
$$(3.25) (-3.21)$$

$$+ 0.00258 \text{ CIGS}$$
$$(1.17)$$

$$R^2 = 0.764 \quad D.F. = 50.$$

No heteroscedasticity could be detected in plotting the
residuals against the variables in the equation above.
Thus, the use of ordinary least squares estimates is satisfactory in this case.

The only notable multicollinearity problems are those
between nutrients. Of these, the most important are between
PROT and each of VITA, COFF, and ALCO, and between VITC and
SFAT (see table 2). Considered as alternatives, however,
these other variables do not test out significantly in the
equation. Vitamin C, however, loses its significance if
either NTRI or PROT is removed from the equation. This was
not surprising since each of these variables explains a substantial portion of the residual variation in cancer
mortality.

This equation rather strongly associates both
nitrites and protein in the diet with cancer. In addition,
vitamin C (ascorbic acid) appears with a significant negative correlation. It should, however, be kept in mind in
interpreting these results that correlation does not prove
causation. In fact, spurious results are often found when

---

* Specifically, median age in our cities will, of course,
   be negatively related to heart disease, that is, earlier
   death lowers median age. Heart disease is most likely
   positively related to cholesterol and saturated fats.
   Thus, since cancer rates are positively affected by
   median age, one might expect cancer to show negative
   correlations with saturated fats and cholesterol even if
   these have no direct causal relationship with cancer.

Table 2. Correlation Matrix for Variables Having Correlations $\geq$ 0.80.

	NTRI	NTRA	SFAT	PROT	CHOL	FIBR	CALO	VITA	VITC	COFF	ALCO
Nitrite	1.0										
Nitrate	.68	1.0									
Saturated fat	-.03		1.0								
Protein	-.57	-.76	.82	1.0							
Cholesteral	-.03		.74	.72	1.0						
Fiber			.86	.80	.86	1.0					
Calories	.86						1.0				
Vitamin A	-.75	-.84	.93	.95	.86	.72		1.0			
Vitamin C	.06		.93	.75	.86	.81			1.0		
Coffee	-.40	-.79	.91	.93	.66	.88		.89	.78	1.0	
Alcohol	-.69	-.89	.73	.94	.74	.74		.98			1.0

unknown collinearity occurs. However, the hypotheses' relation to nitrites in diet cannot be rejected on the basis of
this analysis. If the hypotheses on vitamin C and nitrites
are, in fact, true and if the regressions specified above are
not biased, then the estimated equations may provide values
for the incremental risk of cancer due to dietary exposure to
nitrites. It should also be noted that in both regressions,
nitrite is the second most significant explanatory variable
(t-values exceed 99 percent confidence level) after median
age of the population. This is a relatively important result
in spite of all the caveats given because a correlation between meat consumption (often high in added nitrite) and
cancer rates has been long recognized. This association,
however, is consistent with a number of hypotheses relating
nitrites, protein, fat, and a substantial list of other
possible factors, such as use of DES, and other drugs used
in animal husbandry in the United States, to cancer. The
fact that protein and nitrites remain positively correlated
in competition with other factors that are negatively or in-
significantly correlated (for example, fat) suggests, at
least, directions for future research.

CONCLUSION

        The importance of understanding the role of environ-
mental, including dietary factors in cancer, can be shown by
applying the economic methodology discussed in the first part
of this paper. Since our sample of 60 cities represents
urban populations, we will take the population at risk (N in
the previous section) to be 150 million individuals. To stay
on the conservative side, we will take the incremental cost
of risk $(U/U \, (1-\pi))$ from the Thaler-Rosen study to be
$340,000. Finally, using the second regression equation (9),
estimates of the incremental risk from various environmental
factors (X's from the first part of the paper) are shown in
table 3, along with the incremental benefits of a reduction
in exposure $(N \cdot \pi_X \cdot (U/U'(1-\pi))$.

        Because the units of measure in table 3 are not readily
understandable, table 4 presents the benefits of a 10 percent
reduction in exposure to the factors of table 3, except for
vitamin C for which a 10 percent increase in exposure is assumed. The base exposures are taken to be the sample means
from our data set, as shown in table 1. The implications of
table 4 are perhaps not meaningful in terms of the specific
causal factors listed--about which great question remains--
but rather in terms of the result that a 10 percent variation
in exposure patterns, which quite possibly is achievable with
minor lifestyle changes and control efforts, could result in
benefits of nearly $9 billion per year.

Table 3. Estimates of Environmental Factors.

Environmental factor (units)	Incremental risk of death/unit exposure	Incremental benefits $/unit decrease in exposure to U.S. urban population
Ammonium (ug/m^3)	$.065 \times 10^{-4}$	332×10^6
Gama Radiation (mrem)	$.0042 \times 10^{-4}$	21×10^6
Nitrite (g/cap)	2.7×10^{-4}	$13{,}719 \times 10^6$
Protein (g/cap)	$.00034 \times 10^{-4}$	1.7×10^6
Vitamin C (g/cap)	$-.25 \times 10^{-4}$	-1270×10^6
Cigarettes (packs/cap)	$.0026 \times 10^{-4}$	13×10^6

Table 4. Benefits of a 10 Percent Change in Environmental Factors.

Millions of dollars

Ammonium	$ 38
Gamma Radiation	210
Nitrite	1,742
Protein	4,578
Vitamin C	2,154
Cigarettes	143
Total	$8,865

Acknowledgments.

This research was funded in part by USEPA Grant No. 805059010.
Thanks go to Ralph d'Arge and Berry Ives for their contributions and comments.

REFERENCES

Kneese, Allen and William Schulze
     1977   "Environment, health and economics - the case
             of cancer." American Economic Review 67:1.

Lave, Lester and Eugene Seskin
     1970   "Air pollution and human health." Science 169
             (August 21).

Mishan, E. J.
     1971   "Evaluation of life and limb: A theoretical
             approach." Journal of Political Economy 79:4.

Thaler, R. H. and S. Rosen
     1976   "The value of saving a life: Evidence from the
             labor market." In Terleckyj, N. E. (ed.),
             Household Production and Consumption. New York:
             Columbia University Press.

Health Resource
Allocations

10 Allocation and Priority Setting in Research

Solomon Schneyer

Many discussions of the allocation of research funds for biomedical research seem to make several implicit assumptions without any recognition of the implications of those assumptions for the problem of allocation.

The first assumption comes in two parts, almost like two sides of the same coin, thus:

a. that health issues can be placed into neat categories for purposes of resource allocation (or for any other purpose), and

b. that there is a simple relationship between the purposes for which resources are allocated and eventual program outcomes.

The second assumption is that you can buy particular results in basic science. These assumptions involve many problems.

On another level, often there is no clear distinction made between research and the delivery of service. Statements are made in terms of the allocation of resources for research, but the context of the discussion makes it clear that what was really being addressed was service delivery. These are two very different problems and solutions for one are probably not relevant for the other.

This paper will discuss the problems of allocation within the National Institutes of Health (NIH). Since the NIH is the largest element in the federal biomedical research sector and the non-federal fraction is not subject to any central control, the problems of NIH allocation are most important. In addition, it is the area in which I have the most personal knowledge.

237

THE ALLOCATION PROCESS

The basic organization of the NIH is in terms of
disease categories and the allocation process boils down to
the development of appropriations for the individual institutes. Very briefly, the administration makes proposals
which the Congress digests and then translates into an appropriation. That process is significantly influenced by a
wide range of organizations in the private sector. Common
mythology has it that since this process is political, it is
erratic, non-rational, and could be much improved. I wonder
sometimes if it is really all that bad. The following data
might be instructive.

Many people believe that funding for biomedical research should be directly related to the "significance" of
the health problem at which the research is aimed. Last
year, the Division of Program Analysis at the NIH received
a request from a member of Congress for data which would compare funding levels of the research institutes of the NIH
with measures of mortality and morbidity. We tried to do as
complete a job as existing data would permit and we assembled
some material, with the help of the Public Services Laboratory at Georgetown University. One of the real problems in
putting together this kind of data is that of assigning
disease costs to particular research programs. Each individual institute of the NIH is concerned with research on
particular diseases, but the diseases have the distressing
habit of not staying in the boxes to which we assign them.
This is related to the first "assumption" mentioned earlier.
Diabetes, for example, is one of the major concerns of the
National Institute of Arthritis, Metabolism, and Digestive
Diseases (NIAMD). At the same time, diabetes is often a
factor in heart disease and in blindness. Significant
portions of the budgets of both the National Heart, Lung,
and Blood Institute (NHLBI) and the National Eye Institute
(NEI) are devoted to diabetes-related research. How do we
split the cost of diabetes among these institutes? Diabetes
is not unique. At the present time, a national commission
is examining the problems presented by digestive diseases.
Within the NIH, primary responsibility for digestive diseases
resides, again, with the NIAMD. It appears, however, that
one of the major digestive diseases is cancer.

There are many diseases which have implications for
more than one institute and there is no formula that will
permit a distribution satisfactory to all interested parties.
In order to answer the congressman's question before the next
election, an arbitrary although preliminary solution was
reached in which the total cost of a particular disease was
assigned to that institute which was presumed to have a
primary interest in it. Many research specialists at the NIH
were not satisfied with that solution and a work group was
assembled to try to find a better solution. They have not

yet finished their work but their evaluation of the results
of their efforts includes the following observations:

(1)   There is no correct way of allocating ill-
      ness measures to institutes. After a
      lengthy search for an appropriate allo-
      cation, the Committee was presented with
      five alternative algorithms classified by
      three alternative disease indicators--
      a total of 15 different rankings of rel-
      ative shares. A priori there is a
      rationale, medical or economic, for adopt-
      ing any one of them. There is no obvious
      or consistent link, however, between dis-
      eases and institute concerns.

(2)   Even if there were agreement on a par-
      ticular allocation, there is no means
      of selecting the proper illness measure
      or devising a common denominator for
      combining the various measures.

(3)   The three morbidity and mortality mea-
      sures which can actually be employed in
      this sort of allocation by four-digit
      code fall short of representing a
      rounded picture of the impact of dis-
      eases on health status.

        For present purposes, however, the data assembled
last year will make several points, even though one can argue
with them as not "correctly" representing the activity of
the institutes.

MEASURES FOR RESOURCE ALLOCATION

        The kinds of measures which might be used were limited
by the data available. In general, data were available on
mortality, on short-term hospital bed days, on several aspects of restricted activity, and on visits to physicians
and dentists. It turned out that three measures of restricted activity--restricted-activity days, bed-disability
days, and work-loss days--were all highly related to each
other. The table presented here includes only the work-loss
days, which will serve as representative of the three
(table 1). Completing these data threw several issues into
bold relief. To begin with, they make sense for only eight
of the institutes of the NIH. They are not particularly
useful in examining the activities of the National Institute
of General Medical Sciences (NIGMS), the National Institute
of Environmental Health Sciences (NIEHS), the National Institute on Aging (NIA), and the Division of Research Resources (DRR). The issue here is not the parochial one of

Table 1. Appropriations and Preliminary Estimates of Indicators of the Impact of Diseases for Eight Research Institutes at the NIH.

Institute	Appropriations FY 1976 ($ millions)	Deaths (thousands)	Short-term hospital bed days (millions)	Work-loss days (millions)	Visits to physicians and dentists (millions)
NCI	$ 762.6	366	23.4	4.6	50.6
NHLBI	370.3	804	42.4	55.0	230.8
NIAMD	179.8	109	69.8	77.0	373.4
NINCDS	144.7	209	13.3	17.1	80.3
NICHD	136.6	43	26.3	8.0	78.7
NIAID	127.2	100	20.4	149.7	174.8
NIDR	51.4	--	1.4	4.7	328.4
NEI	50.3	--	3.0	4.0	59.4
Subtotal	1,822.9	1,631	200.3	320.1	1,376.3
Not allocated	374.9*	306	44.9	127.1	613.7
Total	2,197.8	1,937	245.2	447.2	1,990.0

* Includes NIGMS, NIEHS, NIA, and DRR.

how to allocate funds to the individual institutes of the
NIH, but that despite the best of intentions, there is more
than one way of looking at the problem of disease. The difficulty of keeping a disease in a single box has already been
mentioned. A few other difficulties are described below.

The NIGMS is primarily charged with funding basic research when its relevance for a specific disease is not clear
or when, ultimately, the research may be relevant for several
diseases. This brings us to the problem of how to provide
for fundamental research in a disease-based allocation
system. The NIA is charged with doing research on the
process of aging. How do we measure the impact of that
process? In 1975, 64 percent of the people who died in the
United States were 65 years old or older. It might be said,
then, that 64 percent of the U.S. population dies of old age,
but that is not a very useful conclusion. The NIEHS is concerned with the ways in which environmental agents affect the
human organism. The agents which they study may ultimately
be involved in cancer, or the diseases of any organ system--
heart, liver, kidney, the nervous system, whatever. NIEHS
picks up one end of a particular stick and a categorical institute holds the other. How do we measure impact and allocate costs?

Disease-related Institutes

The following comments will focus on the eight institutes for which a disease-related distribution is feasible.
Table 2, in order to make the information in table 1 more
useful, shows the rank order from lowest to highest of each
of the institutes on each of the measures. The bottom line
of the table shows the rank order correlation for each of the
measures shown, with the appropriations of the individual institutes. A rank order correlation is a rather gross measure,
but with these data it seems reasonable. With the measures
shown, the highest relation is between deaths and appropriations. It is not perfect, but it certainly suggests that
causes of death are a critical factor in the decisions which
are made regarding NIH appropriations. Short-term hospital
bed days are also a factor, although by no means as significant as deaths. Work-loss days are much less critical, and
visits to physicians are essentially unrelated to research
appropriations measured this way.

Three problems emerge from this data: (1) In the correlation between deaths and appropriations, there is one
glaring discrepancy: The Cancer Institute and the Heart Institute are out-of-pattern. The NCI receives approximately
twice as much money as the NHLBI does, but heart disease
kills about twice as many people a year as cancer. Obviously, even though death rates are a matter of concern in
the development of public policy on health research, other

Table 2. Rank Order of Appropriations and Preliminary Estimates of Indicators of the Impact of Diseases for Eight Research Institutes at the NIH.

Institute	Appropriations FY 1976	Deaths	Short-term hospital bed days (millions)	Work-loss days	Visits to physicians and dentists
NCI	1	2	4	7	8
NHLBI	2	1	2	3	3
NIAMD	3	4	1	2	1
NINCDS	4	3	6	4	5
NICHD	5	6	3	5	6
NIAID	6	5	5	1	4
NIDR	7	7	8	6	2
NEI	8	8	7	8	7
Rank correlation with appropriations		0.93	0.71	0.24	-0.02

factors enter into it. (2) The correlation shown here between deaths and appropriations is an indication of the perceptions of the Congress regarding NIH research programs--
that the names of the categorical institutes clearly identify
where research related to given diseases is carried out.
However, the work group mentioned earlier has tried to develop measures which parcel out diseases among all institutes
concerned with them, rather than assigning a given disease to
the primary institute, as was done here. Using this approach,
the correlation between death rates and institute appropriations drops sharply. (3) The measures available for assessing the impact of disease in the population do not correlate
very well with each other. This is important because it
makes the problem of allocation even more difficult. If allocation is to be "rational," presumably it should be based
on some set of principles. Coherent principles for this
purpose are extremely difficult to develop. It is con-
ceivable that one might be able to convert all of these measures into some dollar measure. Whether the availability of
such a dollar measure would be useful for decision making in
this area, I do not know. Obviously, concerns like the fear
of cancer would still exist regardless of the dollar costs
involved and the country might or might not feel that dollar
cost is an appropriate basis for allocating research funds.

Scientific Opportunity

        There is another problem in allocation which these
kinds of numbers do not even touch upon and that is the matter of scientific opportunity. To propose a measure, such
as mortality or cost, as a basis for allocation implies,
however vaguely, that there is an assumption that one can
buy solutions to problems on demand. Sometimes this is
possible. Often it is not. The country bought a solution
to polio. We have not yet been able to buy a solution to
cancer. Whether we will be able to and how soon remains for
the future. For some problems, we know enough to be able to
predict that the expenditure of some finite amount of money
gives a high probability of producing a solution within a
reasonable period of time. The development of a vaccine
when one knows enough about the disease is probably a type
case of this sort. For disease problems in which we lack
necessary fundamental understanding, allocation should reflect a scientific judgment of the areas in which the opportunity for advances exist.

THE LEVEL OF INVESTMENT

        Apart from the question of how to allocate research
funds, there is the question of how much should be allocated
for research. I want to emphasize here that this paper represents a personal view and not an official statement on the

part of the NIH. It has been suggested that industrial organizations invest some five or six percent of their annual
sales in research activities and that this would be a reasonable level for the health industry. Using five percent,
in 1976 we should have spent something on the order of $7
billion for the total of health research and development
rather than $5 billion and the NIH appropriation should have
been about $1 billion more than it was. This may or may not
have been a desirable increase depending on one's point of
view about the value of research and perhaps about the value
of NIH programs. I am not certain that a parallel between
the health industry, on the one hand, and, for example, the
automobile industry, on the other, is entirely valid and
clearly such an increase in the federal commitment to biomedical research in 1976 was not politically feasible. Dis-
regarding the question of what the particular level should
be, a significant level of investment in these research
activities is probably necessary. I assume that everyone is
concerned about the rate at which health care costs have been
rising in this century. Research offers one significant hope
for containment of these costs.

Consider one problem. The U.S. Census Bureau estimates that by the year 2030, not as far off as it sounds, the
proportion of the population aged 65 or over will have increased from the present level of about 10 percent to about
17 percent--one person in every six. People in this age
group make disproportionately high demands on the health care
system. As their density in the population increases, those
demands will increase. I am not suggesting that research
will prevent aging, but if management of the diseases of the
aged is not significantly improved, the burden of caring for
this part of the population may well become insupportable.
Parenthetically, when I talk about 65 or over I am not talking about "them." With any luck at all, I am talking about
you and me.

As one concrete example of how research might make a
difference, consider the following. It is estimated that in
1972 some 241,000 cataract operations were performed in the
United States. Cataracts are clearly age-related--over 80
percent of these operations were performed in patients who
were 60 years old or more. If some hypothetical procedure
could be developed which would delay the need for cataract
surgery by 10 years, the number of operations required
annually would be reduced to 132,000. It has been estimated that the average cost of cataract surgery is about
$1,550. This includes pre-operative and post-operative care,
hospital costs, and the costs of special eyeglasses, as well
as the surgeon's fee. This multiplies out to a saving of
about $160 million a year on this procedure alone, a saving
which, obviously, increases as the number of older people
in the population increases.

I do not know how much we <u>should</u> spend on biomedical research. This involves a question of social values. When we are dealing with billions of dollars of public funds, it is difficult to see how this decision can be made by any formula. My own feeling is that we should spend as much as we can afford. How much we can afford is a political question which will inevitably have to be answered in the political arena. Unless we develop some major advance in methods of identifying scientific opportunities or in controlling the outcomes of research, the present process for making this decision may be as rational as we can hope for.

11 Returns to Biomedical Research in Chronic Diseases: A Case Study of Resource Allocation

David W. Dunlop

This paper analyzes a case study of resource allocation to diabetes research. The analysis focuses on the extent to which the research programs of the National Institutes of Health (NIH) minimize death from diabetes, reduce the incidence of the disease, and minimize the decline in functional health status.

To begin with, the paper briefly considers the impact of chronic conditions* on the health of the United States population. Second, the prevalence of diabetes (and other important chronic conditions) is analyzed. Issues related to the impact of multiple chronic conditions on the functional health status of diabetics is considered. Next, the economic costs of diabetes and the nature of research on diabetes are analyzed; the specific biomedical questions that this research has addressed are outlined.

The paper then analyzes the extent to which ongoing and future research (through the early 1980s) will address the major functional health problems of diabetes as well as the minimizing of the incidence of the condition. The paper concludes with a suggestion for a new demand-side orientation to biomedical research, particularly for chronic conditions.

DIABETES: A CHRONIC DISEASE

Much of the biomedical research conducted in this country has focused on (1) health problems that lead to death, (2) significant declines in an individual's ability

---

* Chronic conditions here include chronic diseases, such as diabetes, and chronic disabilities, such as skin disorders.

to function, or (3) health problems that are of an acute,
versus chronic, nature, for example, cancer and heart disease.   Increasingly, however, there are large subsets of the
population who report one or more chronic conditions.   These
chronic conditions, at the very least, inhibit an individual's ability to lead a normal life.   While not everyone in
the country has such a health problem, it is significant to
recall that well over 12 percent of the population report
that their major activities are limited because of the
existence of one or more chronic conditions (NCHS, 1977a) and
that many others have one or more chronic conditions that,
over time, reduce their functional health status (NCHS,
1977b).   Given that such a substantial proportion of the population is afflicted by chronic health problems, it is instructive to conduct a case study of the allocation of biomedical research resources to a particularly important
chronic disease, diabetes.

      According to the National Center for Health Statistics,
approximately five million persons in the country report having diabetes (NCHS, 1977b).   Further, according to the National Commission on Diabetes, approximately five million additional persons do not report their diabetes or are afflicted
with it on a subclinical basis (U.S.PHS, 1976).   These figures
are up considerably from the figures reported for the years
1964-65, in which roughly half that number of persons reported being diabetics (NCHS, 1967).

Mortality and Morbidity Analyzed

      The importance of diabetes as a major health problem
and chronic condition is determined when mortality and morbidity figures are analyzed.   Diabetes is the third leading
cause of death, after heart disease and cancer, in the population.   In 1967, over 85,000 deaths involved diabetes, with
about 40 percent of those deaths citing diabetes as the underlying cause (NCHS, 1971).   In addition, diabetes contributes
to the onset of secondary chronic conditions, which exacerbate
the long-term process of debilitation that occurs in the body
of the diabetic, particularly a diabetic who is not well-
controlled.   The prevalence of secondary chronic conditions
in diabetics is very high.   According to a special set of information obtained on diabetes in 1964-65 from the National
Health Interview Survey, only 20 percent of the diabetic
population report that diabetes was their only chronic condition (NCHS, 1971).   Further, nearly 60 percent reported
three or more chronic conditions, that is, two additional
conditions besides diabetes (NCHS, 1967).

      The most prevalent of the other chronic conditions
that diabetics tend to have is shown in table 1.   Nearly 38
percent of the diabetic population has some heart or hypertension problems.   Another 20 percent have some form of eye

Table 1.   Number and Percent of Diabetics with Selected
           Chronic Conditions and Percent of Diabetics
           with Chronic Conditions Who Are Female, by
           Condition: United States, July 1964-June 1965.

Chronic condition	Number of diabetics with chronic condition (in thousands)	Percent of total diabetics (N=3 million)	Percent of diabetics with chronic conditions who are female
Heart conditions	485	21.1%	61.9%
Hypertension without heart involvement	387	16.8	73.9
Impaired vision	238	10.3	70.6
Genitourinary disorders	190	8.3	63.7
Blind, both eyes	151	6.6	66.2
Cataracts	93	4.0	68.8
Gall bladder	84	3.7	89.3
Vascular lesions, CNS	76	3.3	47.4
Skin disorders	75	3.3	69.3
Goiter and thyroid	71	3.1	81.7
Absence of fingers, toes	51	2.2	23.5
Paralysis, complete or partial	50	2.2	48.0
Glaucoma	36	1.6	66.7
Gout, tuberculosis, or senility	35	1.5	54.3
Absence of major extremities	33	1.4	36.4

Source: National Center for Health Statistics, 10-40,
          table F, 1967, p. 6.

problem, either blindness, cataracts, or some impaired vision.
Poor circulation afflicts another 12.8 percent. Given the
prevalence of secondary chronic conditions, it is important
to determine their etiologies; this will clarify the extent
to which the behavior of a diabetic leads to early onset of
such additional chronic conditions.

     Approximately 83 percent of all diabetics in 1964-65
and in 1973 reported no disability days. On the other hand,
approximately four percent to five percent reported more than
15 bed-disability days per year. In table 2, data presented
for the years 1957-59, 1964-65, and 1973 show the number of

Table 2.   Number of Disability Days Per Diabetic Per Year
           Resulting from Diabetes in 1957-59, 1964-65, and
           1973.

	1957-59		1964-65		1973	
	Re-stricted activity	Bed	Re-stricted activity	Bed	Re-stricted activity	Bed
All ages	19.9	8.5	17.3	8.2	14.6	5.8
Under 45 years	11.9	2.9	9.7	5.2	NA	NA
45-54 years	22.5	8.8	13.0	3.3	NA	NA
55-64 years	19.2	7.1	24.4	7.8	NA	NA
65-74 years	21.4	10.8	16.7	11.1	NA	NA
75+	26.1	14.5	19.8	13.3	NA	NA
All men	17.0	6.6	15.8	6.0	NA	NA
All women	22.0	9.9	18.4	9.8	NA	NA

Source: (1) National Health Survey, series B, no. 21,
               table 4, September 1960, p. 10.
          (2) National Health Survey, series 10, no. 40,
               table G, October 1967, p. 7.
          (3) National Health Survey, series 10, no. 109,
               table A, March 1977, p. 5.

restricted activity days and bed-disability days per diabetic
per year resulting solely from diabetes (none of the secondary chronic conditions) by age and sex. In comparing the
rates for these two health status measures for diabetics with
the rates for the entire population, the number of restricted
activity days resulting solely from diabetes does not significantly differ from that reported for the entire population.* However, reported bed-disability days (related to
diabetes) is about 20 percent greater for diabetics than for
the national rate.

     Of greater interest, however, is the number of dis-
ability days per diabetic per year from all conditions af-
flicting diabetics. In table 3, data are presented for
1964-65 which show that total restricted activity days and
bed days for diabetics is between two to three times as great

---

*   Data taken from the relevant series 10 publications of the
    National Center for Health Statistics.

Table 3. Number of Disability Days Per Diabetic Per Year
          from All Conditions and from Diabetes, by Sex
          and Age: United States, July 1964-June 1965.

Sex and age	Restricted activity		Bed disability	
	From all conditions	From diabetes	From all conditions	From diabetes
Both sexes				
All ages	54.0	17.3	23.3	8.2
Under 45 years	33.4	9.7	15.9	5.2
45-54 years	40.4	13.0	19.4	3.3
55-64 years	67.9	24.4	28.4	7.8
65-74 years	56.9	16.7	23.3	11.1
75+	63.9	19.8	27.6	13.3
Males				
All ages	48.1	15.8	17.8	6.0
Under 45 years	25.7	9.5	9.2	5.0
45-54 years	31.3	9.7	16.6	0.2
55-64 years	65.9	20.4	19.7	0.9
65-74 years	55.7	16.0	14.6	8.2
75+	53.3	23.5	35.1	21.6
Female				
All ages	58.2	18.4	27.2	9.8
Under 45 years	40.6	9.9	22.1	5.4
45-54 years	47.2	15.4	21.4	5.5
55-64 years	69.3	27.2	34.5	12.7
65-74 years	57.7	17.1	28.9	12.9
75+	71.1	17.3	22.6	7.8

Source: National Center for Health Statistics, series 10,
         no. 40, table G, 1967, p. 7.

as that reported in table 2. These data obviously highlight
the importance of secondary complications and chronic
conditions.

     The data in tables 2 and 3 also show a striking dif-
ferential between the male and female rate of restricted
activity days, with the female rate being approximately 20
percent greater than the male, particularly in the prime

working ages (25-54).   In addition, a greater percentage of
women (25 percent) report having some restricted activity
days as compared to men (10-12 percent).   Is this finding due
to (a) a differential degree of seriousness of the disease
between men and women or (b) the differential opportunity
cost of time between males and females in these two age
groups, particularly if they are employed?   These are questions for further research; they can be addressed with data
presently available from the National Center for Health
Statistics.

        In the 1964-65 National Health Interview Survey, a
considerable percentage of the diabetic population report one
or more symptoms of the disease.   Such reporting suggests
that the reportees are less than fully-controlled diabetic
patients.   About one and one-half diabetic symptoms per
diabetic were reported during the month prior to investigation, with the figures for females in the population being
considerably greater than for males--again an interesting
implication for research by labor economists (NCHS, 1967).

        In the 1973 National Health Interview Survey, approxi-
mately 50 percent of diabetics were bothered to some extent
by their diabetes, with 21 percent being bothered "often" or
"all the time"; over 12 percent indicated they were bothered
a "great deal" (NCHS, 1977c).   What would be important to
investigate is the relationship between the reporting of
symptoms and the degree or intensity of bother and the movement from one category to another.   Of further interest would
be the extent to which diabetics allocate resources to reduce
the frequency or degree of bothersomeness--an indication of
willingness to pay.

Economic Cost

        In 1975, one of the work groups for the National Com-
mission on Diabetes analyzed the economic cost of diabetes
and conducted a review of previous research.   The methodology
employed in their analysis follows traditional analytical
concepts of the human capital approach (Weisbrod, 1961; Rice,
1966; Jones-Lee, 1976).   Many of the issues raised at a recent conference on the valuation of human life (Acton, 1976b)
were not incorporated into the Commission's discussion of
the state of the art of cost-benefit analysis, nor was it incorporated into the empirical analysis of the cost of the
disease.

        Despite these limitations, the Commission focused on
estimating three costs of diabetes.   The findings are summarized in table 4.   First, the direct cost of morbidity
due to diabetes, such as hospital care, physician services,
drugs, nursing home care, and other professional medical
services was estimated to be approximately $2.5 billion in

Table 4. Estimated Cost of Diabetes, United States, 1975.

	I Cost of of morbid-ity due to diabetes	II Cost of compli-cations among diabetics	III Total direct costs
(A) Direct costs (in millions)			
Hospital care	$1,050.0	$165.0	$1,215.0
Physician services	590.0	45.4	635.4
Drugs	300.0	39.7	339.7
Nursing home care	520.0	36.1	556.1
Other professional services	60.0	9.9	69.9
Total direct costs	$2,520.0	$297.0	$2,817.0
(B) Indirect costs of diabetes (in millions)			
I. Earnings loss for employed diabetics			
Mortality (annual)		63.4	
Morbidity		397.7	461.1
II. Imputed earnings loss for housewives			
Mortality (annual)		17.3	
Morbidity		47.6	64.9
III. Imputed earnings loss for institutionalized diabetics			235.5
IV. Imputed earnings loss for disabled (non-institutional) diabetics			996.4
V. Lifetime earnings loss from mortality of diabetics			1,065.6
Total indirect costs of diabetics			$2,823.5
Total cost of diabetes Direct and indirect costs (A and B)			$5,640.5

Source: National Commission on Diabetes, vol. III, no. 1, tables 7, 8, and 10, pp. 319, 321, and 326.

1975. Second, the direct cost of other disease complications
resulting in additional morbidity in diabetics approximated
an additional $300 million. Finally, the estimated direct
cost of diabetes in 1975 was greater than $2.8 billion. The
indirect cost estimate followed the methodology developed by
Rice (1966) and Cooper and Rice (1976); it includes present
value estimates of lost output due to premature death and
morbidity among diabetics. To summarize, the Commission
found that the total cost of diabetes was at least $5.7
billion in 1975.

While the above-described cost analysis yields some
useful information, in order to (a) improve our understanding
of the cost of chronic conditions, such as diabetes, and
(b) to utilize the information for decision making in resource allocation to biomedical research, there are two other
issues requiring investigation. (1) It is important to
initiate research measuring the dislocation costs to families
as a consequence of having a diabetic member of the household.
To what extent do certain family members allocate their time
to the provision of health and medical care services to the
diabetic? Does a household alter its expenditure pattern,
particularly by constricting its consumption of certain
utility-producing items? In addition, with respect to the
indirect costs of complications in diabetics, it is important
to determine the extent to which diabetics with secondary
chronic conditions are subject to a higher probability of un-
employment, experience more work days lost if employed, and
have lower lifetime earnings streams than diabetics without
complications. (2) It is important to analyze diabetics'
and others' willingness to pay to alter the bother--in terms
of frequency and degree--caused by diabetes.

RESEARCH FUNDING

In fiscal year 1975, approximately $45 million was
spent by the federal government and other sources on research
into the problem of diabetes. Approximately 85 percent ($39
million) of that research support came from the NIH. Other
departments and agencies of the federal government spent
around $3.5 million; voluntary agencies, including such or-
ganizations as the American Diabetes Association and the
Juvenile Diabetes Foundation, contributed another $2.5 mil-
lion. Private industry, particularly drug companies who produce the primary treatment and control agents used by
diabetics, is known to engage in some research. Eli Lily,
Upjohn, and others are undoubtedly allocating resources
toward the development of more efficacious therapeutic

agents.*

At NIH, the National Institute of Arthritis, Metabolism, and Digestive Diseases (NIAMDD) is the source of approximately 40 percent of the extramural research funds for diabetes. It is significant to note that in fiscal year 1975 diabetes research constituted only 11 percent of all extramural research supported by NIAMDD. Other institutes within the NIH, however, also have significant diabetes research programs that focus on complications and secondary conditions, for example, heart and eye-related problems, from which diabetics suffer. The National Eye Institute (NEI) spent nearly $5 million on a program that analyzed the effects of diabetes on the long-term functioning of the eye. The Division of Research Resources (DRR) also had a $5-6 million program under the aegis of its General Clinical Research Centers Branch to determine how treatment and clinical care for diabetes could be improved. Further, the National Heart, Lung, and Blood Institute (NHLBI) spent over $5.5 million on research concerning the heart and related systems in which a large percentage of complications from diabetes manifest themselves (recall table 1). Finally, the National Institute of Child Health and Human Development (NICHD) is allocating over $1 million to study complications during pregnancy and problems of young diabetics. In summary, it is significant to find that about 50 percent of all NIH funds are allocated to studying secondary chronic conditions associated with diabetes. Further research questions include the determination of whether (a) the mix of resources across institutes engaged in research related to secondary chronic conditions is an appropriate one and (b) whether research projects have short-run or long-run payoffs to the existing stock of diabetics.

NIAMDD Funding

In table 5, an analysis of the extramural research program of NIAMDD is presented. Actual expenditures for fiscal years 1975 and 1976 are shown in relationship to the projected 1976 research program and to the recommended funding by the National Commission on Diabetes for 1980. The figures provide an indication of the institute's priorities with respect to diabetes research.

------

* The exact amounts spent by private industry on diabetes-related research is not known, given trade secrecy and other grounds upon which reluctance to discuss such matters is often justified. See National Commission on Diabetes, vol. 1 (U.S.DHEW, 1976), p. 63.

Table 5. National Institute of Arthritis, Metabolism, and Digestive Diseases (NIAMDD) Extramural Research Program.

Primary research area	Fiscal year 1975 1/ Actual		Fiscal year 1976 Projected 1/		Fiscal year 1976 Actual funding 2/				Fiscal year 1980 1/ Projected	
	($000s)	Percent of total	($000s)	Percent of total	Number of studies	($000s)	Percent of studies	Percent of funding	($000s)	Percent
Basic endocrine and metabolic	$ 7,996	54.1%	$10,400	50.0%	165	$11,320.0	76.7%	80.6%	$29,705	59.0%
Etiology (viruses and genetics)	683	4.7	918	4.4	3	483.6	1.4	3.4	2,346	4.6
Angiopathy 3/	389	2.6	750	3.6	32	844.5	14.9	6.0	1,500	3.0
Nutrition and obesity	487	3.3	1,400	6.8	1	126.7	0.5	0.9	2,644	5.2
Transplantation and artificial devices	684	4.6	1,389	6.7	11	1,042.5	5.1	7.4	5,540	11.0
Epidemiology	394	2.7	545	2.6	2	208.6	0.9	1.5	2,000	4.0
Resources and facilities	--	--	750	3.6	--	--	--	--	1,500	3.0
Clinical study of juvenile diabetes	--	--	500	2.4	--	--	--	--	1,000	2.0
Other	4,144	28.0	4,144	19.9	1	12.2	0.5	0.1	4,144	8.2
Total	14,777	100.0	20,796	100.0	215	14,038.0	100.0	99.9	50,379	100.0

1/ National Commission on Diabetes, The Long-Range Plan to Combat Diabetes, U.S.DHEW, vol. 1, no. (NIH) 76-1018, 1976, p. 71.
2/ NIAMDD, "Primary area research report, fiscal year 1976," Internal Document, June 3, 1977, pp. 11-16.
3/ Angiopathy refers to disease of the blood vessels. Kidney problems often represent an underlying cause of angiopathy.

The data presented in table 5 provide several interesting findings:

(1)   It is projected that the level of research
      support for basic endocrine and metabolic
      studies in diabetes will more than triple
      between 1975 and 1980. Between 1975 and
      1976, there was an actual increase in ex-
      penditures of approximately 41 percent in
      this area. Such research deals with all
      mechanisms by which various organs derive
      energy from the metabolism of foodstuffs,
      the regulation of these metabolic pro-
      cesses with hormones such as insulin
      and glucagon and the metabolic abnormal-
      ities that may exist as a consequence of
      having a disease such as diabetes.

(2)   While projected research funding for study-
      ing the etiology of diabetes as related to
      the viral and genetic hypotheses is shown
      to be increasing, the amount spent has de-
      clined between 1975 and 1976. Has the
      probability of conclusive results de-
      teriorated? In addition, while the fund-
      ing for research on obesity and nutrition
      as related to diabetes--another etiological
      hypothesis--was expected to increase dur-
      ing the late 1970s to approximately $2.6
      million by 1980, actual funding between
      1975 and 1976 suggests a substantial decline.

(3)   Epidemiological studies of the prevalence
      and incidence of diabetes in the population,
      as correlated with other social, environ-
      mental, and demographic characteristics,
      have not as yet received significant fund-
      ing nor have projected funding levels been
      attained.

(4)   Experimentation on microangiopathy in
      diabetes requires funding increases well
      over the projected 1976 figures.

(5)   Research on transplantation to monitor
      blood glucose levels indicates substantial
      and greater-than-expected increases in
      funding.

(6)   While both the research on angiopathy, as
      well as those related to transplantation,
      are directly related to treatment and
      potential functional health status improve-
      ment among diabetics, and most of the
      theoretical basis for such treatment

strategies are based on the findings
of basic endocrine and metabolic research; such basic research currently
constitutes approximately 76 percent
of all the studies that were funded,
and 80 percent of the funds.

Despite the great need, it is clear that little research is being funded by NIAMDD to find ways to reduce the
impairments in functional health status caused by diabetes.
The NIAMDD diabetes research program is, and appears as
though it will continue to be, supply-side oriented.

NIH Diabetes Research Funding

Tables 6 and 7 show data on current appropriations
and future recommendations for diabetes research for all NIH
institutes. An analysis of recommended research funding for
the NIH suggests that Congress, the President, and the
National Commission are aware of the substantial complications from diabetes and that a substantial proportion of
the population suffer or die from these complications. Thus,
since the NIAMDD research program is directed at understanding diabetes per se, the 1977 appropriation alternatives
found in table 6, as well as the actual funding support in
1975 and 1976 as shown in table 7, show that this line of
research has received less than 50 percent of all research
funding. Further, the institutes conducting research on
the most prevalent complications of diabetes, that is, NHLBI
and NEI, tend to have the largest funding support.

Table 6 shows three additional pieces of information
worthy of comment: (1) The funding level for diabetes programs of the General Clinic Research Centers constitutes
about 8 to 10 percent of the total. These research funds
are complementary to many other research endeavors and are,
primarily, for the construction of facilities that are often
used to conduct the clinical-based research in studies
funded by NIAMDD. Thus, when analyzing the funding support
for NIAMDD, the resources allocated to DRR can be added to
that institute's support. Therefore, according to table 6,
NIAMDD research endeavors in 1977 accounted for nearly 59
percent of all appropriations for diabetes research. If
the funding recommendations of the National Commission are
followed, the above percentage would increase to approximately 70 percent of all support by 1979 (see table 7).
(2) The National Institute on Aging (NIA) obtains less than
1 percent of all diabetes-related funding. However, both
the prevalence and incidence of diabetes are concentrated
in the older population. While diabetes is, theoretically,
not as difficult to control in older persons, it is often
complicated by the greater prevalence of other chronic conditions. Given the recent origin of the NIA and its general

Table 6. Appropriations for Diabetes Research: NIH. 1/

Institute 2/	1977 Appropriation ($000s)	Percent of total	1978 President's budget ($000s)	Percent of total	House allowance ($000s)	Percent of total	Senate allowance ($000s)	Percent of total
NIAMDD	$35,727	49.7%	$34,012	47.3%	$40,012	47.9%	$63,512	58.3%
NHLBI	11,900	16.5	12,400	17.2	12,800	15.3	14,200	13.0
NEI	9,065	12.6	9,065	12.6	10,565	12.6	11,517	10.6
DRR	6,355	8.8	7,378	10.3	8,253	9.9	7,783	7.1
NICHD	4,619	6.4	4,750	6.6	5,750	6.9	5,900	5.4
NINCDS	1,860	2.6	1,931	2.7	3,380	4.0	3,380	3.1
NIGMS	1,000	1.4	1,000	1.4	1,300	1.6	1,300	1.2
NIDR	600	0.8	600	0.8	600	0.7	800	0.6
NIA	563	0.8	575	0.8	650	0.8	575	0.5
NCI	250	0.4	250	0.3	250	0.3	250	0.2
Total	71,939	100.0	71,961	100.0	83,560	100.0	109,017	100.0

1/ Data from table on pp. S10932 and S10933, U.S. Congress, Congressional Record, June 28, 1977.
2/ See note 2, table 7, for a translation of the institute acronyms.

Table 7. National Commission on Diabetes: Recommended NIH Funding by Institute--Intramural and Extramural (Fiscal Year). 1/

Institute 2/	1975 ($000s)	Percent of total	1976 ($000s)	Percent of total	1977 ($000s)	Percent of total	1978 ($000s)	Percent of total	1979 ($000s)	Percent of total	1980 ($000s)	Percent of total	1981 ($000s)	Percent of total
NIAMDD	$18,373	46.9%	$18,348	43.5%	$39,826	52.9%	$ 64,453	58.5%	$ 87,877	62.3%	$105,032	63.6%	$120,250	63.9%
NHLBI	5,588	14.3	7,070	16.7	9,700	12.9	12,350	11.2	13,585	9.6	14,845	9.0	16,330	8.7
NEI	4,763	12.2	5,246	12.4	10,041	13.3	11,500	10.4	14,000	9.9	15,500	9.4	17,667	9.4
NICHD	1,476	3.8	2,230	5.3	4,340	5.8	6,166	5.6	7,928	5.6	10,300	6.2	12,363	6.6
NINCDS	782	2.0	331	0.8	2,000	2.7	2,400	2.2	2,600	1.8	2,800	1.7	3,000	1.6
NIDR	427	1.1	400	0.9	600	0.8	1,467	1.3	1,866	1.3	2,281	1.4	2,766	1.5
DRR	5,733	14.6	6,075	14.4	6,324	8.4	9,186	8.3	10,284	7.3	11,334	6.9	12,712	6.7
Other	2,053	5.2	2,515	6.0	2,437	3.2	2,661	2.4	2,843	2.0	2,997	1.8	3,160	1.7
Total	39,195	100.1	42,215	100.0	75,268	99.9	110,183	99.9	140,983	99.8	165,089	100.0	188,248	100.1

1/ Data from table on p. S10932, U.S. Congress, Congressional Record, June 28, 1977.
2/ NIAMDD = National Institute of Arthritis, Metabolism, and Digestive Diseases
    NHLBI = National Health, Lung, and Blood Institute
    NEI   = National Eye Institute
    NICHD = National Institute of Child Health and Human Development
    NINCDS = National Institute of Neurological and Communicative Disorders and Stroke
    NIDR   = National Institute of Dental Research
    DRR   = Division of Research Resources
    Other = National Cancer Institute, National Institute on Aging, National Institute
             of Allergy and Infectious Diseases, National Institute of General Medical
             Sciences, and National Institute of Environmental Health Sciences.

lack of a disease-specific focus common to most institutes in
NIH, its lack of funding for research on diabetes among older
people is understandable. However, assuming NIA's continued
existence, it would be reasonable to expect that a greater
share of research support for diabetes would emanate from
that institute. (3) There is considerable variation in
recommended funding levels for 1978. The Senate's approved
figures are approximately 50 percent greater than the President's budget, and over 30 percent greater than the approved
House budget. Most of the differential is concentrated in
the recommended research support of the NIAMDD, whose basic
biomedical research is studying the cause of diabetes (see
table 5). In the Senate-approved budget, the NIAMDD received
approximately 58 percent of the total allocation, whereas in
both the House and President's budget, the NIAMDD figure constitutes about 48 percent. Actually, the President's 1978
budget is slightly less than 1977 appropriation levels.
These differentials in recommended funding between the Senate,
House, and the President's budgets reflect, to some degree,
the differential perceptions of the benefits to be derived
from the research conducted by NIAMDD. Perhaps a resolution
of these differential recommendations could be had through
the demand-revealing procedure suggested by Edward Clarke
in this volume.

     Table 7 shows several interesting trends: (1) nominal
research support for diabetes within NIH has nearly doubled
in two years (1975-77), from about $39 million to over $75
million.* (2) If the National Commission's funding recommendations are adopted, nominal research support will increase
from about $75 million in 1977 to well over $188 million in
1981, a 150 percent increase. While inflation will cut the
actual purchasing power of these future resources, the figures
still represent substantial increased support. (3) The percentage of total expenditures going to NIAMDD will increase
from about 50 percent to nearly 64 percent over the four-year
period 1977-81. During the same period, research support for
the two most prevalent chronic conditions related to diabetes
(heart and eye conditions) are expected to decline from approximately 26 percent of total support in 1977 to 18 percent
in 1981, even though nominal funding recommendations suggest
an approximate 50 percent increase in support of this research. Since there is a much larger proportion of the population contracting diabetes in older age groups, where
chronic conditions are multiple in nature, it is not clear
why NIAMDD is the institute to which additional resources
should flow, unless compelling research evidence there

---

*   Inflation reduces this increase considerably, perhaps by
     as much as 25 percent, depending on the rate of inflation
     for all inputs used in diabetes research.

suggests an imminent breakthrough in the cause of and cure for the disease.

Finally, table 7 shows that the only other signifi-cant recommended increase in funding, as a proportion of the total recommended funding, is for NICHD. Much of the recom-mended NICHD research is related to diabetes-related problems during pregnancy and the increased probability of spontaneous abortions among diabetic women. There is also growing in-terest in investigating the ways in which maternal diabetes impacts negatively on the health of offspring, either in terms of a greater probability of developing diabetes as a child or by reducing the ability of children to grow and de-velop normally.

To summarize, diabetes research has obtained a con-siderable increase in funding support as a consequence of the National Commission's 1976 Report to Congress; it appears the trend will continue during the next three to five years. The support is increasingly oriented to the basic biomedical sciences directly involved in work on (a) the endocrine and metabolic processes of the body among normal and abnormal in-dividuals and (b) the mechanism of insulin production (either natural or through artificially implanted devices) and its effects on the biochemical functioning of the aging process. Though the absolute level of funding will increase, the per-centage of resources allocated to important secondary chronic conditions will decline.

DEMAND VERSUS SUPPLY APPROACH TO RESEARCH FUNDING

One of the most important problems decision makers for biomedical research confront is determining funding priori-ties. The National Commission's 1976 Report was concerned with (a) the state of biomedical research pertaining to dia-betes and (b) what new initiatives might be implemented. These concerns represent a classic supply-side approach to planning and decision making. It should be noted that the planning process in other crucial areas (for example, economic development) has traditionally been supply-oriented, with ex-perts and government officials guiding decision makers to de-termine what the appropriate development strategies and in-vestments should be. Indeed, the working group of the Na-tional Commission used a traditional supply-side approach in estimating the indirect cost of diabetes to society. In ad-dition, they promptly rejected consideration of benefit mea-surement (U.S.PHS, 1976). While the value of labor services in production is not unrelated to the overall structure of de-mand within an economy, the human-capital approach to valua-tion is not based on individual preferences being either ex-plicitly or implicitly revealed on a public or private basis. Further, uncertainty and interpersonal considerations of car-ing and sharing are not incorporated into this valuation

approach (Acton, 1973, 1976a; Jones-Lee, 1976). Since the
supply-side approach to resource allocation has permeated
the biomedical research community and is embodied in the National Commission's work to date, it is not surprising that
its funding recommendations place increasing emphasis on
basic biomedical research in the fields of endocrinology and
metabolism.

Consumer Behavior

     The above suggests that most research programs, de-
signed to understand the consumer behavior of diabetics and
the ways in which they interact with providers and accept
treatment regimes for long-run chronic conditions, are not
obtaining even the modest research support suggested by the
National Commission's 1976 Report. However, it is important
to note that, as a consequence of a revised funding strategy
developed by NIAMDD to support a set of Diabetes Research and
Training Centers, social and medical scientists are now being
trained to either alter their current research careers or use
their newly-acquired skills to analyze the health problems of
diabetics. Input from non-traditional disciplines will
likely alter future funding and research thrusts.

     In order to better understand the importance of a
demand-side approach for some biomedical research support as
it relates to diabetes, it is instructive to review the data
on non-compliance in tables 8, 9, and 10. While it is possible that the current stock of diabetics can, in many cases,
control their disease by proper diet, exercise, the taking of
insulin and other drugs, there are indications that diabetics,
for a variety of different reasons, do not follow the treatment regime prescribed, even when they know that such regimes
can improve their short-run and long-run functional health
status.

     Table 8 shows data on the percentage of diabetics re-
porting one or more symptoms of the disease during the month
preceding their interviews in 1964-65. The reporting of certain diabetic symptoms is one indication of the degree of uncontrolled illness and the likelihood of an increased rate of
functional health status depreciation. Diabetics who report
none or only one symptom are, presumably, under control and
are engaging in better self-care than other diabetics. However, the data in table 8 suggests that less than one-half of
the diabetics report no symptoms of diabetes, and only 62 percent report one or less. Further, there is a significant
variation between males and females, with males reporting considerably fewer symptoms than females. These findings suggest that more than one-third of all diabetics are relatively
uncontrolled, even though almost all (98.8 percent)
diabetics indicated that they had seen a doctor about their

Table 8. Percent Distribution of Diabetics, by Number of
          Diabetic Symptoms during Month Preceding Inter-
          view according to Sex: United States, July 1964-
          June 1965.

Number of symptoms	Both sexes	Male	Female
All diabetics	100.0%	100.0%	100.0%
None	48.2	53.7	44.3
One symptom	14.6	17.0	12.9
Two-three symptoms	18.4	14.4	21.3
Four-five symptoms	11.2	9.5	12.4
Six symptoms	7.5	5.4	9.1

Source: National Center for Health Statistics, series 10,
         no. 40, 1967, table M, p. 10.

Table 9. Percent of Diabetics in Each Age Group Who Were
          Given a Diet and Who Follow Diet, by Sex:
          United States, July 1964-June 1965.

Age group	Given diet			Follow diet		
	Both sexes	Male	Female	Both sexes	Male	Female
All ages	77.1%	72.8%	80.3%	52.7%	48.5%	55.9%
Under 25 years	70.3	61.1	78.9	47.7	38.9	56.1
25-44 years	78.3	77.0	78.2	51.6	49.6	53.1
45-54 years	76.9	71.4	81.2	52.5	53.4	51.6
55-64 years	82.8	78.0	86.0	58.8	53.1	62.8
65-74 years	77.9	72.2	81.5	52.5	45.6	56.8
75+	66.0	64.5	67.0	44.7	41.3	46.9

Source: National Center for Health Statistics, series 10,
         no. 40, 1967, table Q, p. 12.

Table 10.   Percent of Diabetics Who Use Selected Diet
            Items: United States, July 1964-June 1965.

Diet item	Percent of diabetics who use diet items
Special recipes	35.3%
Dietetic foods:	
Soft drinks only	5.7
Canned fruits only	2.0
Artificial sweeteners only	18.7
More than one	55.7
No special recipes or dietetic foods	14.1
Pastry	53.7
Candy	34.7
Pastry and candy	26.9

NOTE.—The data contained in table 10 are not totally comparable due to the way in which the questions eliciting this information were worded. For the last three
dietary items, that is, pastry, candy, and pastry and
candy, the reference period is one week.

Source: National Center for Health Statistics, series 10,
          no. 40, 1967, table R, p. 12.

diabetes, and 85 percent reported seeing a doctor during the
past year (NCHS, S.10-N109, 1977b).

Table 9 shows data that suggest that approximately 77
percent of the diabetics were prescribed a specific diet. Of
those who were given a prescribed diet to follow, females
tended to follow the diet more often than males. However, a
considerable percentage of both sexes were not following the
diet. Further, the proportion of diabetics who follow the
diet does not increase with age, and this is critical because
complications from the illness that lead to a more rapid reduction in health status are more prevalent among the aged.

Finally, table 10 shows that the percentage of diabetics who consume inappropriate diet items is quite high.
For example, over half the diabetics report consuming
pastries, one-third consume candy, and one-fourth consume
both. To a certain degree, such consumption is important for
the controlling of hypoglycemia or low blood sugar. However,
regular use of such items directly conflicts with standard
medical practice on long-term maintenance of good health in
diabetics.

While it is important to analyze the biochemical aspects of diabetes, an understanding of the way diabetics cope with their disease and relate to other people may be as important an area for research as basic research related to perfecting treatment and cure. That over five million people, approximately one-half of all the estimated diabetics in the country, do not report having the disease is indicative of the negative psychological aspects of living with, and controlling, a chronic condition such as diabetes. It is significant to note that there was one report embodied in the National Commission's 1976 Report that addressed the psychosocial problems of diabetes. However, systematic review of all fiscal year 1977 NIAMDD research projects revealed no project that addresses issues of consumer behavior, particularly how diabetics process information received from providers and how diabetics use that information in maintaining their functional health status. Although the returns on such psychological research cannot be calculated at present, a priori assessment would indicate that the returns would be substantial.

FURTHER ISSUES AND PROBLEMS

Traditional economic theory suggests that optimal resource allocation to alternative programs occurs at the point where the ratios of marginal benefits to marginal costs for each program is equated. For biomedical research, estimates of marginal cost can be obtained, but it is most difficult to obtain an accurate estimate of marginal benefits. Economists previously utilized estimates of earnings foregone as a measure of the productivity benefits that society would derive as a consequence of one resource allocation strategy versus another. Recently, use of the strict human-capital approach for evaluating alternative resource uses in the public sector and for alternative human resource investment has been questioned. For example, in 1976, as mentioned in the first part of this paper, an entire conference focused on the issues of valuing human life.

Perhaps more important for those with chronic health problems is not the valuing of human life per se, but the valuing of alternative states of health based on functioning levels and capacities. There has been a rapid expansion in alternative measures of health status, as well as in the literature on it.* However, little research has focused on attempting to measure preferences between alternative states of functional health (Jones-Lee, 1976; Ware, 1979). The

_____

* See, for example, the set of papers published in Health
   Services Research (Winter 1976) on measuring health
   status.

development of criteria for defining alternative states of functional health status is still in its infancy. It might be proposed that the following criteria be used as a basis in defining alternative health states:

(1)   the extent to which a particular disease or injury restricts normal activity;

(2)   the extent to which it limits mobility; and

(3)   the extent of an individual's pain and disfigurement.

In the 1973 National Health Interview Survey, questions were asked about the frequency and "degree of bother" of chronic conditions. Such questions are key ones for further delineation of alternative functional health states. These questions focus attention on how the individual may alter his behavior at the margin, but not so significantly as to change an entire life style. Such marginal changes in behavior leading to changes in health status are particularly significant in analyzing the demand for particular types of health services in terms of both over-the-counter drug consumption and visits to health care providers. Further, analyzing changes in the consumption of health services in response to changes in the frequency or degree of bother can provide an improved estimate of an individual's willingness to pay to minimize the decline in health status brought on by chronic conditions. While this measure of willingness to pay does not provide an estimate of the extent to which others (members of household and friends) are willing to pay for improvement of an individual's health status, at least a more theoretically sound measure, and one related to consumer choice versus production foregone, can be used. Finally, by incorporating a measure that monitors marginal health status changes, the theoretical tools of economic analysis can be more appropriately used.

Another difficult issue in biomedical research resource allocation is determining the probability of successful implementation of research findings into a program of treatment, prevention, or cure that leads to an improvement in health status. A related problem is to estimate how much time is required before current research will yield an implementable idea. To what extent should resources be allocated to research on complex disease entities which must continue for a considerable period before there is a high probability of an implementable idea? Diabetes certainly is a complex disease entity.

Research on diabetes and other chronic diseases must become more demand-side focused. Well over half of the diabetic population do not follow treatment regimes with which they have been provided. Why? Significant resources are

currently allocated to questions such as understanding how
the pancreas operates, but little information exists about
appropriate intervention strategies when treatment regimes
are not followed. As additional resources are made available to biomedical research in diabetes, a certain proportion of these resources could be fruitfully used to address consumer behavior and its role as a determinant of
functional health status in chronic conditions such as
diabetes.

Acknowledgments.

The author wishes to acknowledge the assistance and comments
of Dr. Oscar B. Crofford, Director, Vanderbilt Diabetes-
Endocrinology Research Center, and Chairman, National Commission on Diabetes. The editorial assistance of
Mrs. Holly R. Caldwell also is greatly appreciated.

REFERENCES

Acton, Jan Paul
    1976a   "Health status indexes--work in progress."
             Paper presented at conference in Health
             Services Research 11(4), Phoenix, Arizona
             (October 25-28).

    1976b   "Valuing lifesaving alternatives and some
             measurements." Paper prepared for Law and
             Contemporary Problems Conference on the
             Value of Human Life, Amelia Island
             (March 11-13).

    1973   Evaluating Public Programs to Save Lives:
             The Case of Heart Attacks. Santa Monica:
             The RAND Corporation (January).

Clarke, Edward H.
    1979   "Social valuation of life- and health-saving
             activities by the demand-revealing process."
             In Mushkin, Selma J. and David W. Dunlop (eds.),
             Health: What is it Worth? (this volume).

Cooper, Barbara S. and Dorothy P. Rice
    1976   "The economic cost revisited." Social Security
             Bulletin (February):21-39.

Jones-Lee, M. W.
    1976   The Value of Life: An Economic Analysis.
             Chicago: The University of Chicago Press.

Mushkin, Selma J.
    1962   "Health as an investment." Journal of Political
             Economy 70(5) (October):129-157 (supplement).

National Center for Health Statistics
U.S. Department of Health, Education, and Welfare
    1977a   Limitation of Activity Due to Chronic Con-
             ditions, United States, 1974, series 10,
             no. 111, U.S.DHEW publication no. (HRA)
             77-1537, Rockville, Md. (June).

    1977b   Problems of Chronic Conditions of the Geni-
             tourinary, Nervous, Endocrine, Metabolic,
             and Blood and Blood-Forming Systems and
             Selected Chronic Conditions, United States,
             1973, series 10, no. 109, U.S.DHEW publication
             no. (HRA) 77-1537, Rockville, Md. (March).

National Center for Health Statistics
U.S. Department of Health, Education, and Welfare
    1977c   Current Estimates from the Health Interview
           Survey, United States, 1975, series 10, no.
           115, U.S.DHEW publication no. (HRA) 77-1543,
           Rockville, Md. (March).

    1976   Health Characteristics of Persons with Chronic
           Activity Limitation, United States, 1974,
           series 10, no. 112, U.S.DHEW publication no.
           (HRA) 77-1539, Rockville, Md. (October).

    1974   Limitation of Activity and Mobility Due to
           Chronic Conditions, United States, 1972,
           Rockville, Md. (November).

    1973   Limitation of Activity Due to Chronic Con-
           ditions, United States, 1969-1070, series 10,
           no. 80, U.S.DHEW publication no. (HSM)
           73-1506, Rockville, Md. (April).

    1971   Diabetes-Mellitus, Mortality in the United
           States, 1950-1967, series 20, no. 10, p. 10,
           Rockville, Md. (July).

    1967   Characteristics of Persons with Diabetes in
           the United States, July 1964-June 1965,
           series 10, no. 40, Rockville, Md. (October).

Public Health Service
U.S. Department of Health, Education, and Welfare
    1977   Report of the National Commission on Diabetes
           to the Congress of the United States, The
           Long-Range Plan to Combat Diabetes, 1976,
           U.S.DHEW publication no. (NIH) 77-1229.

    1976a   Report of the National Commission on Diabetes
           to the Congress of the United States, Vol. I,
           The Long-Range Plan to Combat Diabetes,
           U.S.DHEW publication no. (NIH) 76-1018.

    1976b   Report of the National Commission on Diabetes
           to the Congress of the United States, Vol.
           III, Reports of Committees, Subcommittees and
           Work Groups, Part I, Scope and Impact of
           Diabetes I, U.S.DHEW publication no. (NIH)
           76-1021.

    1976c   Report of the National Commission on Diabetes
           to the Congress of the United States, Vol.
           III, Reports of Committees, Subcommittees and
           Work Groups, Part VI, Group Reports,
           U.S.DHEW publication no. (NIH) 76-1032.

Public Health Service
U.S. Department of Health, Education, and Welfare
    1976d   Report of the National Commission on Diabetes
             to the Congress of the United States, Vol. IV,
             Supporting Material to the Commission Reports,
             U.S.DHEW publication no. (NIH) 76-1033.

Rice, Dorothy P.
    1966   Estimating the Cost of Illness. Health
             Economics series no. 6. Washington, D.C.:
             U.S. Government Printing Office (May).

U.S. Congress
    1977   Congressional Record, vol. 123, no. 112,
             S10932, S10933 (June 27).

U.S. Department of Health, Education, and Welfare
    1960   "Diabetes reported in interviews, United
             States, July 1957-June 1959," series B, no. 21,
             Health Statistics from the U.S. National
             Health Survey, Washington, D.C. (September).

Ware, John E., Jr. and JoAnne Young
    1979   "Issues in the conceptualization and measurement
             of value placed on health." In Mushkin, Selma J.
             and David W. Dunlop (eds.), Health: What is it
             Worth? (this volume).

Weisbrod, Burton
    1961   The Economics of Public Health. Philadelphia:
             The University of Pennsylvania Press.

12 The Relationship Between Children's Health and Intellectual Development

Linda N. Edwards
Michael Grossman

The focus of this paper is on functional health status
of children in the population. More specifically, we examine
a single aspect of functional health status--intellectual development of children.* In a multivariate context, we examine
the relationships between the health indexes and cognitive development of children from six to 11 years of age in Cycle II
of the U.S. Health Examination Survey (HES). We present the
first set of such estimates for a representative sample of
non-institutionalized white children in the United States.
We compare them with existing findings for underdeveloped
countries, Great Britain, and low income families in the
United States.

In choosing to study intellectual development, we are
adopting the view (similar to Haggerty and others, 1975;
Mushkin 1977) that the benefits from investments in children's health should not be restricted to the usual narrow
list of increases in longevity, decreases in morbidity, and
reductions in curative medical care outlays. Indeed, we have
come to believe that enhanced intellectual development is an
important source of benefits from investments in children's
health. While our results do not themselves provide sufficient information for a full cost-benefit analysis of expenditures on child health, they do contain policy-relevant
insights about potential benefits in terms of "physical"
(cognitive development) units.

---

* For a partial survey of the literature on relationships
among earnings, schooling, health, and intelligence of
adults and children, see Grossman (1975).

I. ANALYTICAL FRAMEWORK AND CURRENT LITERATURE

Whenever decision makers, such as firms or households, must allocate scarce resources among competing goals, economists can provide useful insights into their behavior. Parent-child relationships clearly involve such allocation. While it is not easy to define what is meant by the "well-being" of children, factors such as their health, intelligence, school performance, school attainment, social behavior, and lifetime earnings undoubtedly play an important role. To enhance any of these components of children's welfare, parents must allocate to their children some part of their own limited resources--their own time or goods and services purchased in the market.

Our analytical framework is based on two propositions. One is the above notion that parents must allocate scarce resources between a child's well-being (the child's life "quality") and other competing goals. These competing goals include not only the parents' own consumption, but also the consumption of other children in the family. This framework builds upon the important distinction between the quantity and "quality" of children that is stressed in much of the literature on the economics of fertility and optimum family size (for example, Becker and Lewis, 1973; Willis, 1973; O'Hara, 1975). The second proposition, embedded in the household production function approach to consumer behavior, is that consumers produce their basic objects of choice with their own time and inputs of goods and services purchased in the market (Becker, 1965; Lancaster, 1966; Muth, 1966). This insight is of particular relevance in dealing with children's health and cognitive development because parents do not buy these objects of choice directly in the market.

Cognitive development of children can be perceived by applying a multivariate production function. This production function would involve such factors as time inputs of the child and of his parents and teachers; the child's genetic endowment; his current and past health; and various aspects of the child's school and home environment, the latter shaped to a large extent by parents. For example, it has been suggested that an increase in parents' schooling (one important aspect of the home environment) makes parents more efficient in the transmission of knowledge to their children (see Grossman, 1975, 1972; Leibowitz, 1974; Michael, 1972). The production function of cognitive development interacts with parents' income and their preferences at various prices to determine the level of cognitive development of each of their children.

With regard to the specific role of children's health in the above framework, it is widely recognized that poor health can pose a threat to the cognitive development of children (Wallace, 1962; Birch and Gussow, 1970). Health

problems can limit the amount of information acquired in the
home and in school by reducing the amount of time available
to acquire such information, as well as by reducing the amount
acquired in a given period of time. Ultimately, intelligence,
years of formal schooling completed, earnings, and other
measures of well-being in adulthood can be affected by poor
health in childhood. Yet the empirical work in this area is
sparse. In fact, Birch and Gussow (1970), whose book focuses
on the effects of health on learning, point out that most of
the evidence they bring to bear on the issue is indirect because "...there has been little investigation of the specific
relationships between the physical status of poor children
and either their mental development or their school achievement" (p. 10). In the rest of this section, we highlight the
literature that suggests a relationship between various aspects of children's health and their cognitive development.
The studies cited here, as well as others, are discussed in
greater detail in section III.

     Most of the literature relating health to the intel-
lectual development of children focuses on the effects of malnutrition. Pediatricians argue that malnutrition in early
childhood can inhibit intellectual development because a brain
growth spurt occurs in the first two years of human life, during which time the interneural network is formed (Scrimshaw
and Gordon, 1968; Lewin, 1975). Deficient diets at this time
can slow the spurt and thereby permanently affect intellectual
development. Since early brain growth is largely a process
of protein synthesis, a diet that is deficient in this
nutrient may be especially damaging. In fact, a number of
studies in underdeveloped and developing economies show that
children who were severely malnourished in infancy have below
average mental capacity (as measured by intelligence quotient
(IQ) or similar tests), language proficiency, school performance, and adaptive capacity at subsequent ages (Scrimshaw
and Gordon, 1968; Birch and Gussow, 1970; Correa, 1975;
Stoch and Smythe, 1976). Moreover, members of the malnourished group tend to be shorter and thinner and to have
smaller head circumferences than their well-nourished peers,
sometimes even after having recovered from the spell of malnutrition. Richardson (1976) and others caution, however,
that conclusions drawn from these studies are suggestive,
rather than definitive, because malnourished children grow
up in an environment with a substantial number of obstacles
besides inadequate nutrient intake that could slow intellectual growth.

     Mild or moderate malnutrition in school age children
has been less frequently studied and has less dramatic effects. It has been associated with poor judgment, inat-
tention, and a heightened risk of illness, all of which might
ultimately affect intellectual development (Birch and Gussow,
1970; Heller and Drake, 1976; Popkin and Lim-Ybanez, 1977).
These findings are especially relevant for the United States
because, while we do not experience much severe malnutrition,

researchers still report substantial variations in nutritional adequacy (Christakis, 1968; Center for Disease Control, 1972; Acosta, 1974; Driskel and Price, 1974; Owen, 1974; Sims and Morris, 1974; Endozien and others, 1976).

The relationship between intellectual development and other dimensions of children's health is documented in a variety of studies. Birch and Gussow (1970) reviewed the evidence that low birth weight and prematurity can have detrimental effects on the later intellectual development of children. Wallace (1962) and Kessner (1974) mentioned a few small studies that relate health problems, such as hearing loss, to poor school achievement. Haggerty, Roghmann, and Pless (1975) discussed the impact of chronic conditions on school attendance and performance in a sample of Rochester, New York children (but reached few definitive conclusions). Leveson, Ullman, and Wassall (1969) cited a number of studies indicating that about five to seven percent of persons dropping out of high school in the United States have done so primarily because of illness. Grossman (1975) found that the self-rated status of students during years of high school attendance has a positive effect on years of college completed. Cooney (1977) summarized evidence tentatively suggesting that deficient intellectual development due to poor health might lead, ultimately, to juvenile delinquency and other forms of deviant behavior. In sum, these studies strongly suggest the existence of positive effects of good health and nutrition on intellectual development.

In the above brief review of the literature, we have repeatedly used the phrase "effect of health on intellectual development"; further, in section III we employ health measures as independent variables in ordinary least squares multiple regressions with IQ or school achievement as the dependent variable. Yet it would be a mistake to interpret the findings that we have mentioned in this section, or the statistically significant health effects that we report in section III, as indisputable evidence of causal relationships running from health to cognitive development. There are at least three plausible alternative interpretations. (1) Our statistical results might partially reflect causality that runs from cognitive development to health. For example, Miller (1974) reports a negative correlation between intelligence and accidents, a major cause of morbidity and mortality in children, in his study of children in Newcastle Upon Tyne, England. He interprets IQ as the causal agent in this correlation. (2) Statistically significant effects of health on IQ might be due to the omission from the regression analysis of genetic and environmental factors that are common to both health and cognitive development (although in our work we try to control for as many of these as possible). (3) Certain relationships that we report might not partially or even totally reflect health effects at all. To cite one illustration, breast-feeding might foster the development of the brain and the central nervous system and

reduce the risk of illness, thus promoting intellectual
development during the first year of life.* On the other
hand, breast-feeding might simply serve as a proxy measure of
both the amount of time mothers spend with their children and
families' preferences for children.

It would also be a mistake to interpret the findings
in this section solely on the basis of environmental effect
as opposed to genetic effect. Without becoming involved in
the controversy concerning the relative importance of
heredity and environment in the determination of IQ, we wish
to point out that our health indexes have both genetic and
environmental components. For instance, part of the variation in birth weight can be attributed to a woman's knowledge
of appropriate practices during pregnancy and to the amount
and quality of the prenatal care she receives, while part of
the variation is genetic. In addition, genetic differences
may induce environmental changes. That is, parents may respond to the inherited characteristics of children by either
compensating or reinforcing the effects of a favorable or un-
favorable inheritance.** In the empirical work reported below, we make only a modest effort to sort out the separate
effects of heredity and environment. Nevertheless, as long
as some portion of the variability in our health indexes and
IQ measures can be attributed to environmental influences,
our findings will have relevance for public policy.
Bloom's (1964) penetrating survey of studies of the development of various human characteristics provides a compelling
reason to believe that the relationships we uncover are not
solely genetic, but reflect environmental influences as well.
Bloom also points out that the development of IQ and achievement occurs early in the life cycle, but he summarizes evidence that suggests that 50 percent of the development of IQ
measured at age 17 takes place after age four, while 67 percent of the development of general achievement measured at
age 18 takes place after age six.

In summary, the aim of our empirical research is to
uncover significant health-IQ and health-achievement relationships rather than to establish causality or to provide definitive interpretations of these relationships. We adopt this
strategy because none of our techniques represents a controlled experiment and because we lack knowledge about the
underlying structure that generates the sample observations.
The causal nature of the relationships that we uncover can be
established by other persons with different samples and
methods. However, our findings can serve as a useful first
step in an assessment of government policies with respect to

---

*   See section III for references.

** For more detailed discussions of the effects of endow-
    ments on optimal investments in children by parents, see
    Becker and Tomes (1976) and Edwards and Grossman (1977).

children. Our task is to fill a gap in the existing literature by documenting relationships, in a multivariate context,
between health and cognitive development for a representative
sample of white children in the United States.

II.   DATA AND MEASUREMENT OF VARIABLES

The Data Set

      As mentioned before, our data set is Cycle II of the
HES conducted by the National Center for Health Statistics
(NCHS, 1967a). Cycle II is a nationally representative
sample of 7,119 non-institutionalized children aged six
to 11 years, examined over the 1963-65 period.* This sample
is an exceptionally rich source of information about children's health, their intellectual development, and the characteristics of their families. More specifically, the data
comprise each child's complete medical and developmental his-
tories provided by the parent, birth certificate facts, information on family socioeconomic characteristics, and a
school report with information on current school performance
and classroom behavior provided by teachers or other school
officials. Most important, there are objective measures of
health from detailed physical examinations, and there are also
scores on psychological (including vocabulary and achievement)
tests. The physical examinations and the psychological tests
were administered by the Public Health Service.

      Although the sample contains children of all races, we
restrict our analysis to white children only. This procedure
allows us to avoid the problem associated with potential
"cultural biases" in IQ and achievement tests. These biases
could also be dealt with by separately analyzing the data for
white and black children. (Indeed, in preliminary estimation,
there were statistically significant racial differences in the
set of variable coefficients so that separate estimates by
race would be called for in any case.) Separate analysis is
not undertaken for blacks, however, because the black sample
is too small to permit reliable coefficient estimates. The
full Cycle II sample contains 6,100 whites, 987 blacks, and
32 "others."

      Our sample is further limited by excluding children
who do not live with both of their natural or adoptive
parents or for whom there were missing data. (Information
most typically absent were birth weight, school absenteeism,
and income, with a disproportionate number of missing data
from families where a foreign language is spoken in the home.)

_____

*   For a full description of the sample, the sampling techni-
    que, and the data collection, see NCHS (1967a).

Children who live with foster parents, stepparents, guardians, or single, widowed, or divorced parents are excluded to control for the effects of marital instability. Examination of the excluded observations indicates that they have lower IQ and achievement scores and poorer health. Thus, our final sample of 3,599 children may be regarded as an advantaged subgroup of the Cycle II data set. Regression results are reported for boys and girls pooled because coefficient estimates were not found to differ significantly by sex.

The IQ, achievement, and health variables are defined in table 1. Means and standard deviations of these variables are shown in Appendix table A-2.

Measures of Health

The issue of how to measure children's health is very much an unresolved one, even among professionals in the area of public health.* Recent studies of children's health in the United States have used data taken from one or more of the following categories: measures of disability, measures related to the incidence of abnormal conditions, and measures derived from parental assessments of children's health (Wallace, 1962; Mechanic, 1964; Mindlin and Lobach, 1971; Talbot and others, 1971; Kaplan and others, 1972; Hu, 1973; Schack and Starfield, 1973; Kessner, 1974; Haggerty and others, 1975; Inman, 1976). Although we followed the precedent of these earlier studies, some of the above measures (disability and the incidence of certain physical conditions) are not entirely appropriate because we wanted measures of the child's "permanent" state of health (his prospect for life preservation and normal functioning) rather than short-run deviations from that permanent state. Much childhood disability results from the natural sequence of childhood diseases and acute conditions that do not reflect on the child's permanent state of health. Of course, there is a positive correlation between the two in the sense that a child with poor permanent health is more likely to contract acute conditions and to have them for a more extended time period.**

---

*   This is true not only for children's health, but also for adult's health. Sullivan (1966), Berg (1973), and Ware (1976) discuss the general issue of measuring health; and Starfield (1975) and Schack and Starfield (1973) focus on the specific problem of measuring children's health.

** Birch and Gussow (1970) discuss how nutrition (clearly a determinant of permanent health status) and disease are intimately related.

Table 1.   Definition of Health Variables and Cognitive
           Development.

Variable name	Definition	Source a/

A. Cognitive development

WISC   Child's IQ as measured by vocabu-
              lary and block design of the
              Wechsler Intelligence Scale for
              Children, standardized by the mean
              and standard deviation of four-
              month age cohorts   4

WRAT   Child's school achievement as mea-
              sured by the reading and arithmetic
              subtests of the Wide Range Achieve-
              ment Test, standardized by the mean
              and standard deviation of six-month
              age cohorts   4

B. Past health

LIGHT1   Dummy variable that equals one if
              child's birth weight was under 2,000
              grams (4.4 pounds)   2

LIGHT2   Dummy variable that equals one if
              child's birth weight was equal to
              or greater than 2,000 grams but
              under 2,500 grams (5.5 pounds)   2

BFED   Dummy variable that equals one if
              the child was breast-fed   1

LMAG   Dummy variable that equals one if
              the mother was less than 20 years
              old at birth of child   1

HMAG35   Dummy variable that equals one if
              the mother was more than 35 years
              old at birth of child   1

HMAG40   Dummy variable that equals one if
              the mother was 40 years old or more
              at birth of child   1

Table 1. Definition of Health Variables and Cognitive
          Development. (Continued)

Variable name	Definition	Source a/
FYPH	Dummy variable that equals one if parental assessment of child's health at one year was poor or fair, and zero if it was good	1

C. Current health

Variable name	Definition	Source a/
SEEG	Dummy variable that equals one if uncorrected binocular distance is abnormal and child usually wears glasses	3,1
NSEEG	Dummy variable that equals one if uncorrected binocular distance vision is normal and child usually wears glasses	3,1
NRMAL	Dummy variable that equals one if uncorrected binocular distance vision is normal and child does not wear glasses	3,1
IHEAR	Dummy variable that equals one if hearing is abnormal	3
ABN	Dummy variable that equals one if physician finds a "significant abnormality" in examining the child (other than an abnormality resulting from an accident or injury)	
IHEIGHT	Height, standardized by the mean and standard deviation of one-year age-sex cohorts	3
IWEIGHT	Weight, standardized by the mean and standard deviation of one-year age-sex cohorts	3
IDECAY	Number of decayed primary and permanent teeth, standardized by the mean and standard deviation of one-year age-sex cohorts	3

Table 1.   Definition of Health Variables and Cognitive
           Development.   (Continued)

Variable name	Definition	Source a/
PFHEALTH	Dummy variable that equals one if parental assessment of child's health is poor or fair and zero if assessment is good or very good	1
PFGHEALTH	Dummy variable that equals one if parental assessment of child's health is poor, fair, or good and zero if assessment is very good	1
ACC	Dummy variable that equals one if parent reported that the child had one or more accidents from infancy to the present	1
SCHABS	Dummy variable that equals one if child has been excessively absent from school for health reasons during the past six months	5
D. Alternative current health and current weight measures		
TALL	Dummy variable that equals one if child's height is greater than two standard deviations above the mean for the relevant age-sex cohort	3
SHORT	Dummy variable that equals one if child's height is two standard deviations or more below the mean for the relevant age-sex cohort	3
FAT	Dummy variable that equals one if child's weight is greater than two standard deviations above the mean for the relevant age-sex cohort	3
THIN	Dummy variable that equals one if child's weight is two standard deviations or more below the mean for the relevant age-sex cohort	3

a/   The sources are 1 = medical history form completed by
     parent, 2 = birth certificate, 3 = physical examination,
     4 = psychological examination, 5 = school form.

In some situations, a single overall health index might be desired--to parsimoniously describe the health status of a population, or to provide a guide for the allocation of public funds, for example. However, use of a single health index in this study would conceal, rather than reveal, a number of important associations of special policy relevance. This is because the various components of health that we studied (described below) reflect different dimensions of overall health status, and there is no reason to believe that these components of health status all interact with IQ and achievement in exactly the same way.

A total of 13 dimensions are used as descriptive of health status and these are represented by 19 health variables. These variables are defined precisely in table 1. They are divided into two subsets: a set of past health measures and a set of current health measures. Past health measures refer to the child's health prior to the health examination survey (they relate primarily to the child's infancy), while the current measures refer to health at the time of the examination. Some of these variables are self-explanatory and some are further clarified below:

(1) Breast-feeding contributes to the nutritional status of infants and, therefore, is used as an index of early nutrition (see, for example, Mata, 1978). In addition, infants receive from their mothers' milk antibodies that help protect them from acute illnesses during infancy. Whether or not the child was breast-fed is denoted by the dummy variable MBFED.

(2) Mother's age at the time of birth, represented by three dummy variables (LMAG, HMAG35, and HMAG40), is considered a measure of health in infancy because relatively older mothers have been found to have a greater frequency of infants in poor health, while relatively younger mothers, though they may be in better physical health, are more likely to have unwanted conceptions and consequently seek less prenatal care.

(3) Uncorrected binocular distance vision is defined as abnormal if it is worse than 20/30 (NCHS, 1972a). All children were examined without glasses. Therefore, the vision variables (SEEG, NSEEG, NRMAL) distinguish four categories of children: those with abnormal vision who wear glasses (SEEG), those with normal vision who wear glasses (NSEEG), those with normal vision who do not wear glasses (NRMAL), and those with abnormal vision who do not wear glasses (the omitted category).

(4) A child is defined as having abnormal hearing (denoted IHEAR) if, in his best ear, the average threshold decibel reading over the range of 500, 1,000, and 2,000 cycles per second (cps) is greater than 15. These are the

frequencies that occur most frequently in normal speech. A
threshold of less than 15 decibels above audiometric zero at
these frequencies is classified as corresponding to "no significant difficulty with faint speech" by the Committee on
Conservation of Hearing of the American Academy of Ophthal-
mology and Otolaryngology (NCHS, 1970a).

     (5) "Significant abnormalities" reported by the ex-
amining physician include heart disease (congenital or acquired); neurological; muscular, or joint conditions; other
congenital abnormalities; and other major diseases. The
presence of one or more of these abnormalities is denoted by
the variable ABN.

     (6) Current height and weight are standard indicators
of children's nutritional status (for example, NCHS, 1970b,
1975; Seoane and Latham, 1971); and good nutrition is an obvious and natural vehicle for maintaining children's health.
It is well-known that physical growth rates differ by age
and sex. Therefore, for any observation, our height variable
(denoted IHEIGHT) is the difference between the child's actual
height and the mean height for his age-sex group divided by
the standard deviation of height for that age-sex group.
Current weight (denoted IWEIGHT) is computed in a similar
manner. The use of the variables IHEIGHT and IWEIGHT is consistent with the view that the relationships among nutrition,
IQ, and achievement are continuous ones; these variables make
our results comparable with those of several other studies
discussed in section III. We do, however, show how the estimated effects are altered when discrete height and weight
dummy variables (TALL, SHORT, FAT, THIN) replace the continuous variables. An advantage of using the discrete forms
of these variables is that it allows for non-monotonic relationships between height or weight and IQ.

     (7) The number of decayed permanent and primary teeth
(denoted IDECAY), adjusted for age and sex, as are height and
weight, is interpreted as an additional measure of nutrition
and a correlate of basic components of health that affect
cognitive development but are difficult to measure.

Measures of Cognitive Development

     In relating health indexes to cognitive development,
two measures are used as alternative dependent variables: an
IQ measure derived from two subtests of the Wechsler Intelligence Scale for Children (WISC) and a school achievement
measure derived from the reading and arithmetic subtests of
the Wide Range Achievement Test (WRAT). Both measures are
scaled to have means of 100 and standard deviations of 15 for
each age-group (four-month cohorts are used for WISC and six-
month cohorts are used for WRAT). The inadequacies of these
variables as indexes of overall intellectual development are

well-known. Nevertheless, they continue to be widely used because they provide readily obtainable tests that are roughly
comparable across a diverse population.

        WISC is a common IQ test, similar to (and highly cor-
related with results from) the Stanford-Binet IQ test (NCHS,
1972b). The full test consists of 12 subtests, but only two
of these were administered in the HES. The IQ estimates,
based on the vocabulary and block design subtests, are very
highly correlated with those based on all 12 subtests (NCHS,
1972b). WRAT is a single achievement test that can be given
to children of varying ages. In particular, the same test
was given to all children in the HES except the 12-year olds.
The latter group is excluded from our sample. The two tests
used in the HES were found to "...have reasonably good construct validity as judged by their relationship to conventional achievement tests" (NCHS, 1967b).

Other Independent Variables

        All regressions include a basic set of non-health-
related variables. These variables are sex of child, whether
the child is the first born in the family, whether the child
is a twin, whether the child attended kindergarten or nursery
school; other variables include size of family, years of
formal schooling completed by the mother and by the father,
labor force status of the mother, family income, whether a
foreign language is spoken in the home, region of residence,
and size of place of residence. These variables are defined
in more detail in Appendix table A-2. We do not discuss their
effects on IQ or school achievement in this paper, but it
should be realized that all estimated health effects control
for (hold constant) the effects of these variables.

III. RESULTS

Overview

        Ordinary least squares multiple regression equations
for the dependent variables WISC (IQ) and WRAT (school
achievement) are given in Appendix table A-3. When WRAT is
the dependent variable, two equations are estimated. The
first contains the same set of independent variables as the
WISC regression, while the second includes WISC as an additional independent variable. If variations in IQ as measured by WISC are due mainly to genetic factors, the second
regression will give a more accurate picture of the effect
of environmental factors on school achievement than the
first. Of course, WISC has both an environmental and a
genetic component. Therefore, the two WRAT regressions may
be regarded as estimates, both upper and lower bound, of

the impact of environmental factors on school achievement.*

Table 2 contains coefficient estimates of the 19 past
and current health indexes. In general, IQ and achievement
are positively related to positive correlates of health, and
many have statistically significant effects on IQ and school
achievement. The effects of health on school achievement
are reduced in absolute value when IQ is held constant, but
the pattern of statistical significance is not dramatically
altered. In particular, only the coefficients of the number
of decayed permanent and primary teeth (IDECAY) and of birth
weight between 2,000 and 2,500 grams (LIGHT2) become
insignificant.

Past Health Effects

Birth weight.--The results in table 2 suggest that low
birth weight, especially under 2,000 grams (under 4.4 pounds),
is damaging to subsequent intellectual development. For example, these coefficients imply that everything else being
equal, a child who weighed under 2,000 grams at birth has an
IQ four to five points lower on average than a child of normal
weight at birth.** This magnitude is about one-third of a
standard deviation in the WISC measure. Corresponding coefficients for WRAT imply that low birth weight is associated
with a deficiency of more than one-half a standard deviation
in the achievement measure. Somewhat surprisingly, absolute
effects are at least as large in the high income sample as in
the low income sample (see table 3).

The important effects of birth weight have been noted
in a number of studies (see Birch and Gussow, 1970, for a
review), though not in a multivariate context using a large
representative sample. Studies of the effects of birth weight
on IQ or achievement by income or social class are less common. Examples are Drillien (1964); Wiener (1965); and Davie
and others (1972). In general, these studies report

---

*   If WRAT embodies genetic variations in ability that are
     not captured by WISC, the equation with WISC held constant
     would no longer provide a lower bound estimate of the
     effect of environmental factors on WRAT.

**   Cycle II does not distinguish children who are born pre-
     maturely, so we cannot determine to what extent low
     birth weight is a result of prematurity or of other
     factors. The coefficients of LIGHT1 and LIGHT2 reflect
     the average effects of prematurity and of low birth
     weight for full-term infants.

Table 2. Coefficients of Health Variables in WISC or WRAT Regressions. a/

Independent variable	WISC Regression coefficient	F	WRAT Regression coefficient	F	WRAT b/ Regression coefficient	F
FYPH	-.37	(0.24)	-.29	(0.17)	-.13	(0.04)
LMAG	-1.87	(4.98)	-.82	(1.08)	.00	(0.00)
HMAG35	1.68	(4.75)	.48	(0.43)	-.27	(0.17)
HMAG40	-.56	(0.17)	-.30	(0.05)	-.05	(0.00)
BFED	1.84	(16.57)	1.50	(12.54)	.70	(3.42)
LIGHT1	-5.17	(8.03)	-9.33	(29.40)	-7.05	(21.44)
LIGHT2	-2.46	(5.73)	-1.96	(4.09)	-.88	(1.04)
SEEG	1.00	(0.74)	.40	(0.13)	-.04	(0.00)
NSEEG	-2.86	(4.70)	-1.66	(1.78)	-.40	(0.13)
NRMAL	-.93	(0.99)	-1.33	(2.29)	-.92	(1.40)
IHEAR	-3.65	(1.93)	-9.20	(13.84)	-7.60	(12.06)
ABN	-2.31	(9.74)	-3.46	(24.44)	-2.44	(15.49)
IWEIGHT	-.22	(0.63)	.112	(0.18)	-.01	(0.00)
IHEIGHT	1.23	(17.81)	1.32	(23.22)	.78	(10.31)
IDECAY	-.79	(12.16)	-.40	(3.47)	-.05	(0.07)
PFHEALTH	-1.13	(1.12)	-2.68	(7.06)	-2.18	(5.98)
PFGHEALTH	.06	(0.02)	-.34	(0.70)	-.37	(1.06)
ACC	-.22	(0.17)	-.27	(0.29)	-.18	(0.15)
SCHABS	-.09	(0.01)	-.70	(0.56)	-.66	(0.03)

a/ Source: Appendix, table A-3. The critical F values at the five percent level of significance are 2.69 on a one-tailed test and 3.84 on a two-tailed test.

b/ Based on a regression that includes WISC as an independent variable.

Table 3. Coefficients of Health Variables in WISC or WRAT Regressions with Family Income--
          Health Interactions. a/

Dependent variable	FYPH	LMAG	HMAG35	HMAG40	MBFED	LIGHT1	LIGHT2	SEEG	NSEEG
				Family income < $7,000					
WISC	.78 (0.62)	-1.95 (3.96)	2.40 (4.74)	-1.35 (0.56)	1.70 (7.65)	-3.74 (2.08)	-1.37 (1.07)	.04 (0.991)	-3.11 (2.76)
WRAT	.08 (0.01)	-.41 (0.20)	1.23 (1.40)	-.36 (0.04)	1.73 (8.97)	-8.18 (11.17)	-1.84 (2.18)	-1.63 (0.?6)	-2.62 (2.20)
WRAT b/	-.26 (0.10)	-.44 (0.29)	.17 (0.04)	.24 (0.03)	.99 (3.70)	-6.54 (9.10)	-1.24 (1.27)	-1.65 (1.26)	-1.25 (0.64)
				Family income ≥ $7,000					
WISC	-2.05 (2.99)	-1.38 (0.84)	.95 (0.78)	.15 (0.01)	2.07 (10.11)	-6.20 (6.01)	-4.42 (7.39)	1.84 (1.35)	-2.40 (1.65)
WRAT	-.91 (0.66)	-1.67 (1.38)	-.20 (0.04)	-.85 (0.19)	1.31 (4.58)	-10.38 (18.94)	-2.36 (2.78)	1.91 (1.63)	-.63 (0.13)
WRAT b/	-.004 (0.00)	-1.06 (0.72)	-.61 (0.46)	-.92 (0.28)	.40 (0.55)	-7.65 (13.13)	-.42 (0.10)	1.10 (0.69)	.43 (0.08)

Table 3. Coefficients of Health Variables in WISC or WRAT Regressions with Family Income-- Health Interactions. a/ (Continued)

Dependent variable	NRMAL	IHEAR	ABN	IWEIGHT	IHEIGHT	IDECAY	PFHEALTH	PFGHEALTH	ACC	SCHABS
					Family income < $7,000					
WISC	-1.31 (0.94)	-1.64 (0.26)	-2.14 (4.64)	-.59 (2.18)	1.78 (19.18)	-.94 (11.51)	-1.88 (2.13)	.002 (0.00)	-.47 (0.38)	1.51 (1.39)
WRAT	-1.49 (1.37)	-7.36 (5.80)	-3.32 (12.56)	-.34 (0.81)	1.90 (24.65)	-.68 (6.78)	-2.55 (4.40)	-.44 (0.62)	-.26 (0.13)	.65 (0.29)
WRAT b/	-.91 (0.66)	-6.65 (6.04)	-2.38 (8.23)	-.08 (0.06)	1.12 (10.86)	-.27 (1.33)	-1.72 (2.57)	-.44 (0.79)	-.05 (0.01)	-.01 (0.00)
					Family income $\geq$ $7,000					
WISC	-.45 (0.12)	-8.57 (3.59)	-2.57 (5.27)	.16 (0.16)	.63 (2.27)	-.56 (2.15)	-.08 (0.002)	.27 (0.18)	.04 (0.002)	-2.57 (2.62)
WRAT	-1.14 (0.87)	-13.28 (9.70)	-3.65 (11.98)	.10 (0.07)	.73 (3.48)	.07 (0.04)	-3.52 (3.72)	-.07 (0.01)	-.25 (0.13)	-2.85 (3.64)
WRAT b/	-.94 (0.75)	-9.51 (6.35)	-2.52 (7.29)	.03 (0.01)	.46 (1.73)	.32 (1.01)	-3.49 (4.66)	-.19 (0.13)	-.27 (0.18)	-1.72 (1.70)

a/ F statistics are in parentheses. The critical F values at the five percent level of significance are 2.69 for a one-tailed test and 3.84 for a two-tailed test.
b/ Based on a regression that includes WISC as an explanatory variable.

findings similar to ours.* An exception is Illsley
(1966), who finds no relationship between birth weight and IQ
in children from the highest socioeconomic class families in
Aberdeen, Scotland. He defines low birth weight, however, as
under 2,500 grams (under 5.5 pounds). We show that birth
weight under 2,000 grams has a much larger effect than birth
weight between 2,000 and 2,500 grams.

Breast-feeding.--Our estimates indicate that everything else being equal, the IQ and achievement test scores of
breast-fed children are one to two points higher on average
than those of children who had never been breast-fed. While
this effect is not as large as that reported for low birth
weight, it is statistically significant. Differences by
family income level are not great and do not follow any
particular pattern.

The premise mechanism by which breast-feeding affects
cognitive development is not clear, but a number of possible
links have been discussed. Physicians focus on the benefits
due to improved nutrition during early infancy, a time of
maximal brain growth. Gaull (cited in Brody, 1977) and Mata
(1978) suggest that, compared to cow's milk, human milk has a
chemical composition that promotes the development of the
brain and central nervous system in the first year of life.
The main evidence of such a nutrition effect is inferential:
breast-feeding has been found to have a positive effect on
head circumference which is related, in turn, to cognitive
development (see Chernichovsky and Coate, 1977; Broman
and others, 1975; Stoch and Smythe, 1976). Breast-
feeding may also affect cognitive development by improving
the general health of infants. Both Cunningham (cited in
Brody, 1977) and Mata (1978) report that breast-fed babies
have fewer illnesses than bottle-fed babies, even after
nursing ends. In addition to these purely physical effects,
there are psychological benefits of breast-feeding (see, for
example, Mata, 1978). Finally, breast-feeding may serve
as a proxy measure of both the amount and quality of interaction between mother and child during infancy and reflect
the mother's preferences for children.

Mother's age at the time of birth.--Two of the three
dummy variables for mother's age at the time of the birth of
the child have significant effects on WISC, but none of these
variables has a significant effect on WRAT. The coefficient
of LMAC implies that IQ scores of children whose mothers were

---

* Birch and Gussow (1970) question the validity of the
  Wiener study because children are not analyzed separately
  according to race. Our results, which pertain to white
  children only, indicate that birth weight effects appear
  in both high and low income (or social) classes even
  within the white sample.

less than 20 years old at birth are about two points less
than those of children whose mothers were between the ages of
20 and 35 at birth. Similarly, the coefficient of HMAG35 implies that IQ scores of children whose mothers were over the
age of 35 at birth are about 1.5 points higher than those of
children whose mothers were between the ages of 20 and 35 at
birth. The last result and the failure to uncover a negative
IQ differential for children whose mothers were at least 40
years old at birth are somewhat puzzling. One possible explanation is that women who give birth later in life spend
more time with their children. A second possibility is that
the health risks associated with birth at later ages (documented by Birch and Gussow, 1970) are already accounted for
by variables such as low birth weight. The coefficients in
table 3 reveal that the effects of mother's age at birth in
the low income sample are similar to those in the combined
sample. On the other hand, in the high income sample, no
significant effects are observed. We offer no explanation of
these results, except to note that the prevalence of births
to young mothers is twice as high in the low income sample as
in the high income sample (9.70 percent versus 4.10 percent).

Broman and others (1975) report a non-linear relationship between IQ and mother's age in the U.S. Collaborative
Perinatal Project. Their finding that those children whose
mothers were relatively young have lower IQ scores is consistent with ours. The same comment applies to their finding that children of older women do not exhibit impaired
intellectual development.

Parental assessment of infant health status.--The
parents' assessment of the overall health status of their
children at age one year (FYPH) does not have a significant
relationship with either the IQ or achievement measure. This
statement holds, with one exception, for estimates computed
both with and without income interactions. We offer two explanations for the lack of significant effects of this
variable. First, since FYPH reports the response to a rather
general question concerning past health status (as opposed to
MBFED, which refers to a very specific past event, or
PFHEALTH and PFGHEALTH, which refer to current health status),
it is plausible that it contains a relatively large amount of
measurement error. Second, FYPH may reflect aspects of infant
health status that are more accurately measured by the other
past health measures.

Current Health Effects

Height and weight.--The continuous current height
variable (IHEIGHT) has positive and statistically significant
coefficients in the three cognitive development regressions
in table 2. Children who are one standard deviation above
average in height for their age score more than one point

higher on average on IQ and achievement tests. On the other
hand, there is essentially no relationship between the continuous current weight variable (IWEIGHT) and cognitive development. This is not an altogether surprising result;
height is a better summary measure of the lifetime nutritional
status of the child, while weight primarily conveys information about his current nutritional status.

Even though height (adjusted for age) is a standard
measure of nutritional status, it has been argued that the
effect of height on IQ does not reflect nutritional effects
at all but rather unmeasured genetic factors that simultaneously affect both height and IQ. Evidence concerning the
validity of this argument can be gleaned from the separate
estimates by income class. If the relationship between
height and IQ was due primarily to unmeasured genetic effects,
there would be no reason to observe differences in the
strength of the relationship between income classes.* On the
other hand, if height does reflect nutritional status, and if
high income children as a group were better able to achieve
their genetic potential because they were better nourished on
average, variations in height would be associated with larger
IQ effects in the low income sample than in the high income
sample. This is exactly what we do find (see table 3). The
height coefficients in the low income sample are more than
twice as large as those in the high income sample.

These differences in the height coefficients by income
class can also be used to provide a rough estimate of the
"pure" effect of height on IQ due to nutrition. If all of the
variation in height in the high income sample was caused by
genetic factors (some of which simultaneously affect both
height and IQ), while variation in height in the low income
sample was caused by both genetic and nutritional variations,
the difference in the height coefficients in the two samples
would provide an estimate of the pure height effect due to
nutrition. Under these assumptions, comparison of the coefficients in the samples of both high and low income suggest
that, in the low income sample, the nutrition effect accounts
for two-thirds of the value of the coefficient of height. An
alternative rough estimate of the relative nutritional (or
non-genetic) effect in the case of achievement is obtained
by comparing the relationships between height and WRAT in the
regressions where WISC is and is not held constant. If the
unmeasured genetic factors common to height and achievement
are held constant by including WISC in the regression, the
ratio of the height coefficients in the alternative WRAT

---

*   It is also possible to obtain a lower coefficient of
    height in the high income samples simply because the un-
    measured genetic factors have a diminishing effect as IQ
    rises (average IQ as measured by WISC is higher in the high
    income sample than in the low income sample).

equations will indicate what proportion of the height effect
on WRAT is accounted for by variations in nutrition. The
ratio of these two coefficients equals three-fifths. The
agreement between alternative estimates of the relative contribution of nutrition is striking.

Another interpretation of the height-IQ relationship
is given by Tanner (1966), who claims that their positive
correlation results partially from common individual patterns
of both physical growth and the development of mental ability.
He argues that the relationship between height and IQ would
attenuate if adults were observed rather than children. While
our data do not allow us to determine to what extent our results are caused by individual differences in patterns of development, Douglas, Ross, and Simpson (1965) analyze the relationship between cognitive development and height for 15-
year-olds, holding constant stage of puberty as well as social
class and family size, and still report strong positive
associations.

A number of studies have examined relationships among
height, weight, and intellectual development in both developed
and developing countries.* Most of these studies have employed continuous height and weight measures. We review the
findings for developed countries. Miller (1974) reports a
positive relationship between IQ and achievement scores at
age 11 and height at age five in Newcastle Upon Tyne, England.
Douglas, Ross, and Simpson (1965) find positive relationships
between height and cognitive development not only for British
15-year-olds, but also for seven and 11-year-olds. Broman,
Nichols, and Kennedy (1975) do not uncover significant relationships between concurrent height and IQ measures in the
U.S. Collaborative Perinatal Project. Yet their findings
are not inconsistent with ours because they control for head
circumference, which is highly correlated with height. They
do uncover positive and significant relationships between IQ
at four years of age and weight at one year of age for whites,
and between IQ at four years and weight at four months
and at four years of age for blacks.

In addition to our work with continuous height and
weight measures, we estimate our basic equations replacing
these variables with discrete indexes that identify very
tall, very short, very heavy, and very thin children. A
somewhat different pattern of relationships among height,
weight, IQ, and school achievement emerges (see table 4). In
particular, very thin children have very low WISC and WRAT

---

*   A number of major studies have been carried out in the
    developing countries. These include the research of
    Selowsky and Taylor (1973), Richardson (1976), Popkin and
    Lim-Ybanez (1977), and Klein and others (1972).

Table 4.   Coefficients of Dummy Variables for Current Height
           Current Weight in WISC or WRAT Regressions. a/

Dependent variable	Tall	Short	Fat	Thin
Combined				
WISC	.67 (0.20)	-2.19 (1.65)	-.23 (0.05)	-12.55 (6.04)
WRAT	2.59 (3.46)	-2.04 (1.61)	-.52 (0.30)	-15.25 (10.01)
WRAT b/	2.30 (3.48)	-1.07 (0.57)	-.42 (0.25)	-9.68 (5.17)
Family income < $7,000				
WISC	1.53 (0.42)	-2.44 (1.43)	-1.29 (0.91)	-13.16 (5.44)
WRAT	1.07 (0.23)	-2.24 (1.37)	-.35 (0.07)	-14.32 (7.23)
WRAT b/	.39 (0.04)	-1.16 (0.47)	.22 (0.03)	-8.48 (3.25)
Family income $\geq$ $7,000				
WISC	-.001 (0.00)	-.72 (0.05)	.96 (0.47)	-15.09 (1.48)
WRAT	3.78 (4.41)	-1.51 (0.26)	-.40 (0.09)	-23.70 (4.10)
WRAT b/	3.79 (5.67)	-1.19 (0.20)	-.83 (0.50)	-17.01 (2.71)

a/ F statistics in parentheses. The critical F values at the
    five percent level of significance are 2.69 on a one-
    tailed test and 3.84 on a two-tailed test.
b/ Based on a regression that includes WISC as an independent
    variable.

scores. Although the height coefficients are not always statistically significant, taller children have above average scores, while shorter children have below average scores. In interpreting these results, the reader is cautioned that the prevalence of thin children is extremely small (.17). We leave the question of whether height and weight relationships are discrete, continuous, or a mixture of the two as an issue for future research.

Number of decayed primary and permanent teeth.--We find that the number of decayed primary and permanent teeth, adjusted for age and sex (IDECAY), has negative significant effects on cognitive development, except when WRAT is the dependent variable and WISC is held constant. There are several alternative ways to interpret this finding. Some part of the relationship may result from reverse causality; that is, more intelligent children may be more compliant with a program of preventive dental care. Some part of the relationship may reflect unmeasured variations in the family's interest (preferences) in caring for both the physical health and mental development of the child. Finally, the estimated coefficients may reflect the effects of nutrition.

Differences in the coefficients of IDECAY by income class (see table 3) provide some evidence that nutrition is indeed an important explanatory factor. If IDECAY reflects solely the effects of reverse causality and preferences, there would be no reason for its coefficients to vary by income class. However, if IDECAY also reflects nutritional status, and if a larger proportion of the variation in IDECAY in the low income sample (as compared to the high income sample) results from variation in nutrition, the coefficient of IDECAY would be larger in the low income sample. Both for WISC and WRAT, the coefficients of IDECAY indicate a larger negative effect in the low income sample, suggesting that nutrition is at work.

Abnormal hearing.--All three regression coefficients of abnormal hearing (IHEAR) are negative in table 2, and are statistically significant when WRAT is the dependent variable. The importance of poor hearing in the determination of school achievement is revealed by the following comparison. When all other variables, including WISC, are held constant, children with poor hearing have a WRAT score that is approximately 7.5 points lower than children with normal hearing. This difference exceeds the seven-point difference in the mean WRAT score in the high income sample as compared to the low income sample. As shown in table 3, the preceding comparison is even more dramatic when the effect of poor hearing is allowed to interact with family income. Based on the last line in this table, in the high income sample, children with poor hearing have a WRAT score that is approximately 9.5 points lower than children with normal hearing. One explanation for the relatively strong relationship between

poor hearing and WRAT in the high income sample is that high
income children attend schools of higher average quality and
that poor hearing and school quality interact in their effects
on IQ and achievement. Clearly, this explanation is speculative. It could be tested, however, by means of a controlled
experiment in which attempts were made to improve hearing
levels of children in different school environments, and the
subsequent trends in cognitive development compared.

Hu (1973) finds an insignificant, positive effect of
hearing correction on IQ in a sample of children from low
income families in Pennsylvania (see table 3). Our results
are not directly comparable with his because children with
abnormal hearing who have had their hearing corrected cannot
be identified in the health examination survey (HES).*
Further, Hu's analysis suffers from the difficulty that
his coding scheme gives children with a corrected defect
a higher score than children with no defect.

Binocular distance vision.--The set of three dummy
variables denoting whether or not the child has normal vision
and whether or not he wears glasses are, in general, not
statistically significant. This is true both for the full
sample and for the two income classes. The one exception is
the variable NSEEG in the WISC equation. That is, children
with normal vision who wear glasses have WISC scores almost
three points lower, on average, than children with abnormal
vision who do not wear glasses. This effect persists in each
income class, although it is no longer statistically significant. A possible explanation for this puzzling result is
that NSEEG might partially measure the quality of medical
care received by children; that is, children who receive
prescriptions for glasses when their eyesight is normal may
be receiving the lowest quality care among all children in
the sample.

It might seem surprising that children with abnormal
uncorrected distance vision who wear glasses do not have
higher IQ and achievement scores than children with abnormal
uncorrected distance vision who do not wear glasses (see
the coefficients of SEEG). One explanation of this result
is that the effects of poor vision on school learning might
not manifest themselves until ages beyond the age range in
Cycle II of the HES. A related point is that the prevalence of abnormal uncorrected binocular distance vision
is higher at ages 12 through 17, for example, than at
ages six through 11 (NCHS, 1973b). Finally, poor medical care for vision problems has been documented by

---

* In particular, children who wore hearing aids were examined without them. To the extent that these aids are
  beneficial, we understate the impact of abnormal uncorrected hearing on IQ and school achievement.

Kessner (1974), who finds that 40 percent of children in a
low income sample who were tested with their glasses failed a
visual acuity test.

In contrast to our findings, Hu (1973) uncovers a positive and significant relationship between IQ and vision correction, though his study is marred by a coding scheme that
gives children with corrected vision a higher score than
children with no defect. Douglas, Ross, and Simpson's (1967)
findings are more similar to our own. They report that in
the British National Survey of Health and Development, children
with abnormal distance vision have higher IQ and achievement
scores than children with normal vision. They argue that
this is because nearsighted children are more interested in
intellectual activities and less interested in physical activities than their peers with normal vision. As shown by the
difference between the coefficient of SEEG and the coefficient
of NRMAL, a similar tendency is present in the Health
Examination Survey.*

Significant abnormalities.--The presence of significant
abnormalities (ABN) has large negative and significant effects
on both IQ and achievement (except when WISC is held constant
in the WRAT equation). Children with such abnormalities have
IQ scores on average nine points lower than children without
abnormalities. Examination of the coefficients by income
class indicates that the effects are about the same in both
income classes.

Excessive school absence due to illness.--The coefficients of the dichotomous variable for excessive school absence due to illness in the past six months (SCHABS) are negative, but not statistically significant, in table 2. The
estimates by income class (table 3), however, do reveal that
excessive absence for health reasons is damaging to the IQ
and achievement of children from high income families but not
to children from low income families. It is possible to attribute this result, as in the case of poor hearing, to the
effects of higher average school quality in the high income
sample.

Douglas and Ross (1965) also examine the effects of
school absenteeism. They report a negative association between achievement and the incidence of school absence due to
illness except for children from upper middle class families.
We have no explanation of the difference between our results
and theirs.

---

*   This result might also reflect reverse causality from IQ
    and achievement to poor vision due to excessive use of
    the eyes.

Parental assessment of children's current health
status.--Parents' assessment of their child's current health
as poor or fair as compared to good or very good (measured by
the variable PFHEALTH) is associated with significantly lower
achievement scores. These scores are from two to three points
lower for children whose current health is assessed as poor or
fair. In contrast, no significant effects are reported for
IQ. The above results hold for the separate income classes,
as well as for the full sample. The finding that current
health assessment has an effect on achievement and not on IQ
makes sense because the latter is not likely to respond to
the transitory variations in health represented by the
parents' current assessment (remember that these estimates
hold constant variables that represent many aspects of the
child's permanent health status).

Accidents.--The dichotomous variable indicating
whether or not the child has had one or more accidents since
infancy has very small negative coefficients, not
significantly different from zero in all cases. The aspects
of health that are independently reflected by this variable
do not appear to interact with IQ and school achievement.

Income and Race Differences
in IQ and Achievement

To assess the overall impact of health on IQ and
achievement, a measure summarizing the combined effects of all
health variables is needed. Such a measure cannot be
constructed for an abstract case. Rather, two specific cases
are examined: differences between children from high and low
income families and between children from black and white
families. More precisely, we use the coefficients in table 2
and Appendix table A-3 to calculate what proportion of low
income-high income and black-white differences in WISC and
WRAT can be accounted for by differences in the average health
characteristics of these groups.

The resulting computations are summarized in tables 5
and 6. Table 5 shows how many of the gross differences in
WISC and WRAT between the two income classes disappear if the
low income class is given the income distribution, the mean
parents' schooling, mean family size, and mean health levels
of the high income sample, and if the relationship between
WISC (or WRAT) and the explanatory variables was the same in
both income classes. Similarly, table 6 shows how the gross
black-white differentials in WISC and WRAT scores change if
blacks are given the white values of the socioeconomic and
health variables and if the effects of these variables on
WISC and WRAT are the same for blacks and whites. The family
income calculations are based on the six income dummy variables defined in Appendix table A-1. The parents' schooling calculations are based on the separate effects of

Table 5. Children's Health, Family Size, Family Income, and Parents' Schooling Components of Differences in WISC and WRAT between Children from High and Low Income Families. a/

Component	Absolute	Percentage b/ of gross difference
WISC (gross difference = 8.084)		
Children's health	.840	10.39
Family size	.262	3.24
Family income	2.652	32.81
Parents' schooling	3.971	49.12
WRAT (gross difference = 6.508)		
Children's health	.814	12.51
Family size	.246	3.78
Family income	1.902	29.23
Parents' schooling	3.447	52.97
WRAT (with WISC)		
Children's health	.393	6.04
Family size	.130	2.00
Family income	.724	11.12
Parents' schooling	1.688	25.94
WISC	3.581	55.02

a/ Computations are based on a regression that uses the continuous current height and weight variables and does not allow for interaction effects between family income and children's health.

b/ These percentages will not, in general, add up to 100 for two reasons. First, the calculations do not incorporate the effects of the entire set of explanatory variables (indeed, these percentages could sum to more than 100 if the variables excluded from the calculations made a negative contribution to the difference in WISC or WRAT). Second, even if all variables in the regression equation were used, there is still random variation in WISC and WRAT that our equations cannot explain or predict.

Table 6. Children's Health, Parents' Schooling, and Family
          Income Components of Difference in WISC between
          White and Black Children. a/

Component	Absolute	Percentage b/ of gross difference
WISC (gross difference = 14.778)		
Children's health	.179	1.21
Family size	.501	3.39
Family income	1.548	10.48
Parents' schooling	2.990	20.23
WRAT (gross difference = 10.910)		
Children's health	.132	1.21
Family size	.470	4.31
Family income	1.392	12.76
Parents' schooling	2.642	24.22
WRAT (with WISC)		
Children's health	.054	.50
Family size	.249	2.28
Family income	.708	6.49
Parents' schooling	1.316	12.06
WISC	4.833	44.30

a/ Computations are based on a regression that uses the
    continuous current height and weight variables and
    does not allow for interaction effects between family
    income and children's health.

b/ These percentages will not, in general, add up to 100
    for two reasons. First, the calculations do not in-
    corporate the effects of the entire set of explanatory
    variables (indeed, these percentages could sum to more
    than 100 if the variables excluded from the calcula-
    tions made a negative contribution to the difference
    in WISC or WRAT). Second, even if all variables in
    the regression equation were used, there is still
    random variation in WISC and WRAT that our equations
    cannot explain or predict.

mother's schooling and father's schooling. These are crude
estimates to the extent that variations in parents' education
and income and family size lead to variations in health
levels, the full effects of parents' education, income, and
family size will be larger than those given in the tables.

From table 5, it is clear that almost all of the differences in WISC and WRAT between the high and low income
subsamples can be accounted for by differences in the socioeconomic and health variables included in the calculations.
Moreover, it is noteworthy that about 10 percent of the gross
difference is related to health factors alone. These results
are to be contrasted with the case of black-white differentials.* In the latter case, a much smaller percentage of
the gross difference in WISC or WRAT is accounted for by the
variables in our table, and only about one percent of the difference can be attributed to the set of health variables.
Thus, health differences as measured in this study do not appear to provide an important explanation for racial differences in IQ and achievement. Clearly, a complete explanation
of the black children's 15 point deficit in IQ and 11 point
deficit in school achievement would constitute an extremely
important accomplishment for both social science and public
policy.

In conclusion, we view the estimates in tables 5 and 6
as little more than one way to summarize regression results.
These estimates convey three tentative results: (1) differences in IQ and achievement between children in high and
low income classes are due in part to differences in health,
(2) the health component of the IQ or achievement difference
is much less important than either the family income component or the parents' schooling component, and (3) black-
white differences in IQ and achievement scores are much
harder to explain than are income differences, with black-
white health differences playing a minimal role.

IV. SUMMARY AND IMPLICATIONS

Does poor health, as measured by the indicators we have
employed, contribute to retarding the cognitive development
of children? Based on a representative sample of white children in the United States, our tentative answer is that it
does. With family background and home environment variables
held constant, many of the health measures that we have used
in this paper have significant effects on IQ and school
achievement. In addition, either taken as a single set or in
two separate subsets (the health variables measured in infancy

---

* The black sample, like the white sample, includes only
  children who live with both of their natural (or
  adoptive) parents.

and those measured currently), the health variables make a statistically significant contribution to the explanation of variations in school achievement, even when IQ is held constant.

With regard to the effects of specific health indicators, birth weight, breast-feeding, nutritional status (as reflected by height and by the number of decayed permanent and primary teeth), and poor hearing stand out as important correlates of IQ and achievement. Low birth weight is as damaging to children from high income families as to children from low income families. Nutritional status effects are more important in the low income sample, while poor hearing and excessive school absence due to illness are more important in the high income sample.

Our results are useful whether or not the mechanism by which a given health variable alters cognitive development is fully understood. In the case where the mechanism is known, our results can be used to identify the appropriate kinds of government intervention. A case in point is the role of poor hearing in the determination of school achievement. Here we feel confident that the basic force at work is a causal relationship running from hearing problems to school learning. Alternatively, when effects of certain variables are large, but mechanisms are not well-understood, our findings suggest the nature of additional research that is required to formulate public policy, rather than the appropriate policies per se. Consider, for example, our result that current height is an important determinant of cognitive development in children from low income families. This result has a very definite policy implication if the mechanism at work is a positive correlation between height and nutritional status. The policy implication is much less clearcut if the mechanism at work is a common genetic inheritance of height and mental ability.

We view the empirical work in this paper as preliminary or ongoing rather than definitive or final. Due to the preliminary nature of the work, we have not hesitated to suggest alternative explanations of certain findings, to speculate and to be provocative in discussion results, and to propose a partial agenda for future research. Instead of repeating the items on this agenda that were mentioned in section III, we conclude the paper by suggesting two new ones. The first is an investigation of health and cognitive development relationships at later stages in the child's life cycle. In particular, one could determine if some of the strong relationships between indicators of early health and IQ and achievement taper off as the child grows. The second is a longitudinal study of the change in cognitive development for the same child between two different ages as it relates to initial levels of health or to changes in health. The latter study would be particularly useful because of evidence summarized by Bloom (1964) that the rate of growth of cognitive development is more responsive to environmental factors than to the initial level of cognitive development.

Acknowledgments.

Research for this paper was supported by grants from the Ford Foundation and the Robert Wood Johnson Foundation to the National Bureau of Economic Research. We would like to thank Sol Chafkin, Dov Chernichovsky, Douglas Coate, Thomas Cooney, Victor Fuchs, Ruth Gross, M.D., Teh-Wei Hu, Herbert Klarman, Robert Michael, Barry Popkin, and Donald Yett for helpful comments and suggestions; and Ann Colle and Jacob Gesthalter for research assistance. This paper has not undergone the review accorded official NBER publications; in particular, it has not yet been submitted for approval by the Board of Directors.

Table A-1.   Definition of Basic Variables in WISC or WRAT
             Regressions.

Variable name	Definition
TWIN	Dummy variable that equals one if child is a twin
FIRST	Dummy variable that equals one if child is the first born in the family
KIND	Dummy variable that equals one if child attended kindergarten or nursery school
MWORKPT MWORKFT	Dummy variables that equal one if the mother works part-time or full-time, respectively
MALE	Dummy variable that equals one if child is male
FLANG	Dummy variable that equals one if a foreign language is spoken in the home
MEDUCAT	Years of formal schooling completed by mother
FEDUCAT	Years of formal schooling completed by father
Y1 Y2 Y3 Y4 Y5 Y6	Dummy variables that equal one if family income is greater than or equal to $3,000 (Y1); greater than or equal to $4,000 (Y2); greater than or equal to $5,000 (Y3); greater than or equal to $7,000 (Y4); greater than or equal to $10,000 (Y5); greater than or equal to $15,000 (Y6)
NEAST MWEST SOUTH	Dummy variables that equal one if child lives in Northeast, Midwest, or South, respectively
URB1 URB2 URB3 NURB	Dummy variables that equal one if child lives in an urban area with a population of three million or more (URB1); in an urban area with a population between one million and three million (URB2); in an urban area with a population less than one million (URB3); or in a non-rural and non-urbanized area (NURB); omitted class is residence in a rural area
LESS20	Number of persons in the household 20 years of age of less

Table A-2. Means and Standard Deviations of Dependent and
            Independent Variables, Whites, Ages 6-11, Mother
            and Father Present. (n = 3599)

Variable	Mean	Standard deviation
WISC	103.1937	13.9535
WRAT	103.1773	12.8378
LIGHT1	.0128	.1123
LIGHT2	.0411	.1986
BFED	.3037	.4599
LMAG	.0697	.2547
HMAG35	.1042	.3056
HMAG40	.0308	.1729
FYPH	.0839	.2773
LESS20	3.6163	1.6371
SEEG	.0709	.2566
NSEEG	.0431	.2030
NRMAL	.8377	.3687
IHEAR	.0058	.0762
ABN	.0806	.2722
IHEIGHT	.0371	.9673
IWEIGHT	.0596	.9982
IDECAY	-.0674	.9643
PFHEALTH	.0417	.1999
PFGHEALTH	.4451	.4970
ACC	.1678	.3738
SCHABS	.0428	.2024
TALL	.0206	.1419
SHORT	.0153	.1227
FAT	.0464	.2104
THIN	.0017	.0408
TWIN	.0233	.1510
FIRST	.2895	.4536
KIND	.7313	.4433
MWORKPT	.1373	.3422
MWORKFT	.1373	.3422
MALE	.5115	.4999
FLANG	.1020	.3027
MEDUCAT	11.2431	2.7456
FEDUCAT	11.2698	3.4444
Y1	.9011	.2986
Y2	.8361	.3703
Y3	.7497	.4333
Y4	.4793	.4996
Y5	.2212	.4151
Y6	.0614	.2401
NEAST	.2390	.4265
MWEST	.3279	.4695
SOUTH	.1759	.3808
URB1	.1976	.3982
URB2	.1256	.3314
URB3	.1814	.3854
NURB	.1500	.3572

Table A-3. Ordinary Least Squares Regressions of WISC and WRAT. a/

Independent variable	WISC Regression coefficient	F	WRAT Regression coefficient	F	WRAT Regression coefficient	F
TWIN	-3.04	4.92	-1.08	0.70	.26	0.05
MWORKFT	-1.92	10.26	-1.25	4.91	-.41	0.66
MWORKPT	.59	0.99	.38	0.46	.12	0.06
MEDUCAT	.92	77.82	.72	54.08	.32	13.07
FEDUCAT	.63	52.95	.60	54.17	.32	19.76
MALE	3.05	57.96	-2.69	50.74	-4.03	143.61
FLANG	-1.73	6.08	.53	0.64	1.29	4.86
FIRST	-.01	0.00	.66	2.02	.67	2.61
KIND	1.03	3.51	-.31	0.35	-.76	2.75
Y1	1.62	2.53	-1.83	3.64	-2.55	9.00
Y2	.66	0.40	3.04	9.53	2.76	9.98
Y3	1.08	1.92	1.86	6.34	1.38	4.47
Y4	.72	1.66	.09	0.03	-.23	0.23
Y5	1.75	7.28	.78	1.64	.01	0.00
Y6	.69	0.52	-.56	0.39	-.87	1.19
LESS20	-.59	18.76	-.56	18.68	-.30	6.72
FYPH	-.37	0.24	-.29	0.17	-.13	0.04
LMAG	-1.87	4.98	-.82	1.08	.00	0.00
HMAG35	1.68	4.75	.48	0.43	-.27	0.17
HMAG40	-.56	0.17	-.30	0.05	-.05	0.00
BFED	1.84	16.57	1.50	12.54	.70	3.42
LIGHT1	-5.17	8.03	-9.33	29.40	-7.05	21.44
LIGHT2	-2.46	5.73	-1.96	4.09	-.88	1.04
SEEG	1.00	0.74	.40	0.13	-.04	0.00
NSEEG	-2.86	4.70	-1.66	1.78	-.40	0.13
NRMAL	-.93	0.99	-1.33	2.29	-.92	1.40
IHEAR	-3.65	1.93	-9.20	13.84	-7.60	12.06
ABN	-2.31	9.74	-3.46	24.44	-2.44	15.49
IWEIGHT	-.22	0.63	-.11	0.18	-.01	0.00
IHEIGHT	1.23	17.81	1.32	23.22	.78	10.31
IDECAY	-.79	12.16	-.40	3.47	-.05	0.07
PFHEALTH	-1.13	1.12	-2.68	7.06	-2.18	5.98
PFGHEALTH	.06	0.02	-.34	0.70	-.37	1.06
ACC	-.22	0.17	-.27	0.29	-.18	0.15
SCHABS	-.09	0.01	-.70	0.56	-.66	0.63
WISC					.44	993.82
CONSTANT	85.06		89.71		52.21	
Adj.R^2	.27		.25		.40	
F	33.37		27.67		57.68	
n	35.99		35.99		35.99	

a/ Regressions include three region and four residence variables. The critical
F values at the five percent level of significance are 2.69 on a one-tailed
test and 3.84 on a two-tailed test.

REFERENCES

Acosta, Phyllis B.
    1974   "Nutritional status of Mexican American preschool
            children in a border town." American Journal of
            Clinical Nutrition 27 (December).

Becker, Gary S.
    1965   "A theory of the allocation of time." Economic
            Journal 75 (September):299.

Becker, Gary S. and H. Gregg Lewis
    1973   "On the interaction between the quantity and
            quality of children." In Schultz, T. W. (ed.),
            New Economic Approaches to Fertility. Proceed-
            ings of a conference sponsored by the National
            Bureau of Economic Research and the Population
            Council. Journal of Political Economy 81
            (March/April):2, part II.

Becker, Gary S. and Nigel Tomes
    1976   "Child endowments and the quantity and quality
            of children." Journal of Political Economy 84
            (August):4, part II.

Berg, Robert L.
    1973   Health Status Indexes. Proceedings of a con-
            ference conducted by Health Services Research,
            Tucson, Arizona, October 1972. Chicago: Hos-
            pital Research and Educational Trust.

Birch, Herbert G. and Joan Dye Gussow
    1970   Disadvantaged Children: Health, Nutrition, and
            School Failure. (p. 10). New York: Harcourt,
            Brace, and World, Inc.

Bloom, Benjamin S.
    1964   Stability and Change in Human Characteristics.
            New York: John Wiley and Sons, Inc.

Brody, Jane E.
    1977   "Personal health: Breast-feeding may help an
            infant to a better life." The New York Times
            (March 9).

Broman, Sarah H., Paul L. Nichols, and Wallace A. Kennedy
    1975   Preschool IQ: Prenatal and Early Developmental
            Correlates. Hillsdale, N.J.: Lawrence Erlbaum
            Associates.

Center for Disease Control
   1972   Ten-State Nutrition Survey in the United States,
          1968-1970. I - Historical Development; II -
          Demographic Data, U.S.DHEW publication no. (HSM)
          72-8130; III - Clinical, Anthropometry, Dental,
          U.S.DHEW publication no. (HSM) 72-8131; IV -
          Biochemical, U.S.DHEW publication no. (HSM) 72-
          8132; V - Dietary, U.S.DHEW publication no.
          (HSM) 72-8133; Highlights, U.S.DHEW publication
          no. (HSM) 72-8134. Atlanta, Ga.: Health Serv-
          ices and Mental Health Association.

Chernichovsky, Dov and Douglas Coate
   1977   "The choice of diet for young children and its
          relation to children's growth." Unpublished
          paper.

Christakis, George
   1968   "Nutritional epidemiologic investigation of 642
          New York City children." American Journal of
          Clinical Nutrition 21 (January).

Cooney, Jr., Thomas E.
   1977   "Health and nutrition as possible factors in
          juvenile anti-social behavior." Prepared for
          the Ford Foundation.

Correa, H.
   1975   "Measured influence of nutrition on socioeconomic
          development." World Review of Nutrition and
          Dietetics 20.

Davie, Ronald, Neville Butler, and Harvey Goldstein
   1972   From Birth to Seven. New York: Humanities
          Press, Inc.

Douglas, J.W.B. and J. M. Ross
   1965   "The effects of absence on primary school per-
          formance." British Journal of Educational
          Psychology 35, part I.

Douglas, J.W.B., J. M. Ross, and H. R. Simpson
   1967   "The ability and attainment of short-sighted
          pupils." Journal of the Royal Statistical
          Society 130, part 4.

   1965   "The relation between height and measured edu-
          cational ability in school children of the same
          social class, family size, and stage of sexual
          development." Human Biology 37:2.

Drillien, Cecil M.
   1964   The Growth and Development of the Prematurely
          Born Infant. Baltimore: Williams and Wilkins.

Driskel, Judy A. and Claudia S. Price
    1974   "Nutritional status of preschoolers from low-
            income Alabama families." Journal of American
            Dietetic Association 65 (September).

Edwards, Linda Nasif
    1975   "The economics of schooling decisions: Teenage
            enrollment rates." The Journal of Human
            Resources 10 (Spring):2.

Edwards, Linda Nasif and Michael Grossman
    1977   "An economic analysis of children's health and
            intellectual development." National Bureau of
            Economic Research Working Paper no. 180 (May).

Endozien, J. C., B. R. Switzer, and R. B. Bryan
    1976   Medical Evaluation of the Special Supplemental
            Food Program for Women, Infants, and Children
            (WIC): Summary and Conclusions. Department of
            Nutrition, School of Public Health, University of
            North Carolina (July).

Grossman, Michael
    1975   "The correlation between health and schooling."
            In Terleckyj, Nestor E. (ed.), Household Pro-
            duction and Consumption. New York: Columbia
            University Press for the National Bureau of
            Economic Research.

    1972   The Demand for Health: A Theoretical and Empiri-
            cal Investigation. New York: Columbia Univer-
            sity Press for the National Bureau of Economic
            Research.

Haggerty, Robert J., Klaus J. Roghmann, and Ivan B. Pless
    1975   Child Health and the Community. New York:
            John Wiley and Sons.

Heller, Peter S. and William D. Drake
    1976   Malnutrition, Child Morbidity, and the Family
            Decision Process. Discussion Paper no. 58.
            Center for Research on Economic Development,
            The University of Michigan (September).

Hu, Teh-Wei
    1973   "Effectiveness of child health and welfare
            programs: A simultaneous equations approach."
            Socio-Economic Planning Sciences 7.

Illsley, Raymond
    1966   "Preventive medicine in the perinatal period."
            Proceedings of the Royal Society of Medicine
            59 (March).

Inman, Robert P.
    1976   "The family provision of children's health: An
            economic analysis." In Rosett, Richard (ed.),
            The Role of Health Insurance in the Health
            Services Sector. New York: Columbia University
            Press for the National Bureau of Economic
            Research.

Kaplan, Robert S., Lester B. Lave, and Samuel Leinhardt
    1972   "The efficacy of a comprehensive health care
            project: An empirical analysis." American
            Journal of Public Health 62 (July):7.

Kessner, David M.
    1974   Assessment of Medical Care for Children:
            Contrasts in Health Status, vol. 3. Washington,
            D.C.: Institute of Medicine.

Klein, Robert E.
    1972   "Is big smart? The relation of growth to
            cognition." Journal of Health and Social
            Behavior 13 (September).

Lancaster, Kelvin J.
    1966   "A new approach to consumer theory." Journal of
            Political Economy 74 (April):2.

Leibowitz, Arleen
    1974   "Home investment in children." In Schultz, T.W.
            (ed.), Economics of the Family. New York:
            Columbia University Press for the National
            Bureau of Economic Research.

Leveson, Irving, Doris Ullman, and Gregory Wassall
    1969   "Effects of health on education and productiv-
            ity." Inquiry 5 (December):4.

Lewin, Roger
    1975   "Starved brains." Psychology Today 9 (Septem-
            ber):4.

Mata, Leonardo
    1978   "Breast feeding: Main promoter of infant
            health." American Journal of Clinical
            Nutrition 31 (May).

Mechanic, David
    1964   "The influence of mothers on their children's
            health, attitudes, and behavior." Pediatrics
            33 (March).

Michael, Robert T.
    1972   The Effect of Education on Efficiency in Con-
            sumption. New York: Columbia University Press
            for the National Bureau of Economic Research.

Miller, F. J.
    1974   The School Years in Newcastle Upon Tyne 1952-
            62: Being a Further Contribution to the Study
            of a Thousand Families. New York: Oxford
            University Press.

Mushkin, Selma J.
    1977   "Knowledge and choices in health policy." Paper
            prepared for delivery at National Health Forum
            (March 23).

Muth, Richard F.
    1966   "Household production and consumer demand
            functions." Econometrica 34 (July):3.

National Center for Health Statistics
U.S. Department of Health, Education, and Welfare
    1975   Eye Examination Findings Among Youths Aged
            12-17 Years: United States. Public Health
            Service publication no. 1000, series 11,
            no. 155.

    1973   Body Weight, Stature, and Sitting Height:
            White and Negro Youths 12-17 Years,
            United States. Vital and Health Statistics,
            series 11, no. 126.

    1972a   Binocular Visual Acuity of Children:
            Demographic and Socioeconomic Characteristics -
            United States. Vital and Health Statistics,
            series 11, no. 112.

    1972b   Periodontal Disease and Oral Hygiene Among
            Children: United States. Vital and Health
            Statistics, series 11, no. 117.

    1970a   Hearing Levels of Children by Age and Sex:
            United States. Public Health Service
            publication no. 1000, series 11, no. 102.

National Center for Health Statistics
U.S. Department of Health, Education, and Welfare
    1970b   Height and Weight of Children: United States.
             Public Health Service publication no. 1000,
             series 11, no. 119.

    1967a   Plan, Operation, and Response Results of a Pro-
             gram of Children's Examinations. Public Health
             Service publication no. 1000, series 1, no. 5.

    1967b   A Study of the Achievement Test Used in the
             Health Examination Survey of Persons Aged 6-17
             Years. Public Health Service publication no.
             1000, series 2, no. 24.

O'Hara, Donald J.
    1975   "Microeconomic aspects of the demographic
             transition." Journal of Political Economy 83
             (December):6.

Owen, George M.
    1974   "A study of nutritional status of preschool
             children in the United States, 1968-1970."
             Pediatrics 53 (April):supplement.

Popkin, Barry M. and Marisol Lim-Ybanez
    1977   "Nutrition and learning: An economic analysis."
             Unpublished paper.

Richardson, Stephen A.
    1976   "The influence of severe malnutrition in infancy
             on the intelligence of children at school age:
             An ecological perspective." In Walsh, Roger N.
             and William T. Greenough (eds.), Environments
             as Therapy for Brain Dysfunction. New York:
             Plenum Publishing Corporation.

Schack, Elisabeth and Barbara Starfield
    1973   "Acute disability in childhood examination of
             agreement between various measures." Medical
             Care 11 (July/August):4.

Scrimshaw, Nevin S. and John E. Gordon
    1968   Malnutrition, Learning, and Behavior. Cambridge,
             Mass.: The M.I.T. Press.

Selowsky, Marcelo and Lance Taylor
    1973   "The economics of malnourished children: An
             example of disinvestment in human capital."
             Economic Development and Cultural Change 22
             (October):1.

Seoane, Nicole and Michael C. Latham
    1971   "National anthropometry in the identification of
            malnutrition in childhood." Journal of Tropical
            Pediatric and Environmental Child Health
            (September).

Sims, Laura S. and Portia M. Morris
    1974   "Nutritional status of preschoolers." Journal
            of American Dietetic Association 64 (May).

Starfield, Barbara
    1975   "Health needs of children." Prepared for the
            Robert Wood Johnson Foundation.

Stoch, M. B. and P. M. Smythe
    1976   "15-year developmental study on effects of
            severe undernutrition during infancy on subse-
            quent physical growth and intellectual func-
            tioning." Archives of Disease in Childhood 51.

Sullivan, Daniel F.
    1966   "Conceptual problems in developing an index of
            health." Public Health Service publication no.
            1000. Vital and Health Statistics, series 2,
            no. 17. Rockville, Md.: National Center for
            Health Statistics.

Talbot, Nathan B., Jerome Kagan, and Leon Eisenberg (eds.)
    1971   Behavioral Science in Pediatric Medicine.
            Philadelphia: W. B. Saunders Company.

Tanner, J. M.
    1966   "Galtonian eugenics and the study of growth."
            Eugenics Review 58.

Wallace, Helen M.
    1962   Health Services for Mothers and Children.
            Philadelphia: W. B. Saunders Company.

Ware, Jr., John E.
    1976   "The conceptualization and measurement of health
            for policy-relevant research in medical care
            delivery." Presented at the annual meetings of
            the American Association for the Advancement of
            Science, Boston, Massachusetts (February).

Wiener, Gerald
    1965   "Correlates of low birth weight: Psychological
            status at six to seven years of age." Pediatrics
            35 (March):3, part I.

Willis, Robert
     1973   "A new approach to the economic theory of
             fertility behavior." In Schultz, T. W. (ed.),
             New Economic Approaches to Fertility. Proceed-
             ings of a conference sponsored by the National
             Bureau of Economic Research and the Population
             Council. Journal of Political Economy 81
             (March/April):2, part II.

13 Health Indexes for Health Assessments
Selma J. Mushkin

It has become customary to emphasize the outcomes of
health programs, which are achieved by the expenditure of
scarce resources. The focus is on cost and the "product."
Are people healthier as a consequence of health expenditures?
Is the pain of those afflicted reduced? Is the quality of
life improved? Are costs reduced by introduction of new
technology? Or are they increased? The link between cost
and outcomes is itself perplexing. A routine of inquiry is
sought on the outcomes and probabilities of success of given
therapies or research efforts.

Despite the emphasis on the importance of outcomes
or benefits and costs, the plaint, with the repetitiveness
of a Greek chorus, is the lack of acceptable measurements
(indexes) of outcome. Three questions, in particular, about
health outcomes which press for resolution are addressed in
the following sections of this concluding paper:

(1) What are the most important and relevant
gradations in levels of health and well-
being that represent outcomes or benefits
of health programs?

(2) What is the value of desirable outcomes?
What would the public be willing to pay
for improved chances of being in a higher
functional level upon contracting a chronic
disease? Practically, how can this willingness be measured?

(3) Given public preferences, how should health
funds, including biomedical research funds,
be distributed among disease problems?

315

LEVELS OF HEALTH STATUS

The record of past progress in medicine is familiar.
Death rates have declined and illness from infectious and communicable diseases has been reduced markedly.* In the United
States, a number of the major killers and cripplers of years
ago have been largely wiped out, including smallpox, typhoid,
diphtheria, malaria, hookwork, and pellagra. Particularly impressive in the record of progress is the dramatic reduction
in infant and early childhood deaths and in maternity deaths.
An epoch of miracle medicine was ushered in with antibiotics,
which helped to reduce the duration of sickness and mortality
further (including death rates of the adult population).
Most health policies today, including research activities, are
built on the considerable progress of the past. These policies are designed to alleviate a disease condition or to provide "half-way technologies" (Thomas, 1975) that generally
allow a person with a disease to function but do not cure the
disease. The major research institutes of the National Institutes of Health deal mainly with chronic diseases, such as
heart diseases, cancer, and chronic obstructive lung diseases; the aim of these institutes is the basic research
and the development of new therapies to treat and control
chronic conditions.

In the past, health statistics concentrated on mortality and morbidity. Developed mainly as general indicators
of the health of the nation or community, these mortality and
morbidity statistics have come to be used as outcome measures.
However, they do not capture the essential impacts of biomedical research; they do not provide operational need-
assessment or evaluation criteria for health programs. Alternative measures of health status are needed. This need
has stimulated much research on health status. Studies of
new measures of health status and function are being carried
out in increasing numbers. These studies include the important work of Bush and his colleagues who have formulated
measures of functional years (well years) or value-adjusted
life expectancy (Fanshel and Bush, 1970). The measure is
derived by weighting functional level expectancies to yield
a scalar value. Zeckhauser and Shepard (1976) have adopted
a quality-adjusted life year as an evaluative criterion.
Wylie and White (1964) earlier developed the "Maryland Disability Index" for measuring the effectiveness of rehabilitation services. Jones, McNitt, and Densen (1979) have applied to nursing home care the "Index of Independence in
Activities of Daily Living," developed by Katz (1963), for
measuring the functional states of the elderly and
chronically ill. The National Cancer Institute has applied

---

* For instance, the probability of living from age 45 to
  age 46 for the average U.S. citizen is 99.6 percent
  (Public Health Service, U.S.DHEW, 1975).

a "Sickness Impact Profile" (SIP) to clinic trials, as a
component in a quality of life assessment (Gilson and
others, 1975). Martin Chen has done considerable work
on indexing of health status (Chen, M. K., 1976, 1973).
These examples are only illustrative. The Chen-Bush
paper in this volume reviews the studies at greater length.

    Measurements run the gamut from a few selected indexes
of individuals' functioning capacity to complex sociomedical
health indicators and measurements of quality of life. The
simple measures rely on a few measures of function that are
easy to collect and interpret. The more complex measurements
seek to incorporate gradations of physical, psychological, and
social dysfunction. In addition, the more complex measurements often include time-specific states of function that
yield transition probabilities, based on time spent in a defined condition and subsequent prognosis. The number of components in these complex indexes vary; as the number increases, the indexes become more technical and complicated.

Criteria for Health Status Measurements

    Choosing among the many measurements of health status
that have, or might, become available, using all kinds of
techniques and applying a variety of concepts, can be a monumental task. The choice will be guided by the desired use of
the measure; the most important use of any health status
measure is in deciding which policies and treatments are most
effective. Among other things, one would like a measure that
is easy to comprehend, unlikely to be misunderstood or mis-
interpreted, and for which data can be collected without in-
ordinate expense. The following is a list of desirable criteria that an index of health status and function should be
able to meet:

    (1) Simple: The index should be easy to under-
         stand and to present to policy makers.

    (2) Comprehensive: The index needs to provide
         an assessment of the degree to which in-
         tended public purposes are being met by
         resource allocations or program decisions.

    (3) Able to isolate impacts: The index should
         change if, and only if, a change in health or
         functional states occurs due to intervention.
         In addition, it should record adverse as well
         as positive impacts.

    (4) Able to identify target groups: The index
         should facilitate the identification of im-
         pact on special target groups; for example,
         changes in functional capacity of children.

(5) Reproducible: Index information should be
     collected in a sufficiently simple manner
     to facilitate repeated samples. Each time
     that the procedure is reproduced, the same
     type of information should be gathered; in
     this way, the information obtained can be
     compared with that for other groups of in-
     dividuals or with that for the same in-
     dividuals in different time periods.

(6) Low cost: Collection of information needs
     to be kept at a cost commensurate with the
     usefulness of the data.

(7) Reasonable: Measures need to be "reasonable"
     to the diverse groups whose interests are
     involved in the health policy, for example,
     consumers, policy officials, health providers,
     and research scientists.

In addition to these criteria, there is the need for a
measure that allows for each disease's special characteristics. Practitioners and research scientists often need to
measure their progress toward prevention or control in terms
of those special characteristics. For example, in the case
of lung disease, this may mean measurements related specifically to lung function; in the case of heart disease, results of EKGs may be important. However, in order to use an
index for choices about health policy, the index must be comparable across diseases and usable from one health problem
to another. Only by such a single set of measurements can
options be compared. Thus, the commonality of measures of
outcome in terms of functional states must be stressed.
Precision measuring of outcomes with regard to each disease
will clearly be lost; however, the sacrifice allows appli-
cability of the index to a wide range of purposes, as well
as a lower initial cost.

A Desirable Functional Measure

An example of a functional measure that has many of
the above attributes is presented below. Developed initially
for use in an evaluation scheme for lung disease, the functional states identified appear to meet the need for a set of
health indicators that reflect the real outcomes of current
health programs. These health indicators are also useful for
policy analysis and evaluation (Mushkin, 1977). The functional states identified are these:

(1) Cured or in remission

     This category includes persons considered
     to be cured of disease, subsequent to a
     recommended intervention. They can perform

all major activities that are normal for
their age and sex, and have no remaining
detectable signs of disease.

(2) Fully-functioning despite disease or
     impairment

This category includes persons with disease
or impairment who engage in such activities
as keeping house, working, shopping; attending school, church, or clubs; and taking
part in sports or other recreational activities.
To be considered "fully functioning despite
disease or impairment," the person must be
free of pain most of the time and must not
be affected in ways that are an embarrass-
ment to the patient or a cause for rejection
by friends, acquaintances, or employers.
Persons may be included in this category
even if they have some minor limitations
in mobility or are on medication that requires a limited number of hours a week
away from work or school. The National
Center for Health Statistics data on whether
the disease condition is a bother come as
close as existing statistics gets to this
concept.

(3) Functioning with some limitations

This category, as defined by the National
Center for Health Statistics, includes persons with the following limitations:

a. unable to carry on major activities
    in which persons of their age and
    sex normally engage;

b. limited in the amount or kind of major
    activity performed; and

c. not limited in major activity but other-
    wise limited in athletics, extracurricular
    activities, church, hobbies, shopping,
    civic projects, or other usual activities.

(4) Capable of self-care but major and other
     activities severely limited

This category includes persons with disease
or impairment who are capable of self-care
(for example, eating, dressing, and bathing),
but who are unable, most of the time, to
leave their homes and are unable to work

(including keeping house), shop, go to
school, churches or clubs, or engage in
sports and other recreational activities.
Persons included in this category can care
for themselves, but their mobility is limited to the point that they need help in
leaving their homes.

(5)   Not capable of self-care

This category includes persons in institu-
tions and requiring care by others because
their physical or mental capacity is so impaired that they are unable to perform all
or most self-care activities (for example,
eating, bathing, dressing, and going to the
toilet).

Persons are included in this category if
they are in nursing homes or other long-
term care or extended-care facilities,
even if they might otherwise be able to
care for themselves. Persons are also included in this category if they require
assistance from professional nurses or
paid homemakers for an extended period,
or if such assistance is provided by
family members or friends who devote
substantial time to such care.

Data on the functional states of a population would
permit comparisons to be made between the results of current
practices, without a new intervention, and the changes in
functional states attributable to interventions. To illustrate the uses of quantification of functional states, table 1
represents the assumed distribution among the functional
states of the population with a disease, before any new program intervention or new therapy, and after two optional interventions. The costs of each intervention, as well as the
prevalence of functional states, are presented. (It is assumed that there is no difference in death rates between the
options.)

The illustration underscores some choice problems.
The differences in cost between the two interventions are
large in relation to the differences in impact. A first $100
million of added cost yields a 10 percentage-point gain in
numbers cured and a 20 percentage-point gain in those fully
functioning, and it moves all persons with the disease to at
least a self-care position. The program or policy official
choosing whether to intervene by the first method, with an
expenditure of $100 million, can judge the importance of the
change. The second intervention also costs $100 million.
Compared to intervention 1, it changes those with the disease

Table 1. Proportion of the Population with Disease A by Functional States.

(After 6-month duration)

Intervention	Cost of intervention	Cured	Fully function- ing despite disease (bothered little or not at all)	Limited function- ing (activity limitation)	Confined but capable of self-care	Confined and requiring care by others
Before new intervention	--	10%	10%	50%	20%	10%
After intervention 1	$100M	20	30	40	10	--
After intervention 2	$100M	20	40	30	5	5

10 percentage points from limited to fully functioning, the
same as intervention 1; however, the gain is at the cost of
more persons requiring care by others compared to the first
intervention. The decision as to which of the alternative
interventions is better will depend on the relative valuation
placed on changes in functional states. What value should be
placed on moving from limited functioning to fully functioning? What value should be placed on moving from requiring
care to self-care? Policy officials, responsible for fund
allocation, must decide which intervention is better as a step
toward accountability to the public for their decisions.

        This example can be expanded in many ways to incor-
porate more information. The time period under consideration
can be varied. Outcomes for a designated patient group may
be assessed over intervals of specified months, or there may
be followups through longitudinal studies over a long term.
Cross-sectional outcome analysis may be used. Here the intent
is to assess the likely change in the functional states of a
population group--those healthy and those with disease--given
diverse programs and different commitments of health resources. Severe pain or disfigurement due to the available
therapies can be added to the functional state measurements.
Functional states might be shown separately by age of individual, with special reference to children. While each
characteristic provides more information, it also adds complexity, making it more difficult to display and evaluate.
Therefore, the use of additional information must be balanced
against additional complexity.

        In contrast to indexes of quality of life or of func-
tional years, such as Bush's or Zeckhauser's, functional state
measurement permits public officials to identify the types of
changes occurring in function because of interventions
changes are not buried by incorporation into an overall index.
In addition, the concept of functional states, while requiring
new data collection, relies to a maximum extent on preexisting data from the National Center for Health Statistics and
restricts the additional data collection required to an essential minimum. The use of preexisting data is extremely
desirable because of its efficiency; it reduces the
costs and takes advantage of past research and data collection. Another advantage is that, in concept, functional
state measurement has various evaluation applications that
range from clinical testing of therapies to analysis of optional congressional policies on health insurance programs'
health benefits. Commonality of measurement would permit
the compilation of data, for example, on the change in distribution among functional states of the patient population
due to (1) a chemotherapy agent for cancer, (2) a curtailing
of smoking, (3) greater compliance with physician-prescribed
regimens in hypertension, or (4) health services quality
controls under various monitoring plans.

If a single, composite index is considered more useful than the separate measures, the indexes of Bush and Zeckhauser or others become most appropriate. Alternatively, efforts can be made to translate "days," at each level of functioning, into a single index: Groups of individuals who are well can be asked, for example, about the days of dependent bed care they would accept in order to achieve a higher level of functioning. The number of days of dependent bed care becomes, in essence, the common unit of measurement.*

Measured changes in the distribution of cases among functional states facilitate answering these questions: What difference does one therapy as contrasted with another make in functioning? For how long does one therapy work compared to another? What is the probability of success as measured by a shift from bed care to fully functioning, for example? Is psychological or emotional support in serious illness more (or less) important than physical medicine in terms of functional states? What medical care can make a difference in functional status? Does a particular eligibility test or method of payment for care encourage (or discourage) self-care and use of those health services that might make a difference in functional status?

Data on functional states can supply information adequate to sufficiently inform policy officials about program effectiveness. Indeed, the data on specific measures of functional states often serve policy purposes better than any composite summary figure. However, for other purposes, composite estimates of health gains, which can be compared with cost and can provide the comparability of monetary measures from one program to another, are highly useful.

CONSUMER PREFERENCES

In the past, "pricing" of health benefits has relied on measurement of human capital gained through reductions in disability or death; for example, see Weisbrod (1961), Mushkin (1962), Klarman (1965), and Cooper and Rice (1967). By analogy to physical capital, human capital has been measured in terms of gains in the length of time at work and the productivity while at work. The human capital approach is now being challenged both conceptually and practically. The facts about health intervention in recent years, when based only on

---

* In a trial, with limited number of respondents from the health professions, made by the Public Services Laboratory, most indicated a willingness, when ill, to accept 10 days of dependent care to gain one fully functioning day, and five days of confinement to bed while capable of self-care for one day of full functioning. To one respondent, "Each day has an equal value."

death rates and disability indexes, do not appear to provide
much optimism about the benefits of further research and medical treatment. This does not mean that benefits will not be
achieved; the measurements are simply not sensitive enough to
the current and future changes.

It is also charged that the conceptual notion of human
capital does not fit the basic economic idea of consumer
satisfaction as a guiding mechanism in the economy; this
notion of human capital does not reflect the desire of individuals to improve their own chances of survival (Schelling,
1968; Mishan, 1971), or of functioning fully, when disease
strikes. Indeed, the concept has been challenged as being
appropriate only to a slave state. A method that better
fits the conceptual framework of economic efficiency
analysis and consumer preferences than that of the human
capital approach is to measure benefits as the sum of
individuals' willingness to pay. What, for example, is
the price individuals would be willing to pay to improve
the ratio of quality-adjusted life years to total life
years (longevity)? What would individuals pay to reduce
the probability of years in bed, dependent upon others
for care when illness strikes, in favor of greater self-
care and self-dependency, to draw an illustration from
the evaluation criteria discussed earlier?

Willingness to pay, as a conceptual method of putting
dollar values on benefits or program outcomes that can then
permit benefit and cost comparisons, has gained acceptance
for application to health program analysis. However, problems
of operational application continue to pose real difficulties.
A primary question is the following: What analytical approaches may be followed to give reality to the theoretical
concepts, recognizing that many of these approaches remain
controversial? Different methods of determining willingness
to pay and problems of measurement are discussed by Clarke,
Fischer, Lipscomb, Schulze, and other contributors to this
volume. The various optional measures include direct response
from consumers through surveys, imputations of value from market behavior, and the application of demand-revealing processes. In all cases, the benefits that are being priced by
determinations of willingness to pay are benefits to all persons in the population. Benefits are specified in terms of a
reduction in the risk, for example, of being confined to bed
when chronic illness strikes. If the chance that one per
1,000 persons will be confined to bed with a chronic ailment
next year could be reduced to 0.3 per 1,000 as a consequence
of new biomedical research, what would each person and, in
sum, all persons together be willing to pay to reduce the
probability of bed confinement? The price that individuals
would be willing to pay for a change in the probability of
being in a less desirable state, or in that state for a
longer period of time, is likely to vary according to age,
income, and risk aversion.

In the literature on willingness to pay, three classes
of benefits flowing from health interventions have been dis-
tinguished, each of which requires pricing. These benefits
include (1) the benefit to the individual, (2) benefits to
family and friends, and (3) net benefits to society. The most
direct benefit comes from the individual's reduced risk of
severity of functional impairment. How much would an average
person be willing to pay for a given reduction in this risk?

Surveys of Preferences

Seemingly, the most direct method of determining individuals' preferences is to ask them by surveys. The
question to be posed is the following: What is the dollar
value of other consumption that the individual consumer would
give up for some defined reduction in the probability of impairment or illness in a defined period? Acton (1976,
1973) has pioneered in work on surveys along these
lines, particularly in a study of the risk of heart attacks.

As Fischer indicates elsewhere in this volume,
a number of difficult issues are encountered in the
survey method of deriving preferences. There is no
reason to assume that the responses are accurate or even
that the hypothetical question is really understood. When
eliciting willingness-to-pay responses for actual implementation of policy, there is no way to monitor the truthfulness
of response nor to penalize strategic behavior that involves
representation of preferences. The validity of the survey
instrument, stability of response, and replicability of result
--all are of technical concern. Response behavior on surveys
of willingness to pay is not yet well researched. Up to now,
the survey technique has not yielded a practical measurement
tool that is acceptable in guiding policy officials on public
decisions. Optional methods, however, are available to assess
willingness to pay and consumer preferences about resource
allocations in health programs. One such method is suggested
by the work of Martin Bailey.

Present Market Values

Bailey (1977) obtains a lower bound for the "value of
life" by measuring the discounted present value of the stream
of lifetime earnings. According to him, the lower bound for
the "value of life" (an individual's willingness to pay for
maintaining earnings for his family in event of death) is the
discounted present value of the expected stream of lifetime
earnings. The argument is advanced that if an individual
were assured that at death his family would continue to receive income equivalent to his earnings, he would not purchase life insurance. Life insurance purchases, accordingly,
are a market indication of the preference of the individual

for protection for his family. They represent a lower bound
and an underestimate when you consider both the value to life,
above and beyond that of merely consuming, and the amounts
paid additionally for risk aversion. Individuals manifest
their aversion to risk by their behavior in a number of ways,
including the purchase of insurance with a loading factor that
calls for premiums in excess of claims paid.

Bailey measures the willingness to pay for risk avoidance by using the Thaler-Rosen (1974) study's estimates of
wage premium paid for increased risk. In attempting to separate the premiums for risk of death from premiums for the
risk of injury, he asks: How much compensation is required
to induce a worker to accept a .001 per year risk of
permanent disability as compared to the .001 percent risk of
death? In making this comparison, it is assumed, based on
Social Security data, that accidental death at work causes
a loss of 24 years of work and earnings, and accidents resulting in permanent disability lead to an average of five years
inability to work plus partial disability for the rest of the
life. The amount of extra compensation for the risk of disability is considered by Bailey somewhat arbitrarily (based on
the ratio of five years of disability to 24 years of work
lost due to death) to be 1/5 (0.2) of the compensation for the
risk of death. Thus, a .001 per year extra risk of work dis-
ablement would require 1/5 the compensation of a .001 per
year probability of death.

In contrast to Bailey's examples of accidental death
and disability due to work injuries, general health and biomedical research policies are concerned with chronic illnesses
in which years of illness may precede death, resulting in a
larger number of impaired lives in the population. Instead
of deaths among young persons, there is an increase in illness. Relatively young persons may live on with a chronic
problem. For instance, instead of five years loss due to
disability, consider a risk per 1,000 of living 30 or 40 more
years of remaining life expectancy with an illness such as
diabetes. This option may be considered less desirable than
the option of five years of loss, followed by a slightly impaired life. Thus, instead of a market value of .2 for the
extra compensation due to premature death, it could be perhaps .5 to .9 that of death. In the Bailey example, updated
to 1978, the premium for the risk of accidental death would
be $180 per year at a probability level of one per 1,000
workers.

For any individual and group average, there are
"function level expectancies," to use the terminology of
Chen, Bush, and Patrick (1975). That is, given existing
medical knowledge and practices for defined disease conditions, the distribution of remaining years of life among
functional states is indicative of the experience in transition from one state to another. Diabetes or cancer of the
skin, given existing therapies (and assuming adherence to

those therapies) at different ages, moves along defined
transition courses from functional state to state, within more
or less defined time frames. The probabilities of the average
length of each transition need to be quantified for known al-
terative therapies.

The concept of willingness to pay, measured by
wage differences as a market valuation of risk, can be
so applied as to permit quantification by functional
states and, accordingly, quantification of benefits
from expenditures on improvement of knowledge about
disease and therapies.

Suppose that $180 is the added compensation for a .001
probability of death, as in table 2. The corresponding average annual premium per accidental injury at the probability
level of one per 1,000 would be $36, or 1/5 of $180. Some
fraction or ratio of the $180 compensation for a .001 risk
would represent the premium for the additional risk to individuals of functional states short of ultimate death. For
example, the functional state of "confined to dependent bed
care" may require a premium equal to 9/10 of $180, that is,
the added compensation required for the risk of dependent bed
care would be $162, compared to the .001 risk of death at
$180 per year. The risk of having the disease, yet being able
to function fully with the disease, might require a premium
equal to 2/10 of $180 or require additional compensation equal
to $36. The cost of the risk of a functional state would in
each case be the added compensation required for the risk and
the willingness to pay to avoid that added risk.

Given information on the average probability of contracting a chronic disease that will affect functioning for a
period, it is possible to quantify the benefits in terms of
yearly willingness to pay for improvement in functional state.
It is also practical to quantify the present value of annual
amounts that would continue for a substantial length of time
by discounting those annual payments over the length of time
the improved functional state is expected to last.

Benefits to family.--If, following Bailey, we accept
the notion that an individual's willingness to pay to reduce
his own risk of loss in function is measured in relation to
the earnings difference attributable to risk, there remains
the problem of assessing willingness to pay for the other
two classes of benefits identified by Dorfman (1979), namely,
reduction in risk for family members and neighbors and net
financial gain to society. It may be argued that the willingness to pay for family members is linked to the consumption
value of earnings. As indicated earlier, in the case of life
insurance, the protection is for the surviving beneficiary.
Except for survivors, there would be no need for life insurance and no risk of loss of consumption by survivors. The
willingness to buy such protection is dependent upon, and

Table 2. Cost of the Risk of a Functional State.

Functional state	Hypothetical percentage of added death compensation	Added compensation (willingness to pay) to avoid "extra" risk
Death	100%	$180
Confined to dependent bed care	90	162
Confined but caring for self	80	144
Partially functioning	50	90
Fully functioning	20	36

may be measured by, the present value of future earnings.
Similarly, when the potential beneficiary is the family of a
disabled wage earner rather than a survivor, willingness to
pay for a reduction in the chances of the disability may be
considered as some share of the chief wage earner's income.
Certainly, members of families are willing to pay to improve
the chances of greater function for those they love. If we
think of the family as a unit with a combined income, the
wage adjustments made by the market for greater risk of illness or accident can be considered to measure the benefit of
improved functioning as a benefit to self (class 1) and,
also, as a benefit to family (class 2) (see p. 325).
(The underlying concept of the assumptions made here requires
further analyses beyond the scope of this discussion.)

    Benefits to society.--Net benefits to society (class 3)
are the costs of chronic illnesses that confine patients to
bed; these costs and the lost resources that they represent
can be avoided and diverted to other more productive or desirable uses. Several different measures of the price that
persons would willingly pay for such net gains to society
are feasible. One such measure is the net premium paid
(premiums in excess of claims) for disability protections.
These net premiums represent the "savings" individuals are
willing to make available to others for the protection those
premiums provide. Still another measure would be the cost
of bed care averted, a cost that otherwise would have to be
financed out of the common insurance pool, less health insurance premiums paid by the individual himself.

Weakness of approach.--Using market wage differences
as the key to imputing values has its weaknesses, as well as
its strengths: (1) To establish wage differences that reflect differences in risk, market wage differences depend
upon markets that operate on an unfettered and competitive
basis. (2) Market wage differences presume relatively informed wage earners. (3) Market wage differences do not take
account of the likelihood that workers who take risky jobs
are less averse to risks than others. (4) Market wage differences, as measured, reflect existing earnings differentials between races and between men and women. (5) Market
wage differences have the tremendous advantage, however, of
using preexisting measures and complete abstracts from actual
strategic behavior on the part of individuals. Measurement
of benefits of health programs in terms of earnings is a
familiar procedure. Indeed, the computation of present value
of future earnings of individuals is now a routine in assessing health outcomes. But Bailey gives to these measurements
a different justification. The indicators are the same; the
theoretical constructs very different. Bailey applies earnings differentials as an indicator of willingness to pay.
Using these risk-compensation estimates, it is now possible
to quantify each function state's value in relation to a
defined rate of risk.

In summary, the valuation of changes in functional
states would require a quantity estimate for (a) benefits to
self from changes in those functional states; (b) benefits
to family, assumed to be essentially measured by the same
quantities as included in (a); and (c) benefits to the rest
of society measured either by net premiums for insurance in
excess of benefits, or by net remaining cost of hospital and
other institutional care, less premiums and charges paid by
the individual himself (excluding employers and governmental
payments). Rough approximations, as indicated earlier, can
be arrived at. What is required is knowledge about changes
in probabilities, with various forms of intervention, of a
population's being in different function states. If quantification by disease is sought, differences in the relative
impact of diseases on function states must be known.

Demand-revealing Processes of Willingness to Pay

Much of the impetus for deriving measures of willingness to pay comes from the desire to implement policy or
public projects. Many of these in turn are public goods.
Public goods are plagued with "free rider" problems, that is,
the use of a public good by one person does not preclude or
inhibit the use by any other persons. If one is told that
one will actually have to pay what one says one is willing
to, there is incentive to underrepresent willingness to pay.
A way to avoid this problem is to derive measures from market behavior, as above, in the use of average differentials

in earnings. Another way has been derived by Clarke (1977).
He developed a system of eliciting responses that incorporates an incentive to reveal true preferences.

As indicated in an earlier chapter in this volume,
Clarke has shown that individuals can be persuaded to reveal
their true preferences for public goods. The conceptual
framework he has formulated overcomes the theoretical
dilemmas that have thwarted pricing for many years. Penalties are exacted for misrepresenting the true preferences.
There are two penalties: The first is that the individual
(or group) would have to pay an amount equal to the value
foregone by others when his vote changes the outcome that
would otherwise have been chosen. The second penalty is the
lost benefit that would occur if a solution other than his
preferred choice were selected. Rather than forego the value
of changing the outcome, he will reveal his values honestly.

The conceptual framework is more complicated than may
be implied above. If individuals were asked to contribute to
biomedical research at a price in terms of their own preferences, we would have a record of those preferences; we
would also have a record of the risks that individuals are
willing to pay to avoid, relative to functional states,
through cures and treatments. However, we do not have
that information. For one thing, the results of biomedical
research are uncertain. In addition, the types of resources
required to achieve prevention, cures, or disease control by
functional state are not known. Guidance on resource allocation by disease or research institutes requires more
knowledge about how to produce changes in such areas as the
probability of bed dependency or limited functionality.
The option exists, however, within the bounds of existing
knowledge, to substitute experts for the consumer in expressing preferences about functional states for resource
allocation decisions.

Voluntary Agencies' Preferences

Essentially, choices are sought. These choices reflect the relative scaling of priorities among classes of
goods and services; governmental support for biomedical research is only one part, and a not very large one, of this
scaling of priorities. Asking consumers to record their
willingness to pay for support of alternative packages of
biomedical research results in many methodological problems,
as indicated earlier. Instead, we might look to those groups
who represent the public on biomedical research issues (for
example, the various health agencies, such as the American
Cancer Society, the American Diabetes Association, the
American Heart Association, and the Epilepsy Foundation) to
be representative of, and record the preferences of, those
who contribute resources to them. The voluntary agencies

have some expertness in the disease problems that are of
concern to them and can call upon research scientists for
further expert assistance. In common with consumers, moreover, the voluntary agencies have restraints on their budgets
so that the choices about priorities can be subjected to the
real life situation of budget constraints.

While knowledge about the role of technology in medical research is most inadequate, it should be understood best
by those voluntary agencies concerned about resources for research and those experts to whom they have easy access.
These agencies have an understanding of the research projects
most likely to be undertaken by various scientists at
different levels of funding. Thus, the voluntary agencies
could be surveyed individually to provide their subjective
opinions on the likely effect different quantities of research effort would have on functional states.

The questionnaire for such a survey would have to be
developed, but the kind of information to be gathered may be
illustrated as follows:

Assume that the indicated amount of research
money is allocated to research on the disease
of special concern to your agency, what is
your best estimate (and that of expert research scientists who advise you) of the
percentage of patients in the functional
states described below?

Disease-specific Research Allocations

(In millions)

Functional state	$0	$100	$200	$300	$400	$500
A Cured	A_0	A_1	A_2	A_3	A_4	A_5
B Fully functioning	B_0	B_1	B_2	B_3	B_4	B_5
C Limited function	C_0	C_1	C_2	C_3	C_4	C_5
D Self-care	D_0	D_1	D_2	D_3	D_4	D_5
E Not capable of self-care	E_0	E_1	E_2	E_3	E_4	E_5

The changes in percents of patients in each functional
state would be combined with changes in research expenditures
for all disease categories. This would be done be weighting
each column of entries for a research sum by the prevalence
of the disease in the population. For example, if with $100

million research outlay for a disease, such as chronic obstructive lung disease, 20 percent of the patients are estimated to be in a limited functional state at a cross-
section of time and 40 percent to be capable of self-care,
these percentages would be combined with reports from those
concerned about cancer research, research on spinal cord injuries, and so forth, in accord with the relative prevalence
of each disease. The result would be a composite distribution of the benefits in changes in functional state as a consequence of changes, based on the judgments of the voluntary
agencies and their experts, in the total budgeted funds for
research. These judgmental estimates would have to be scaled
to the likely appropriations for biomedical research and a
new estimate prepared of the expected changes in functional
state. This process would be carried out by disease and for
all diseases combined. The estimates of changes in the distribution of patients among functional states could be for
some specified time ahead (for example, five years) or for a
number of specified future dates.

To achieve reporting that is reasonably realistic,
after the specified period, voluntary agencies could be
"penalized" for gross inaccuracies in the percentage distribution of patients among functional states at different
research budget levels. As a consequence of the gross in-
accuracy in the estimate of functional state distribution of
patients, voluntary agencies could be required, as a condition for participation in the resource allocation process,
to pledge, let us say, $1 of their own budgeted funds for
each $10 of research fund allocation that is diverted to re-
search on the disease of special concern to them.

The process for resource allocation is based on the
general assumption that the returns to biomedical research
expenditure are decreasing returns. Additional outlays above
some level are not expected to yield equal additional returns.
At any point in time, projects most likely to pay off in
terms of benefits will be undertaken first; those with somewhat lower probability of success will be assigned a lower
claim on resources. The expected payoff of enlarging funds
for research on any disease would be measured by comparing
the change in the distribution of patients among functional
states given changes in aggregate funding levels. For example, the change in expected payoff with research expenditures raised for a specific disease from $200 million to $300
million would be estimated as the difference in percentage
distribution of patients by functional level. In the illustration presented above (p. 331), the difference in each
functional group would be:

<u>Hypothetical</u>

A_3-A_2	10%
B_3-B_2	20%
C_3-C_2	-5%
D_3-D_2	-10%
E_3-E_2	-15%

Without a change in incidence of the disease, the number of new cases would not be altered by the different research funding levels. The improvement, if achieved, would show up in the gains in functional states.

An Experimental Resource Allocation Guide

A somewhat different approach might be tested experimentally. It is an approach that calls for application of a version of the recent theoretical work on demand-revealing processes. We assume for purposes of this experiment that the 40 or so voluntary health agencies are asked to record their preferences about the allocation of an incremental increase of funds among the research institutes of the National Institutes of Health. We assume the incremental amount to be $200 million, equivalent to something below 10 percent of biomedical research funds (U.S.PHS, 1978). We assume further that the $200 million is the equivalent of about 50 cents for each $1 of funds available, in the aggregate, to the approximate 40 voluntary agencies.*

Each voluntary agency would be asked to record its preferences, subject to two constraints, about the allocation of the $200 million among research institutes. Two possible constraints might be:

(1) Not more than 50 percent of all voting power can be allocated to one research institute.

(2) The maximum voting power of a voluntary agency is the lesser of the following:

(a) the volunteer agency's own annual budget, or

---

* Based on estimates provided by Dr. William E. Rhode, Division of Resource Analysis, National Institutes of Health.

(b)   the total amount that is being voted
      on for distribution.

Alternatively, the 50 percent constraint in item (1)
might be removed and other rules set. Within these rules,
choices would be made which would give the voluntary health
agencies a more direct role in the allocation of research
funds and which would, in concept at least, move the allocations closer to the choices of consumers about biomedical
research funds. By the achievement of a closer correspondence to consumer choice, greater efficiency would be
achieved.

An initial simulation experiment, using the above-
defined criteria, was conducted by the Public Services
Laboratory staff to determine how an additional $200 million
would be allocated to the various institutes by the voluntary
agencies. This simulation, whereby the votes were, in concept at least, in accord with an assumed voting pattern of
specified voluntary agencies, indicated that the distribution
of total funds changes only fractionally and the rank order-
ing very little. While this may not be representative of a
real-life vote, certain characteristics of the voting system
have been clarified. The voluntary agency, following
its own self-interest, tends to allocate the maximum
amount that it is permitted to vote, under the rules,
to the research institute with which it is most closely
associated. If the constraint is set below 100 percent,
a voluntary agency would tend to follow this vote
strategically, with a vote of funds to those other research institutes that, in its view, contribute most
to carrying out the voluntary agency's mission.

*   *   *

The entire area of measuring and quantifying preferences is of extreme importance. It is worth grappling with
concepts other than the traditional human capital approach in
order to give greater depth to the information made available to policy officials. We have suggested here some optional methods of measurement. It is the expectation that
out of the work of this conference, new decision-making tools
may be forged, thereby facilitating accountability to the
public.

Acknowledgments.

The author is indebted to J. Steven Landefeld,
Jody Sindelar, and Charles P. Turner for their research
assistance in preparing this study.

REFERENCES

Acton, Jan Paul
    1976   Measuring the Monetary Value of Life-Saving
            Programs, P-5075. Santa Monica: The RAND
            Corporation.

    1975   Measuring the Social Impact of Heart and
            Circulatory Disease Programs: Preliminary
            Framework and Estimates, R-1697-NHLI.
            Santa Monica: The RAND Corporation.

    1973   Evaluating Public Programs to Save Lives:
            The Case of Heart Attacks, R-950-RC.
            Santa Monica: The RAND Corporation.

Bailey, Martin
    1978a   "Safety decisions and insurance." American
            Economic Review 68 (May):295-298.

    1978b   "Measuring the benefits of life-saving."
            Working paper, University of Maryland.

    1977   "Earnings, life valuation, and insurance."
            Working paper, University of Maryland.

Chen, Martin K.
    1976   "The K index: A proxy measure of health care
            quality." Health Services Research 11(4)
            (Winter):452-463.

    1973   "The G index for program priority." In
            Berg, Robert L. (ed.), Health Status Indexes
            28-34. Chicago: Hospital Research and Edu-
            cational Trust.

Chen, Milton M. and James W. Bush
    1979   "Health status measures, policy, and biomedical
            research." In Mushkin, Selma J. and David W.
            Dunlop (eds.), Health: What is it Worth?
            (this volume).

Chen, Milton M., James W. Bush, and Donald L. Patrick
    1975   "Social indicators for health planning and
            policy analysis." Policy Sciences 6 (March):
            71-89.

Clarke, Edward H.
    1979   "Social valuation of life- and health-
            saving activities by the demand-
            revealing process." In Mushkin, Selma J.
            and David W. Dunlop (eds.), Health:
            What is it Worth? (this volume).

Clarke, Edward H.
    1977   Demand Revelation and Public Goods, Woodrow
            Wilson International Center for Scholars,
            Smithsonian Institution (December).

Cooper, Barbara S. and Dorothy P. Rice
    1967   "The economic value of human life." American
            Journal of Public Health 57 (November):
            1954-1966.

Dorfman, Nancy
    1979   "The social value of saving a life." In Mushkin,
            Selma J. and David W. Dunlop (eds.), Health:
            What is it Worth? (this volume).

Fanshel, S. and J. W. Bush
    1970   "A health status index and its application to
            health services outcomes." Operations Research
            18 (November/December):1021-1066.

Fischer, Gregory W.
    1979   "Willingness to pay for probabilistic improve-
            ments in functional health status: A
            psychological perspective." In Mushkin,
            Selma J. and David W. Dunlop (eds.), Health:
            What is it Worth? (this volume).

Gilson, Betty S., M. Berger, R. A. Bobbitt, and W. B. Carter
    1975   "The sickness impact profile: Development of
            an outcome measure of health care." American
            Journal of Public Health 65(12) (December).

Jones, Ellen W., Barbara J. McNitt, and Paul M. Densen
    1979   "An approach to the assessment of long-term
            care." In Mushkin, Selma J. and David W. Dunlop
            (eds.), Health: What is it Worth? (this
            volume).

Katz, S.
    1963   "Studies of illness in the aged. The index of
            ADL: A standardized measure of biological and
            psychosocial function." Journal of the
            American Medical Association 185 (November):
            914-919.

Klarman, Herbert E.
    1965   "Syphilis control programs." In Dorfman,
            Robert (ed.), Measuring Benefits of Government
            Investment. Washington, D.C.: The Brookings
            Institution, pp. 367-414.

Lipscomb, Joseph
    1979   "The willingness-to-pay criterion and public
            program evaluation in health." In Mushkin,
            Selma J. and David W. Dunlop (eds.), Health:
            What is it Worth? (this volume).

Mishan, E. J.
    1971   "Evaluation of life and limb: A theoretical
            approach." Journal of Political Economy 19
            (July/August):687-705.

Mushkin, Selma J.
    1977   "Criteria for program evaluation." In
            Respiratory Diseases: Task Force Report on
            Prevention, Control, Education, U.S.DHEW
            publication no. (NIH) 77-1248, Washington, D.C.
            (March).

    1962   "Health as an investment." Journal of Political
            Economy 70 (October):129-157.

Public Health Service
U.S. Department of Health, Education, and Welfare
    1978   Basic Data Relating to the National Institutes
            of Health, Washington, D.C. (March).

    1975   Vital Statistics of the United States, 1975,
            vol. II, section 5, "Life tables."

Schelling, Thomas C.
    1968   "The life you save may be your own." In Chase,
            S. B. (ed.), Problems in Public Expenditure
            Expenditure Analysis. Washington, D.C.:
            The Brookings Institution, pp. 127-162.

Schulze, William, Shaul Ben-David, Thomas D. Crocker,
and Allen Kneese
    1979   "Economics and epidemiology: Application
            to cancer." In Mushkin, Selma J. and
            David W. Dunlop (eds.), Health: What is
            it Worth? (this volume).

Thaler, Richard and Sherwin Rosen
    1974   "Estimating the value of a life." Paper pre-
            sented at Workshop in Human Resources Economics,
            University of California at Los Angeles
            (February 19).

Thomas, L.
    1975   The Lives of a Cell. New York: Bantam Books,
            p. 37.

Weisbrod, B. A.
    1961   Economics of Public Health. Philadelphia:
            University of Pennsylvania Press.

Wylie, C. M. and B. K. White
    1964   "A measure of disability." Archives of Environ-
            mental Health 8 (June):834-839.

Zeckhauser, Richard and Donald Shepard
    1976   "Where now for saving lives?" Law and
            Contemporary Problems 40 (Autumn):5-45.

Bibliography

Acosta, Phyllis B.
1974   "Nutritional status of Mexican American pre-
school children in a border town." American
Journal of Clinical Nutrition 27 (December).

Acton, Jan Paul
1976   "Health status indexes--work in progress."
Paper presented at a conference in Health
Services Research 11(4), Phoenix, Arizona
(October).

1976   "Valuing lifesaving alternatives and some
measurements." Paper prepared for Law
and Contemporary Problems Conference on the
Value of Human Life, Amelia Island (March
11-13).

1973   Evaluating Public Programs to Save Lives: The
Case of Heart Attacks. Santa Monica: The RAND
Corporation (January).

Ahumada, Jorge
1965   Health Planning: Problems of Concept and
Method. Publication no. 111. Washington, D.C.:
Pan American Health Organization (April).

Akpom, C. A., S. Katz, and P. M. Densen
1973   "Methods of classifying disability and severity
of illness in ambulatory care." Medical Care
11 (Supplement).

American Medical Association
Committee on Rating of Mental and Physical Impairment
1971   Guides to the Evaluation of Permanent Impairment. Chicago: American Medical Association.

Andersen, R.
1968   A Behavioral Model of Families' Use of Health
Services. Research series no. 25. Chicago:
University of Chicago.

Andersen, R. and J. R. Newman
    1973   "Societal and individual determinants of
            medical care utilization in the United States."
            Health and Society 51.

Anderson, N. H.
    1970   "Functional measurement and psychophysical
            judgment." Psychological Review 77.

Armor, D. J.
    1974   "Theta reliability and factor scaling." In
            Costner, H. L. (ed.), Sociological Methodology,
            1973-1974. San Francisco: Jossey-Bass
            Publishers.

Arrow, Kenneth J.
    1973   Optimal Insurance and Generalized Deductibles.
            Santa Monica: The RAND Corporation.

    1965a   "Uncertainty and welfare economics of medical
            care." American Economic Review (March).

    1965b   "Reply." American Economic Review (March).

    1963   Social Choice and Individual Values (second
            edition). New Haven: Yale University Press.

Bailey, Martin
    1978a   "Safety decisions and insurance." American
            Economic Review 68 (May).

    1978b   "Measuring the benefits of life-saving."
            Working paper, University of Maryland.

    1977   "Earnings, life valuation, and insurance."
            Working paper, University of Maryland.

Balch, M. and P. C. Fishburn
    1974   "Subjective expected utility for conditional
            primitives." In Balch, M., D. McFadden, and
            S. Wu (eds.), Essays on Economic Behavior
            Under Uncertainty. Amsterdam: North-Holland.

Balinsky, W. and R. Berger
    1975   "A review of research on general health status
            indexes." Medical Care 13.

Barnoon, Shlomo and Harvey Wolfe
    1972   Measuring the Effectiveness of Medical Decis-
            ions: An Operations Research Approach.
            Springfield, Ill.: Charles C. Thomas.

Baumol, William J.
    1969   Economic Theory and Operations Analysis.
            Englewood Cliffs, N.J.: Prentice-Hall, Inc.

Becker, Gary S.
    1965   "A theory of the allocation of time." Economic
              Journal 75 (September).

    1964   Human Capital. New York: National Bureau of
              Economic Research.

Becker, Gary S. and H. Gregg Lewis
    1973   "On the interaction between the quantity and
              quality of children." In Schultz, T. W. (ed.),
              New Economic Approaches to Fertility. Proceed-
              ings of a conference sponsored by the National
              Bureau of Economic Research and the Population
              Council. Journal of Political Economy 81
              (March/April).

Becker, Gary S. and Nigel Tomes
    1976   "Child endowments and the quantity and quality
              of children." Journal of Political Economy 84
              (August).

Becker, M. H., D. P. Haefner, S. V. Kasl, J. P. Kirscht,
L. A. Maiman, and I. M. Rosenstock
    1977   "Selected psychological models and correlates
              of individual health-related behaviors."
              Medical Care 15.

Berdit, Martin and John W. Williamson
    1973   "Function limitation scale for measuring health
              outcomes." In Berg, Robert L. (ed.), Health
              Status Indexes. Chicago: Hospital Research
              and Educational Trust.

Berg, Robert L.
    1973   Health Status Indexes. Proceedings of a con-
              ference conducted by Health Services Research,
              Tucson, Arizona, October 1972. Chicago:
              Hospital Research and Educational Trust.

    1973   "Weighted life expectancy as a health status
              index." Health Services Research 8(2) (Summer).

Berg, Robert L., Dean S. Hallauer, and Stephen N. Berk
    1976   "Neglected aspects of the quality of life."
              Health Services Research 11(4) (Winter).

Birch, Herbert G. and Joan Dye Gussow
    1970   Disadvantaged Children: Health, Nutrition, and
              School Failure. New York: Harcourt, Brace
              and World, Inc.

Black, D.A.K. and J. D. Pole
    1975   "Priorities in biomedical research: Indices
              of burden." British Journal of Preventive and
              Social Medicine 29(4) (December).

Bloom, Benjamin S.
    1964   Stability and Change in Human Characteristics.
            New York: John Wiley and Sons, Inc.

Bonnet, P. D.
    1969   Increased Production and Better Utilization.
            Report of the National Conference on Medical
            Costs, June 27-28, 1967. Washington, D.C.
            U.S.DHEW.

Brody, Jane E.
    1977   "Personal health: Breast-feeding may help an
            infant to a better life." The New York Times
            (March 9).

Broman, Sarah H., Paul L. Nichols, and Wallace A. Kennedy
    1975   Preschool IQ: Prenatal and Early Developmental
            Correlates. Hillsdale, N.J.: Lawrence Erlbaum
            Associates.

Brook, R. H. and F. A. Appel
    1973   "Quality of care assessment: Choosing a method
            for peer review." New England Journal of
            Medicine 288.

Bruett, T. L. and R. P. Overs
    1969   "A critical review of 12 ADL scales."
            Physical Therapy 49.

Bull, N.
    1941   "The biological basis of value." The Scientific
            Monthly 53.

Bush, James W. and Milton M. Chen
    1970   "Markovian analysis of disease history and the
            problem of equilibrium." Paper presented before
            the Statistics Section of the Annual Meeting of
            the American Public Health Association, Houston,
            Texas (October).

Bush, James W., Milton M. Chen, and Donald L. Patrick
    1973   "Health status index in cost-effectiveness:
            Analysis of PKU program." In Berg, Robert L.
            (ed.), Health Status Indexes. Chicago:
            Hospital Research and Educational Trust.

Bush, James W., Sol Fanshel, and Milton M. Chen
    1972   "Analysis of a tuberculin testing program using
            a health status index." Socio-Economic Planning
            Sciences 6(1) (February).

Caste, Chris
    1976   "Outlook for biomedical research hearings, a
            special report." Washington Report on Health
            Legislation (December 8).

Center for Disease Control
    1972   Ten-State Nutrition Survey in the United States,
            1968-1970. Highlights, U.S.DHEW pub. no.
            (HSM) 72-8134. Atlanta, Ga.: Health Services
            and Mental Health Administration.

Chen, Martin K.
    1976   "The K index: A proxy measure of health care
            quality." Health Services Research 11(4)
            (Winter).

    1973   "The G index for program priority." In Berg,
            Robert L. (ed.), Health Status Indexes.
            Chicago: Hospital Research and Educational
            Trust.

Chen, Milton M.
    1976   "Federal health grants-in-aid to states:
            Rationale and interstate redistributional
            effect." Paper presented at Eastern Economic
            Association meeting, Bloomsburg, Pa. (April).

Chen, Milton M. and James W. Bush
    1977   "Maximizing health system output with political
            and administrative constraints using mathematical
            programming." Inquiry 13.

Chen, Milton M., James W. Bush, and Donald L. Patrick
    1975   "Social indicators for health planning and policy
            analysis." Policy Sciences 6 (March).

Chen, Milton M., James W. Bush, and Joseph Zaremba
    1975   "A critical analysis of effectiveness measures
            for operations research in health services. In
            Shuman, L., R. Speas, and J. Young (eds.),
            Operations Research in Health Care--A Critical
            Analysis. Baltimore: The Johns Hopkins
            University Press.

Chen, Milton M. and D. P. Wagner
    1978   "Gains in mortality from biomedical research,
            1930-1975: An initial assessment." Social
            Science and Medicine (forthcoming).

Chiang, C. L.
    1976   "Making annual indexes of health." Health
            Services Research 11(4) (Winter).

    1965   "An index of health: Mathematical models."
            Vital and Health Statistics, series 2, no. 5.
            Washington, D.C.: National Center for
            Health Statistics.

Chiang, C. L. and R. D. Cohen
    1973   "How to measure health: A stochastic model for
            an index of health." International Journal of
            Epidemiology 2(1) (Spring).

Christakis, George
    1968   "Nutritional epidemiologic investigation of 642
            New York City children." American Journal
            of Clinical Nutrition 21 (January).

Clarke, Edward H.
    1977a   "Social valuation of environmental quality by
            the demand-revealing process." Paper presented
            at Conference on Environmental Benefit Estima-
            tion, University of Chicago (June).

    1977b   "Some aspects of the demand-revealing process."
            Public Choice (Special Spring Supplement).

    1971   "Multipart pricing of public goods." Public
            Choice (Fall).

Cochrane, A. L.
    1972   Effectiveness and Efficiency: Random Reflections
            on Health Services. London: Nuffield Pro-
            vincial Hospital Trust.

Collins, Selwyn D.
            "Cases and days of illness among males and
            females with special reference to confinement
            to bed." Public Health Reports 55(2).

Commission on Chronic Illness
    1956   Chronic Illness in the United States, Vol. II.
            Care of the Long-Term Patient. Cambridge:
            Harvard University Press.

Conley, B. C.
    1973   The Value of Human Life in the Demand for
            Safety. Research Report, Center for Public
            Economics, California State University,
            San Diego.

Coombs, C. H., R. M. Dawes, and A. Tversky
    1970   Mathematical Psychology: An Elementary Intro-
            duction. Englewood Cliffs, N.J. Prentice-
            Hall, Inc.

Cooney, Thomas E., Jr.
    1977   Health and Nutrition as Possible Factors in
            Juvenile Anti-social Behavior. New York:
            The Ford Foundation.

Cooper, Barbara S. and Dorothy P. Rice
    1976   "The economic cost revisited." Social Security
            Bulletin (February).

Correa, H.
    1975   Population, Health, Nutrition, and Development.
            Lexington, Mass.: Lexington Books, D. C.
            Heath Co.

Cronbach, L. J.
    1951   "Coefficient alpha and the internal structure
            of tests." Psychometrika 16.

Davidson, D., P. Suppes, and S. Siegel
    1957   Decision-Making: An Experimental Approach.
            Stanford University Press.

Davie, Ronald, Neville Butler, and Harvey Goldstein
    1972   From Birth to Seven. New York: Humanities
            Press, Inc.

Donabedian, A. D.
    1966   "Evaluating the quality of medical care."
            Milbank Memorial Fund Quarterly 44 (Supplement).

Douglas, J.W.B. and J. M. Ross
    1965   "The effects of absence on primary school per-
            formance." British Journal of Educational
            Psychology 35, part I.

Douglas, J.W.B., J. M. Ross, and H. R. Simpson
    1967   "The ability and attainment of short-sighted
            pupils." Journal of the Royal Statistical
            Society 130, part 4.

    1965   "The relation between height and measured edu-
            cational ability in school children of the
            same social class, family size, and stage of
            sexual development." Human Biology 37.

Drillien, Cecil M.
    1964   The Growth and Development of the Prematurely
            Born Infant. Baltimore: Williams and Wilkins.

Driskel, Judy A. and Claudia S. Price
    1974   "Nutritional status of preschoolers from low-
            income Alabama families." Journal of American
            Dietetic Association 65 (September).

Dublin, Louis I. and A. J. Lotka
    1946   The Money Value of a Man. New York: The
            Ronald Press.

Edwards, Linda Nasif
    1975   "The economics of schooling decisions: Teenage
             enrollment rates."   The Journal of Human Re-
             sources 10 (Spring).

Edwards, Linda Nasif and Michael Grossman
    1977   "An economic analysis of children's health and
             intellectual development."   National Bureau of
             Economic Research Working Paper no. 180 (May).

Ehrlich, Isaac and Gary S. Becker
    1972   "Market insurance, self-insurance, and self-
             protection."   Journal of Political Economy 80.

Endozien, J. C., B. R. Switzer, and R. B. Bryan
    1976   Medical Evaluation of the Special Supplemental
             Food Program for Women, Infants, and Children
             (WIC):   Summary and Conclusions.   Department of
             Nutrition, School of Public Health, University
             of North Carolina (July).

Fabrega, H., Jr. and R. E. Roberts
    1972   "Social-psychological correlates of physician
             use by economically disadvantaged Negro urban
             residents."   Medical Care 10.

Falcone, A. R. and S. M. Bright
    1976   Patient Assessment: A Training Manual for Use
             of Patient Classification in Long-Term Care.
             Prepared by the Harvard Center for Community
             Health and Medical Care, Division of Long-
             Term Care, Health Resources Administration,
             Public Health Service, and the Department of
             Health, Education and Welfare (June).

Feather, N. T.
    1975   Values in Education and Society.   New York:
             The Free Press.

Feldstein, Martin S.
    1968   Economic Analysis for Health Service Efficiency.
             Chicago: Markham Press.

Fischer, Gregory W.
    1977   "Convergent validation of decomposed multi-
             attribute utility procedures for risky and
             riskless decisions."   Organizational Behavior
             and Human Performance 18.

Fischer, Gregory W. and J. Vaupel
    1976   "A lifespan utility model: Assessing prefer-
             ences for consumption and longevity."   In
             Vogt, W. G. and M. H. Mickle (eds.), Modeling
             and Simulation, vol. 7, part 2.

Fischoff, B. and R. Beyth
    1975   "I knew it would happen: Remembered probabil-
            ities of once-future things." Organizational
            Behavior and Human Performance 13.

Fishburn, P. C.
    1965   "Independence in utility theory with whole
            product sets." Operation Research 13.

Forst, Brian E.
    1973   "Quantifying the patient's preferences." In
            Berg, Robert L. (ed.), Health Status Indexes.
            Chicago: Hospital Research and Educational
            Trust.

Freeman, H. E., S. Levine, and L. G. Reeder
    1972   Handbook of Medical Sociology. Englewood Cliffs,
            N.J.: Prentice-Hall, Inc.

Fudenberg, H. H.
    1972   "The dollar benefits of biomedical research: A
            cost analysis." Journal of Laboratory and
            Clinical Medicine 79(3).

Gilson, Betty S., M. Berger, R. A. Bobbitt, and W. B. Carter
    1975   "The sickness impact profile: Development of
            an outcome measure of health care." American
            Journal of Public Health 65(12) (December).

Goldstein, K.
    1959   "Health as a value." In Maslow, A. (ed.),
            New Knowledge in Human Values. Chicago:
            Henry Regnery Co.

Gonnella, J. S. and M. J. Goran
    1975   "Quality of patient care - a measurement of
            change: The staging concept." Medical Care
            13.

Gordon, Gerald and G. Lawrence Fisher
    1975   The Diffusion of Medical Technology: Policy
            and Research Planning Perspectives. Cambridge:
            Ballinger Publishing Co.

Grossman, Michael
    1975   "The correlation between health and schooling."
            In Terleckyj, Nestor E. (ed.), Household
            Production and Consumption. New York:
            Columbia University Press for the National
            Bureau of Economic Research.

    1972   The Demand for Health: A Theoretical and Em-
            pirical Investigation. New York: Columbia
            University Press for the National Bureau of
            Economic Research.

Gruenberg, Ernest M.
    1977   "The failures of success." Milbank Memorial
            Fund Quarterly 55(4) (Winter).

Haggerty, Robert J., Klaus J. Roghmann, and Ivan B. Pless
    1975   Child Health and the Community. New York:
            John Wiley and Sons.

Harberger, A. C.
    1971   "Three basic postulates for applied welfare
            economics: An interpretative essay." Journal
            of Economic Literature 9.

Harvard Center for Community Health and Medical Care
    1974   Summary of Proceedings: Third Invitational Con-
            ference on Nursing Home Care. Boston, Mass.
            (May 30).

    1973   Summary of Proceedings: Second Nursing Home
            Conference. Cambridge, Mass. (December 6).

    1972   Conference Highlights. Nursing Home Care:
            Problems Perceived by Providers, Standard
            Setting Agencies and Fiscal Agencies.
            Cambridge, Mass. (November 28-29).

Heller, Peter S. and William D. Drake
    1976   Malnutrition, Child Morbidity, and the Family
            Decision Process. Center for Research on
            Economic Development, The University of
            Michigan, Discussion Paper no. 58 (September).

Howard, Ronald A.
    1971   Dynamic Probabilistic Systems. Vol. II: Semi-
            Markov and Decision Processes. New York:
            John Wiley and Sons, Inc.

Hu, Teh-Wei
    1973   "Effectiveness of child health and welfare
            programs: A simultaneous equations approach."
            Socio-Economic Planning Sciences 7.

Illich, Evan
    1976   Medical Nemesis (The Expropriation of Health).
            New York: Random House, Inc.

Illsley, Raymond
    1966   "Preventive medicine in the perinatal period."
            Proceedings of the Royal Society of Medicine
            59 (March).

Inman, Robert P.
    1976   "The family provision of children's health: An
            economic analysis." In Rosett, Richard (ed.),
            The Role of Health Insurance in the Health
            Services Sector. New York: Columbia University
            Press for the National Bureau of Economic
            Research.

Johnston, S. A. and J. E. Ware, Jr.
    1976   "Income group differences in relationships
            among survey measures of physical and mental
            health." Health Services Research 11.

Jones, E. W., B. J. McNitt, and E. M. McKnight
    1974   Patient Classification for Long-Term Care:
            User's Manual, U.S.DHEW publication no. (HRA)
            75-3107, Health Resources Administration,
            Bureau of Health Services Research and
            Evaluation, U.S.DHEW.

Jones-Lee, M. W.
    1976   The Value of Life: An Economic Analysis.
            Chicago: University of Chicago Press.

Kaiser, H. F.
    1958   "The Varimax criteria for analytic rotation
            in factor analysis." Psychometrika 23.

Kaiser, H. F. and J. Caffrey
    1965   "Alpha factor analysis." Psychometrika 30.

Kaiser, H. F., S. Hunka, and J. C. Bianchini
    1971   "Relating factors between studies based upon
            different individuals." Multivariate Be-
            havioral Research 6.

Kao, Edward P.C.
    1972   "A semi-Markov model to predict recovery
            progress of coronary patients." Health
            Services Research 8 (Fall).

Kaplan, Robert M., James W. Bush, and Charles C. Berry
    1976   "Health status: Types of validity and the
            index of well-being." Health Services
            Research 11(4) (Winter).

Kaplan, Robert S., Lester B. Lave, and Samuel Leinhardt
    1972   "The efficacy of a comprehensive health care
            project: An empirical analysis." American
            Journal of Public Health 62 (July).

Karnofsky, David A. and J. H. Burchenal
     1949   "The clinical evaluation of chemotherapeutic
              agents in cancer." In McLeod, Colin (ed.),
              Evaluation of Chemotherapeutic Agents.
              New York: Columbia University Press.

Katz, Sidney
     1973   "Measuring the health status of populations."
              In Berg, Robert L. (ed.), Health Status Indexes.
              Chicago: Hospital Research and Educational
              Trust.

     1963   "Studies of illness in the aged." Journal of
              American Medical Association 185(12) (September).

Katz, Sidney and C. A. Akpom
     1976   "A measure of primary sociobiological functions."
              International Journal of Health Services 6.

Katz, Sidney, A. B. Ford, T. D. Downs, M. Adams, and
D. I. Rusby
     1972   Effects of Continued Care: A Study of Chronic
              Illness in the Home. U.S.DHEW publication no.
              (HSM) 73-3010, Health Services and Mental Health
              Administration, National Center for Health
              Services Research and Development, U.S.DHEW.

Keeney, R. L. and H. Raiffa
     1976   Decisions with Multiple Objectives. New York:
              John Wiley and Sons, Inc.

Kenny, M.
     1963   "Social values and health in Spain: Some pre-
              liminary considerations." Human Organizations
              21.

Kessner, David M.
     1974   Assessment of Medical Care for Children. Con-
              trasts in Health Status, Vol. 3. Washington,
              D.C.: Institute of Medicine.

Klarman, Herbert E.
     1965   "Syphilis control programs." In Dorfman,
              Robert (ed.), Measuring Benefits of Government
              Investment. Washington, D.C.: The Brookings
              Institution.

Klein, Robert E.
     1972   "Is big smart? The relation of growth to cog-
              nition." Journal of Health and Social Be-
              havior 13 (September).

Kleinman, J. C.
    1977   "Age-adjusted mortality indexes for small
            areas: Applications to health planning."
            American Journal of Public Health 67(9)
            (September).

Kneese, Allen
    1973   "Benefit-cost analysis and unscheduled events
            in the nuclear fuel cycle." Resources
            (September).

Kneese, Allen and William Schulze
    1977   "Environment, health, and economics - The
            case of cancer." American Economic Review 67(1).

Lancaster, K.
    1971   Consumer Demand: A New Approach. New York:
            Columbia University Press.

Lave, Lester and Eugene Seskin
    1970   "Air pollution and human health." Science 169
            (August).

Lesaurne, J.
    1975   Cost-Benefit Analysis and Economic Theory.
            Amsterdam: North-Holland.

Lichtenstein, S. L., B. Fischoff, and L. D. Phillips
    In   "Calibration of probabilities: The state of
    press   the art." In Jungerman, H. and G. de Zeeum
            (eds.), Decision-Making and Change in Human
            Affairs. Amsterdam: D. Reidl.

Lichtenstein, S. L. and P. Slovic
    1973   "Response-induced reversals of preference in
            gambling: An extended replication in Las
            Vegas." Journal of Experimental Psychology
            101.

    1971   "Reversals of preference between bids and
            choices in gambling decisions." Journal of
            Experimental Psychology 89.

Lipscomb, Joseph
Forthcoming "Health resource allocation and quality of care
            measurement in a social policy framework."
            Policy Sciences.

Lipscomb, Joseph, Lawrence E. Berg, Virginia L. London,
and Paul A. Nutting
    1977   Health Status Maximization and Manpower Alloca-
            tion. Working paper no. 9761, Institute of
            Policy Sciences and Public Affairs, Duke
            University (April).

352   HEALTH: WHAT IS IT WORTH?

Lipscomb, Joseph and Richard M. Scheffler
     1975   "The impact of the expanded duty assistant on
               cost and productivity in dental care delivery."
               Health Services Research 10 (Spring).

Luce, R. Duncan and Howard Raiffa
     1971   Games and Decisions.   New York: John Wiley
               and Sons, Inc.

Luce, R. Duncan and J. W. Tukey
     1964   "Simultaneous conjoint measurement: A new type
               of fundamental measurement."   Journal of Mathe-
               matical Psychology 1.

Mansfield, E., E. Rapoport, R. Wagner, and J. Bearsely
     1977   "Social and private rate of returns from in-
               dustrial innovation."   Quarterly Journal of
               Economics 91.

Mata, Leonardo
     1978   "Breast-feeding: Main promoter of infant
               health."   American Journal of Clinical
               Nutrition 31 (May).

McKown, Thomas, R. G. Record, and R. O. Turner
     1975   "An interpretation of the decline of mortality
               in England and Wales during the twentieth
               century."   Population Studies 29.

McNitt, B. J. and P. C. Brown
     1976   Guide for Completing Patient Appraisal and
               Care Evaluation (PACE) Instrument.   Prepared
               by Harvard Center for Community Health and
               Medical Care for the Office of Long-Term Care,
               U.S.DHEW (July).

Mechanic, D.
     1968   Medical Sociology: A Selective View.   New York:
               The Free Press.

Meyer, R. F.
     1970   "On the relationship among the utility of assets,
               the utility of consumption, and investment
               strategy in an uncertain, but time invariant
               world."   In Lawrence, J. (ed.), Proceedings of
               the Fifth International Conference on Opera-
               tional Research.   Operations Research 69.
               London: Tavistock Publications.

Miller, G. A.
     1956   "The magical number seven plus or minus two:
               Some limits on our capacity to process informa-
               tion."   Psychological Review 63.

Miller, J. E.
    1970   "An indicator to aid management in assigning
            program priorities." Public Health Reports
            85(8) (August).

Mishan, E. J.
    1971   Cost-Benefit Analysis: An Introduction.
            New York: Praeger Press.

    1971   "Evaluation of life and limb: A theoretical
            approach." Journal of Political Economy
            (July/August).

Moriyama, Iwao M.
    1968   "Problems in the measurement of health status."
            In Sheldon, E. B. and W. Moore (eds.),
            Indicators of Social Change: Concepts and
            Measurement. New York: Russell Sage.

Musgrave, Richard A.
    1959   The Theory of Public Finance. New York:
            McGraw-Hill.

Mushkin, Selma J.
    1977   "Criteria for program evaluation," in
            Respiratory Diseases: Task Force Report on
            Prevention, Control, Education, U.S.DHEW
            publication no. (NIH) 77-1248 (March).

    1962   "Health as an investment." Journal of Political
            Economy 70(5) (October) (Supplement).

Mushkin, Selma J., L. Paringer, and M. M. Chen
    1976   Returns to Biomedical Research, 1900-1975:
            An Initial Assessment of Impacts on Health
            Expenditures. Report on NIH contract no.
            N01-00-5-2121. Washington, D.C. Public
            Services Laboratory, Georgetown University
            (October).

National Center for Health Statistics
U.S. Department of Health, Education, and Welfare
    1977   Current Estimates from the Health Interview
            Survey, United States, 1975. Series 10, no.
            115, U.S.DHEW pub. (HRA) 77-1543. Rockville, Md.

    1977   Limitation of Activity Due to Chronic Conditions,
            United States, 1974. Series 10, no. 111, U.S.
            DHEW pub. (HRA) 77-1537. Rockville, Md.

National Center for Health Statistics
U.S. Department of Health, Education, and Welfare
    1977   Problems of Chronic Conditions of the Geni-
            tourinary, Nervous, Endocrine, Metabolic,
            and Blood and Blood-Forming Systems and
            Selected Chronic Conditions, United States,
            1973. Series 10, no. 109, U.S.DHEW pub. no.
            (HRA) 77-1536. Rockville, Md. (March).

    1976   Health Characteristics of Persons with Chronic
            Activity Limitation, United States, 1974.
            Series 10, no. 112, U.S.DHEW pub. no. (HRA)
            77-1539. Rockville, Md. (October).

    1975   Eye Examination Findings among Youths Aged 12-17
            Years: United States. Series 11, no. 155,
            Public Health Service pub. no. 1000.

    1973   Body Weight, Stature, and Sitting Height: White
            and Negro Youths 12-17 Years, United States.
            Series 11, no. 126, Vital and Health Statistics.

    1973   Limitation of Activity Due to Chronic Conditions,
            United States, 1969-1970. Series 10, no. 80,
            U.S.DHEW pub. no. (HSM) 73-1506. Rockville, Md.

    1972a   Binocular Visual Acuity of Children: Demo-
            graphic and Socioeconomic Characteristics -
            United States. Series 11, no. 112, Vital
            and Health Statistics.

    1972b   Periodontal Disease and Oral Hygiene among
            Children: United States. Series 11, no. 117,
            Vital and Health Statistics.

    1971   Diabetes-Mellitus, Mortality in the United
            States, 1950-1967. Series 20, no. 10.
            Rockville, Md. (July).

    1970a   Hearing Levels of Children by Age and Sex:
            United States. Series 11, no. 102, Public
            Health Service pub. no. 1000.

    1970b   Height and Weight of Children: United States.
            Series 11, no. 119, Public Health Service pub.
            no. 1000.

    1967a   Plan, Operation, and Response Results of a
            Program of Children's Examinations. Series 1,
            no. 5, Public Health Service pub. no. 1000.

National Center for Health Statistics
U.S. Department of Health, Education, and Welfare
    1967b   A Study of the Achievement Test Used in the
            Health Examination Survey of Persons Aged 6-17
            Years. Series 2, no. 24, Public Health Service
            pub. no. 1000.

    1967c   Characteristics of Persons with Diabetes in the
            United States, July 1964-June 1965. Series 10,
            no. 40 (October).

    1964   "Health survey procedure: Concepts, question-
            naire development, and definitions in the health
            interview survey." Series 1, no. 2, Vital and
            Health Statistics (May).

Nunnally, J. C.
    1967   Psychometric Theory. New York: McGraw-Hill.

O'Hara, Donald J.
    1975   "Microeconomic aspects of the demographic
            transition." Journal of Political Economy
            83 (December).

Orloff, Marshall J.
    1975   "Contributions of surgical research to health
            care, 1945-1970." In Zuidema, G. (ed.), Study
            on Surgical Services for the United States.
            Baltimore, Md.: Lewis Advertising Co.

Owen, George M.
    1974   "A study of nutritional status of preschool
            children in the United States, 1968-1970."
            Pediatrics 53 (April) (Supplement).

Parsons, Talcott
    1958   "Definitions of health and illness in light of
            American values and social structure." In
            Jaco, E. Gartley (ed.), Patients, Physicians,
            and Illness. New York: The Free Press.

Patrick, Donald L., James W. Bush, and Milton M. Chen
    1973   "Toward an operational definition of health."
            Journal of Health and Social Behavior 14(1)
            (March).

    1973   "Methods for measuring levels of well-being
            for a health status index." Health Services
            Research 8.

Pauly, Mark V.
    1972   Medical Care at Public Expense. New York:
            Praeger Press.

Payne, J.
    1976   "Task complexity and contingent processing in
             decision making: An information search and
             protocol analysis." Organizational Behavior
             and Human Performance 16.

Peltzman, S.
    1973   "The benefits and costs of new drug regulation."
             In Landau, R. L. (ed.), Regulating New Drugs,
             University of Chicago Center for Policy Study.

Public Health Service
U.S. Department of Health, Education, and Welfare
    1977   Respiratory Disease Task Force Report on Pre-
             vention, Control, and Education. Division of
             Lung Diseases, National Institutes of Health
             (March).

    1977   Report of the National Commission on Diabetes to
             the Congress of the United States, The Long
             Range Plan to Combat Diabetes, 1976. U.S.DHEW
             pub. no. (NIH) 77-1229. National Institutes of
             Health.

    1975   Long-Term Care Facility Improvement Study.
             Introductory Report (July).

    1974   P.S.R.O. Program Manual. Prepared by Office of
             Professional Standards Review (March).

    1960   "Diabetes reported in interviews, United States,
             July 1957-June 1959." Series B, no. 21. Health
             Statistics from the U.S. National Health Survey
             (September).

Raiffa, H.
    1968   Decision Analysis. Reading, Mass.: Addison
             Wesley Publishing Co.

Reynolds, W. Jeff, William A. Rushing, and David L. Miles
    1974   "The validation of a function status index."
             Journal of Health and Social Behavior 15(4)
             (December).

Rice, Dorothy P.
    1966   Estimating the Cost of Illness. Health
             Economics series no. 6. Washington, D.C.:
             U.S. Government Printing Office (May).

Rice, Dorothy P. and Barbara S. Cooper
    1967   "The economic value of human life." American
             Journal of Public Health 57(11) (November).

Richard, S. F.
    1972   Optimal Life Insurance Decisions for a Rational
            Economic Man. Unpublished doctoral dissertation,
            Graduate School of Business Administration,
            Harvard University.

Richardson, Elliot L.
    1972   "The inescapable necessity of choice." Los
            Angeles Times, section 5, p. 6 (February 20).

Richardson, Stephen A.
    1976   "The influence of severe malnutrition in infancy
            on the intelligence of children at school age:
            An ecological perspective." In Walsh, Roger N.
            and William T. Greenough (eds.), Environments
            as Therapy for Brain Dysfunction. New York:
            Plenum Publishing Corporation.

Rokeach, M.
    1973   The Nature of Human Values. New York: The
            Free Press.

Rosser, J. M.
    1971   "Values and health." The Journal of School
            Health 41.

Rosser, Rachel M. and Vincent C. Watts
    1972   "The measurement of hospital output." Inter-
            national Journal of Epidemiology 1(4) (Winter).

Ryder, C. F., W. F. Elkin, and D. Doten
    1971   "Patient assessment - An essential tool in
            placement and planning care." U.S.DHEW.
            HSMHA Health Reports 86.

Sackett, David L. and R. Brian Haynes
    1976   Compliance with Therapeutic Regimes.
            Baltimore: Johns Hopkins Press.

Savage, L. J.
    1954   The Foundations of Statistics. New York:
            John Wiley and Sons, Inc.

Schack, Elisabeth and Barbara Starfield
    1973   "Acute disability in childhood examination of
            agreement between various measures." Medical
            Care 11 (July/August).

Schelling, T. C.
    1968   "The life you save may be your own." In Chase,
            Samuel B. (ed.), Problems in Public Expenditure
            Analysis. Washington, D.C.: The Brookings
            Institution.

Scrimshaw, Nevin S. and John E. Gordon
    1968   Malnutrition, Learning, and Behavior.
             Cambridge: The M.I.T. Press.

Selowsky, Marcelo and Lance Taylor
    1973   "The economics of malnourished children: An
             example of disinvestment in human capital."
             Economic Development and Cultural Change 22
             (October).

Seoane, Nicole and Michael C. Latham
    1971   "National anthropometry in the identification
             of malnutrition in childhood." Journal of
             Tropical Pediatric and Environmental Child
             Health (September).

Shapiro, S.
    1967   "End result measurements of quality of medical
             care." Milbank Memorial Fund Quarterly 45:2,
             part 1.

Sheldon, E. B. and H. E. Freeman
    1970   "Notes on social indicators. Promises and
             potential." Policy Sciences 1.

Sims, Laura S. and Portia M. Morris
    1974   "Nutritional status of preschoolers." Journal
             of American Dietetic Association 64 (May).

Slovic, P., B. Fischoff, and S. L. Lichtenstein
    1977   "Behavioral decision theory." Annual Review
             of Psychology.

    1976   "Cognitive processes and societal risk taking."
             In Carroll, J. S. and J. W. Payne (eds.),
             Cognition and Social Behavior. Hillsdale, N.J.:
             Lawrence Erlbaum Associates.

Slovic, P. and S. L. Lichtenstein
    1971   "Comparison of Bayesian and regression approaches
             to the study of information processing in
             judgment." Organizational Behavior and Human
             Performance 6.

Starfield, Barbara
    1975   "Health needs of children." Princeton, N.J.:
             Robert Wood Johnson Foundation.

Stoch, M. B. and P. M. Smythe
    1976   "15-year developmental study on effects of se-
             vere undernutrition during infancy on subse-
             quent physical growth and intellectual func-
             tioning." Archives of Disease in Childhood 51.

Strotz, R. H.
    1957   "The empirical implication of a utility tree."
            Econometrica 25.

Sullivan, Daniel F.
    1971   "A single index of mortality and morbidity."
            U.S.DHEW. HSMHA Health Reports 86(4) (April).

    1966   "Conceptual problems in developing an index of
            health." Series 2, no. 17, Public Health Service
            pub. no. 1000, Vital and Health Statistics.
            Rockville, Md.: National Center for Health
            Statistics.

Talbot, Nathan B., Jerome Kagan, and Leon Eisenberg (eds.)
    1971   Behavioral Science in Pediatric Medicine.
            Philadelphia: W. B. Saunders Company.

Tanner, J. M.
    1966   "Galtonian eugenics and the study of growth."
            Eugenics Review 58.

Thaler, R. H. and S. Rosen
    1976   "The value of saving a life: Evidence from the
            labor market." In Terleckyj, N. E. (ed.),
            Household Production and Consumption. New York:
            Columbia University Press.

Thurston, L. L.
    1959   The Measurement of Value. Chicago: University
            of Chicago Press.

Tideman, T. N. and G. Tullock
    1976   "A new and superior process for making social
            choices." Journal of Political Economy
            (December).

Torrance, George W., David L. Sackett, and Warren H. Thomas
    1973   "Utility maximization model for program evalua-
            tion: A demonstration application." In Berg,
            Robert E. (ed.), Health Status Indexes.
            Chicago: Hospital Research and Educational
            Trust.

Torrance, George W., Warren H. Thomas, and David L. Sackett
    1972   "A utility maximization model for evaluation of
            health care programs." Health Services Re-
            search 7(2) (Summer).

Treuber, Conrad
    1976   "If nobody died of cancer." The Kennedy
            Institute Quarterly Report (Summer). Wash-
            ington, D.C.: Georgetown University.

Tversky, A.
    1967   "Additivity, utility, and subjective pro-
              ability." Journal of Mathematical Psychology 4.

Tversky, A. and D. Kahneman
    1974   "Judgment under uncertainty: Heuristics and
              biases." Science 185.

von Neumann, J. and O. Morgenstern
    1944   Theory of Games and Economic Behavior.
              Princeton, N.J.: Princeton University Press.

Wallace, Helen M.
    1962   Health Services for Mothers and Children.
              Philadelphia: W. B. Saunders Company.

Wallston, K. A., S. A. Maides, and B. A. Wallston
    1974   Health Care Information Seeking as a Function of
              Health Locus of Control and Health Value.
              Nashville, Tenn.: Vanderbilt University
              (Mimeographed).

Ware, John E., Jr.
    1976   "The conceptualization and measurement of health
              for policy relevant research in medical care
              delivery." Presented at the annual meetings of
              the American Association for the Advancement of
              Science, Boston, Mass. (February).

    1976   "Scales for measuring general health percep-
              tions." Health Services Research 11.

Ware, John E., Jr. and J. Young
    1976   Conceptualization and Measurement of Health as
              a Value: Volume III of a Final Report.
              Carbondale, Ill.: Southern Illinois University
              School of Medicine.

Weinstein, M. C., D. S. Shepard, and J. S. Pliskin
    1975   Decision-Theoretic Approaches to Valuing a Year
              of Life. Center for the Analysis of Health
              Practices, Harvard School of Public Health
              (January).

Weisbrod, Burton
    1971   "Cost and benefit of medical research: A cost
              study of poliomyelitis." Journal of Political
              Economy 79.

    1961   The Economics of Public Health. Philadelphia:
              The University of Pennsylvania Press.

    1961   "The valuation of human capital." Journal of
              Political Economy 69 (October).

Wiener, Gerald
     1965   "Correlates of low birth weight: Psychological
             status at six to seven years of age." Pediatrics
             35 (March).

Williamson, John W.
     1968   Prognostic Epidemiology: Concept, Process, and
             Product. Baltimore: The Johns Hopkins School
             of Hygiene and Public Health, Department of
             Medical Care and Hospitals.

Willig, R. D.
     1976   "Consumer surplus without apology." American
             Economics Review 66 (September).

     1973   "Consumer's surplus: A rigorous cashbook."
             Technical Report 98, Economic Series. Institute
             for Mathematical Study in the Social Sciences,
             Stanford University.

Willis, Robert
     1973   "A new approach to the economic theory of
             fertility behavior." In Schultz, T. W. (ed.),
             New Economic Approaches to Fertility. Proceed-
             ings of a conference sponsored by the National
             Bureau of Economic Research and the Population
             Council. Journal of Political Economy 81
             (March/April).

Winterholler, Claire
     1966   "Attack on diabetes." Vanderbilt Alumnus 62(4)
             (Summer).

Wyer, R. S., Jr.
     1975   "The role of probabilistic and syllogistic rea-
             soning in cognitive organization and social in-
             ference." In Kaplan, M. F. and S. Schwartz
             (eds.), Human Judgment and Decision Processes.
             New York: Academic Press, Inc.

Wyler, Allen R., M. Masuda, and T. H. Holmes
     1968   "The seriousness of illness rating scale."
             Journal of Psychosomatic Research 11.

Wylie, Charles M. and Betty K. White
     1964   "A measure of disability." Archives of Environ-
             mental Health 8.

Zeckhauser, Richard and Donald Shepard
     1976   "Where now for saving lives?" Law and Con-
             temporary Problems (Summer).

Index

Pergamon Policy Studies